Instructor's Manual to Accompany Clinical Decision Making

Case Studies in Pharmacology

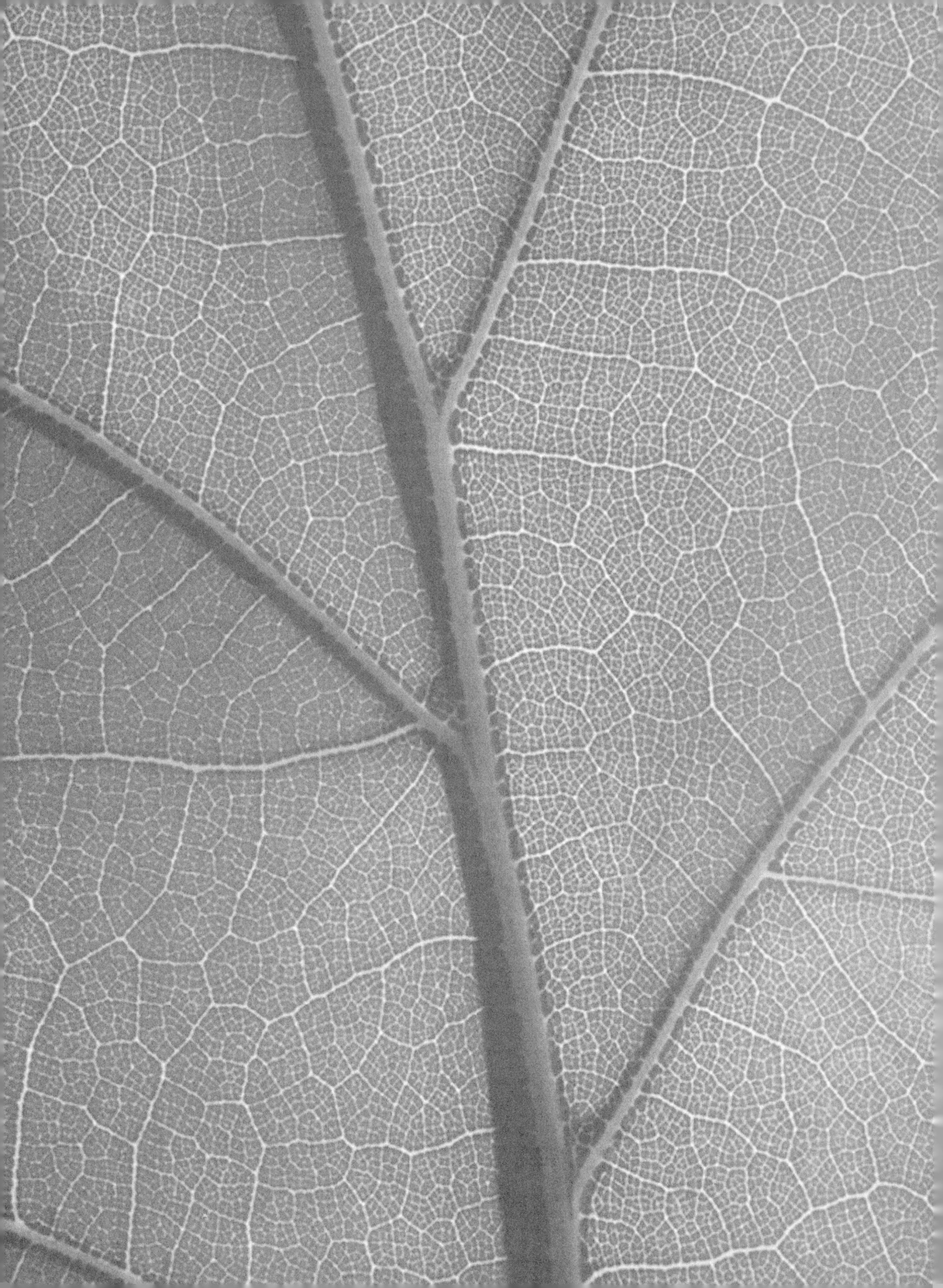

INSTRUCTOR'S MANUAL TO ACCOMPANY CLINICAL DECISION MAKING

Case Studies in Pharmacology

Hyacinth C. Martin
BSN, MA, MSEd, MPS, RNBC

THOMSON
DELMAR LEARNING

Australia Canada Mexico Singapore Spain United Kingdom United States

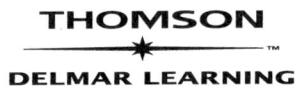

Instructor's Manual to Accompany Clinical Decision Making: Case Studies in Pharmacology
by Hyacinth C. Martin, BSN, MA, MSEd, MPS, RNBC

Vice President,
Health Care Business Unit:
William Brottmiller

Director of Learning Solutions:
Matthew Kane

Acquisitions Editor:
Maureen Rosener

Product Manager:
Elizabeth Howe

Editorial Assistant:
Chelsey Iaquinta

Marketing Director:
Jennifer McAvey

Marketing Manager:
Michele McTighe

Marketing Coordinator:
Danielle Pacella

Production Director:
Carolyn Miller

Content Project Manager:
Jessica McNavich

COPYRIGHT © 2007 by Thomson Delmar Learning, part of The Thomson Corporation. Thomson Delmar Learning, Thomson and the Thomson logo are trademarks used herein under license.

Printed in the United States of America
1 2 3 4 5 6 7 XXX 08 07 06 05 04

For more information, contact Thomson Delmar Learning, 5 Maxwell Drive, Clifton Park, NY 12065-2919

Or you can visit our Internet site at
http://www.delmarlearning.com

ALL RIGHTS RESERVED. No part of this work covered by the copyright hereon may be reproduced or used in any form or by any means—graphic, electronic, or mechanical, including photocopying, recording, taping, Web distribution or information storage and retrieval systems—without the written permission of the publisher.

For permission to use material from this text or product, contact us by
Tel (800) 730-2214
Fax (800) 730-2215
www.thomsonrights.com

ISBN 1-4018-3522-8

Notice to the Reader

Publisher does not warrant or guarantee any of the products described herein or perform any independent analysis in connection with any of the product information contained herein. Publisher does not assume, and expressly disclaims, any obligation to obtain and include information other than that provided to it by the manufacturer.

The reader is expressly warned to consider and adopt all safety precautions that might be indicated by the activities described herein and to avoid all potential hazards. By following the instructions contained herein, the reader willingly assumes all risks in connection with such instructions.

The publisher makes no representations or warranties of any kind, including but not limited to, the warranties of fitness for particular purpose or merchantability, nor are any such representations implied with respect to the material set forth herein, and the publisher takes no responsibility with respect to such material. The publisher shall not be liable for any special, consequential, or exemplary damages resulting, in whole or part, from the readers' use of, or reliance upon, this material.

Contents

Reviewers   vii

Preface   ix

Part 1 — The Digestive and Urinary Systems ... 1

Case Study 1	Cyanocobalamin (Vitamin B_{12} Deficiency Anemia, Pernicious Anemia)	3
Case Study 2	Renal Calculi	9
Case Study 3	Stage IIC Cancer of the Prostate	15
Case Study 4	Ulcerative Colitis	19
Case Study 5	Acute Renal Failure	25
Case Study 6	Appendicitis	35
Case Study 7	Lower Gastrointestinal Bleeding	41
Case Study 8	Chronic Renal Failure (End-Stage Renal Disease)	47

Part 2 — The Respiratory and Immune Systems ... 55

Case Study 1	Chronic Bronchitis	57
Case Study 2	Human Immunodeficiency Virus Infection (CDC Category A)	63
Case Study 3	Pulmonary Tuberculosis	69
Case Study 4	Pulmonary Empyema	75
Case Study 5	Non-Small Cell Adenocarcinoma of the Right Lung	81
Case Study 6	Pulmonary Emphysema	87
Case Study 7	Acute Respiratory Distress Syndrome	93
Case Study 8	Acquired Immunodeficiency Syndrome	99

Part 3 — The Cardiovascular and Lymphatic Systems ... 105

Case Study 1	Primary (Essential) Hypertension	107
Case Study 2	Coronary Artery Disease (Atherosclerosis)	113
Case Study 3	Chronic Vascular Ulcers of the Right Foot	121
Case Study 4	Disseminated Intravascular Coagulation	127
Case Study 5	Unstable Angina Pectoris (Acute Myocardial Ischemia)	133
Case Study 6	Sternal Wound Infection	139
Case Study 7	Valvular Heart Disease – Aortic Stenosis	145
Case Study 8	Hodgkin's Disease	151
Case Study 9	Multiple Myeloma (Plasma Cell Myeloma)	157
Case Study 10	Chronic Myelogenous Leukemia	163

Case Study 11	*Femoral-Popliteal Bypass for Peripheral Vascular Disease*	169
Case Study 12	*Premature Ventricular Contractions*	175

Part 4 — The Nervous System … 183

Case Study 1	*Unilateral Ménière's Disease*	185
Case Study 2	*Multiple Sclerosis*	189
Case Study 3	*Generalized Tonic-Clonic Seizure*	195
Case Study 4	*Subarachnoid Hemorrhage – Grade II*	201

Part 5 — The Endocrine System … 209

Case Study 1	*Hyperthyroidism*	211
Case Study 2	*Hypercortisolism (Cushing's Syndrome)*	217
Case Study 3	*Diabetes Mellitus Type 1*	223
Case Study 4	*Addison's Disease (Acute-Primary Hypocortisolism)*	231
Case Study 5	*Pheochromocytoma*	237

Part 6 — The Musculoskeletal and Reproductive Systems … 243

Case Study 1	*Cervical Cancer Stage IA*	245
Case Study 2	*Closed Femoral Head Fracture (Intracapsular Fracture)*	249
Case Study 3	*Osteomyelitis of Left Foot*	255
Case Study 4	*Osteoarthritis*	259
Case Study 5	*Breast Cancer*	265
Case Study 6	*Myasthenia Gravis*	271

Reviewers

Mary Beth Kiefner, RN, MS
Nursing Program Director
Nursing Faculty, Illinois Central College
East Peoria, Illinois

Joan Piper Mader, RN, MSN
Associate Professor or Nursing
College of the Mainland
Texas City, Texas

Darla R. Ura, MA, RN, APRN, BC
Clinical Associate Professor
Department of Adult and Elder Health Nursing
School of Nursing, Emory University
Atlanta, Georgia

Mari A. Smith, DSN, RN, CCRN
Professor
School of Nursing, Middle Tennessee State University
Murfreesboro, Tennessee

Preface

The *Instructor's Manual to Accompany Clinical Decision Making: Case Studies in Pharmacology* provides all of the cases from the book with their accompanying questions, answers, and rationales. Answers and rationales allow the instructor to facilitate discussion of the critical-thinking questions while using the answers as a guide. Each case includes the table of variables and references.

How to Use This Book

Every case begins with a table of variables that are encountered in practice, and that must be understood by the nurse in order to provide appropriate care to the client. Categories of variables include age, gender, setting, culture, ethnicity, cultural considerations, preexisting conditions, coexisting conditions, communication considerations, disability considerations, socioeconomic considerations, spiritual considerations, pharmacological considerations, psychosocial considerations, legal considerations, ethical considerations, alternative therapy, prioritization considerations, and delegation considerations. If a case involves a variable that is considered to have a significant impact on care, the specific variable is included in the table. This allows the user an "at-a-glance" view of the issues that will need to be considered to provide care to the client in the scenario. The table of variables is followed by a presentation of the case, including the history of the client, current condition, clinical setting, and professionals involved. A series of questions follows each case that ask the user to consider how she would handle the issues presented within the scenario.

Organization

Cases are grouped according to body system. Within each part, cases are organized by difficulty level from easy, to moderate, to difficult. This classification is somewhat subjective, but it is based upon a developed standard. In general, difficulty level has been determined by the number of variables that impact the case and the complexity of the client's condition. Colored tabs are used to allow the user to distinguish the difficulty levels more easily. A comprehensive table of variables is also provided for reference, to allow the user to quickly select cases containing a particular variable of care.

While every effort has been made to group cases into the most applicable body system, the scope of many of the cases may include more than one body system. In such instances, the case will still only appear in the section for one of the body systems addressed. The cases are fictitious; however, they are based on actual problems and/or situations the nurse will encounter. Any resemblance to actual cases or individuals is coincidental.

Praise for Thomson Delmar Learning's Case Study Series

"[This text's] strength is the large variety of case studies – it seemed to be all inclusive. Another strength is the extensiveness built into each case study. You can almost see this person as they enter the ED because of the descriptions that are given."

—MARY BETH KIEFNER, RN, MS
Nursing Program Director/Nursing Faculty,
Illinois Central College

"The cases . . . reflect the complexity of nursing practice. They are an excellent way to refine critical thinking skills."

—DARLA R. URA, MA, RN, APRN, BC
Clinical Associate Professor, Department of Adult and Elder Health Nursing, School of Nursing, Emory University

"This text does an excellent job of reflecting the complexity of nursing practice."

—VICKI NEES, RNC, MSN, APRN-BC
Associate Professor, Ivy Tech State College

". . . the case studies are very comprehensive and allow the undergraduate student an opportunity to apply knowledge gained in the classroom to a potentially real clinical situation."

—TAMELLA LIVENGOOD, APRN, BC, MSN, FNP
Nursing Faculty, Northwestern Michigan College

"These cases and how you have approached them definitely stimulate the students to use critical-thinking skills. I thought the questions asked really pushed the students to think deeply and thoroughly."

—JOANNE SOLCHANY, PhD, ARNP, RN, CS
Assistant Professor, Family & Child Nursing, University of Washington, Seattle

"The use of case studies is pedagogically sound and very appealing to students and instructors. I think that some instructors avoid them because of the challenge of case development. You have provided the material for them."

—NANCY L. OLDENBURG, RN, MS, CPNP
Clinical Instructor, Northern Illinois University

"[The author] has done an excellent job of assisting students to engage in critical thinking. I am very impressed with the cases, questions and content. I rarely ask that students buy more than one . . . book . . . but, in this instance, I can't wait until this book is published."

—DEBORAH J. PERSELL, MSN, RN, CPNP
Assistant Professor, Arkansas State University

"This is a groundbreaking book. . . . This book should be a required text for all undergraduate and graduate nursing programs and should be well-received by faculty."

—JANE H. BARNSTEINER, PhD, RN, FAAN
Professor of Pediatric Nursing, University of Pennsylvania School of Nursing

About the Author

Hyacinth C. Martin was first influenced by her elementary school teacher in choosing nursing as a career. However, the major influential persons in her choice of nursing as a career were nurses who wore white uniforms, white shoes, including nursing hats, and who seemed to have generated the highest respect from those they came in contact with. Hyacinth's nursing career includes staff nurse experiences on medical-surgical units, head nurse/nurse manager for medical-surgical units and critical-care units, administrative nursing supervisor, community nursing, and administrative nursing supervisor in long-term care agencies. Her academic experiences include teaching theory and clinical in a Licensed Practical Nursing program, a Baccalaureate Degree Program and at present in an Associate Degree program. In 1999, Hyacinth was a guest speaker on WMBC-TV (Channel 63, Newton, NJ), discussing issues pertaining to multiculturalism, with a focus on multicultural marriage and its effects on the family.

Publications include two articles for a nursing journal, one manuscript for Continuing Medical Education Resource, and part of a chapter on the endocrine system, published by Thomson Delmar Learning. She has also reviewed a chapter in *Pharmacology for Nursing Care*, Richard A. Lehne (5th ed.), and revised *PowerPoint for Pharmacology for Nursing Care* (6th ed.) and an instructor's manual. She was a contributor for *Gerontological Nursing Textbook* (2006), P. A. Tabloski.

Her contributions to education include recent presentations: "Pulmonary Tuberculosis: Controlling the Transmission of the Disease," at PACE University Conference; "Civic Society, Environmental Responsibility, & Sustainable Development in the United States & Brazil," presented at the Manhattan Veteran's Hospital Medical Center Conference, New York; and "The Effective Use of Unfractionated and Fractionated Heparin Therapy to Patients at Risk for Thrombus Formation" and "Nurse's Nurturing Nurses," presented at Lincoln Hospital Medical Center, New York.

Achievements

Hyacinth Martin was recognized in *Who's Who Among American Teachers* for four successive years. A current recipient of a PSC-CUNY Grant for research on Gender and Career Choice in Nursing, she is a full-time tenured professor in the nursing program at Borough of Manhattan Community College/The City University of New York. Her passion in teaching is to assist in the success of students who enroll in the nursing program at Borough of Manhattan Community College.

Hyacinth's other contributions (along with her husband's) to the welfare of others include adopting a basic school in one of the West Indian islands, and sponsoring a nursing student in Davao City, Philippines. Hyacinth earned a BSN degree and a Master's Degree in Career Guidance and Counseling from Lehman College, a Master's Degree in Nursing Administration from Columbia University, and a Master's Degree in Urban Education/Theology from NYACK College, New York. She is currently pursuing a doctoral degree in theology.

Acknowledgments

I want to express my sincere thanks to Elizabeth Howe, Product Manager, for the professional manner in which she communicated with me both verbally and by e-mail. I also want to thank the entire editorial staff at Thomson Delmar Learning for guidance in writing this text. I wish to record my thanks to the accuracy reviewer,

Bonita E. Broyles, RN, BSN, EdD. Your excellent guidance removed much of the stress that writing the text generated. A special thanks to Reverend Florentina Lapsey and Professor Louise Green for their constant prayers as I pursued the task of research and writing the text. I am grateful to Dr. David Ephraim for his encouragement and the many hours spent making sure computers and laptops were functioning, and lost content restored. Lastly, thank you, Professor Boyle-Egland for that special moment of support as the text was entering its final stage.

This book is dedicated to:
   My granddaughter, Nardia – May you also become the author of many books.
   My husband, Frederick, a retired registered nurse himself, in recognition of all that I owe him for his patience and understanding as he took on the responsibility of most of the household chores to enable me to accomplish this goal. It is my hope and prayer that this modest work will assist nursing students to better understand the content of medical-surgical nursing and, in so doing, help them to appreciate more of the incredible writings of nurse authors.

Hyacinth C. Martin

PART ONE

The Digestive and Urinary Systems

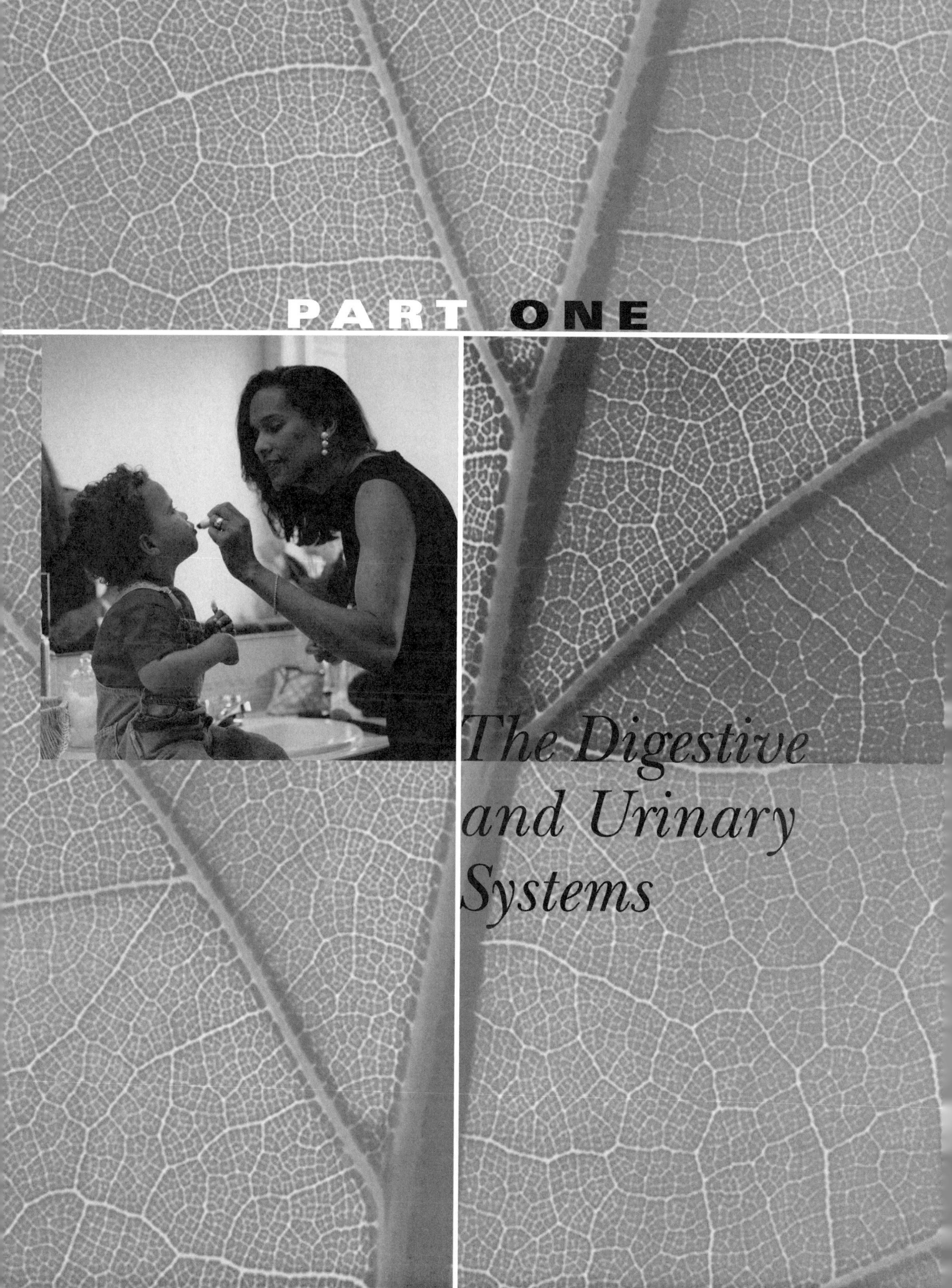

CASE STUDY 1

Cyanocobalamin (Vitamin B₁₂ Deficiency Anemia, Pernicious Anemia)

GENDER
- M

AGE
- 64

SETTING
- Hospital

ETHNICITY/CULTURE
- White

PREEXISTING CONDITIONS
- Zollinger-Ellison syndrome

COEXISTING CONDITIONS
- Total gastrectomy

LIFESTYLE
- Retired

COMMUNICATION

DISABILITY

SOCIOECONOMIC STATUS
- Middle

SPIRITUAL/RELIGIOUS
- Catholic

PHARMACOLOGIC
- Vitamin B₁₂
- Folic acid (Apo-Folic)

PSYCHOSOCIAL
- Periods of irritability and depression

LEGAL

ETHICAL

ALTERNATIVE THERAPY
- Clams
- Frankfurters
- Red beans

PRIORITIZATION
- Monitor for signs of alteration in cognition or irritability

DELEGATION
- RN
- Client education

THE DIGESTIVE AND URINARY SYSTEMS

Level of difficulty: Easy

Overview: This case involves a thorough assessment of the past medical and surgical history. The nurse must observe the client for signs of impaired memory or irritability during the assessment.

Client Profile

Mr. L is a 64-year-old client who had a total gastrectomy of the small and large bowel resection including the ileum two years ago. Mr. L is referred to the hospital inpatient clinic by his primary health care provider for further evaluation after a routine annual examination.

Case Study

During the initial interview, Mr. L complains of having had anorexia, nausea, vomiting, and abdominal pain for the past two days. Physical assessment findings include paresthesia of the hands and feet, reduced vibratory and position senses, ataxia, and muscle weakness. Assessment data on his daily nutritional intake includes frankfurters, brewer's yeast, clams, dried beans, and carrots. Vital signs taken by the nursing assistant are:

Blood pressure: 120/78
Pulse: 78
Respirations: 18
Temperature: 98.4° F

Tentative diagnosis of pernicious anemia is made and the health care provider prescribes serum laboratory data: hematocrit, hemoglobin, methylmalonic acid and homocysteine level, platelet count, red blood cell count, folic acid level, and peripheral blood smear. Mr. L is to return to the clinic in two days for a follow-up on the results of the laboratory data, confirmation of the diagnosis, and prescription as required. Mr. L returns to the clinic as scheduled. His laboratory results are:

Hematocrit (Hct): 38%
Hemoglobin (Hgb): 16 g/dL
Methylmalonic acid and homocysteine levels: elevated
Platelet count: 200,000/mm^3
Red blood cell (RBC) count: 2,500,000/mm^3
Folic acid: 3 ng/mL

Also, the peripheral blood smear shows oval, macrocytic, and hyperchromic RBCs. The health care provider reviews the data, and a diagnosis of pernicious anemia is confirmed.

Questions and Suggested Answers

1. **Explain the pathophysiology of vitamin B_{12} deficiency and its relationship to pernicious anemia.** Vitamin B_{12} performs several metabolic functions, acting as a hydrogen acceptor coenzyme. Its most important function is to act as a coenzyme for reducing ribonucleotides to deoxyribonucleotides, a step that is necessary in the replication of genes. Vitamin B_{12} is one of the two vitamins that is essential for the final maturation of red blood cells (folic acid is the other vitamin). Vitamin B_{12} is needed for the synthesis of deoxyribose nucleic acid (DNA), because it aids in the formation of thymidine triphosphate, one of the essential building blocks of DNA. The lack of this vitamin will therefore cause abnormal and diminished DNA, and, consequently, failure of nuclear maturation and cell division, in the process of erythropoiesis. This failure of nuclear maturation results in the disease pernicious anemia, in which the basic abnormality is an atrophic gastric mucosa that fails to produce normal gastric secretions. The parietal cells of the gastric glands secrete a glycoprotein called intrinsic factor (IF), which combines with vitamin B_{12} in food and makes the B_{12} available for absorption by the gut. This occurs when the intrinsic factor binds tightly with the vitamin B_{12}, and in the bound state, the B_{12} is protected from digestion by the gastrointestinal (GI) secretions. While in the bound state,

the IF binds to specific receptor sites on the brush border membranes of the mucosal cells in the ileum, then vitamin B_{12} is transported into the blood during the next few hours by the process of pinocytosis, carrying the IF and the vitamin together through the membrane. Lack of the IF, therefore, causes diminished availability of vitamin B_{12} because of faulty absorption of the vitamin. Once vitamin B_{12} has been absorbed from the GI tract, it is first stored in large quantities in the liver, then released slowly as needed by the bone marrow. Untreated vitamin B_{12} deficiency can result in progressive neuropathy, which usually begins in the peripheral nerves. Its deficiency causes demyelination of nerve fibers, especially in the posterior columns, and occasionally the lateral columns, of the spinal cord. As a result, many people with pernicious anemia have loss of peripheral sensation and, in severe cases, even become paralyzed.

2. **Why is vitamin B_{12} anemia called megaloblastic anemia?** Vitamin B_{12} is called megaloblastic anemia because it is characterized by the appearance of megaloblasts (large primitive red blood cells). in the blood and bone marrow.

3. **Discuss classic manifestations of vitamin B_{12} deficiency a nurse should expect to observe during assessment of this client.** Classic manifestations of vitamin B_{12} deficiency anemia include pallor, glossitis (a smooth beefy-red tongue), fatigue, weight loss, anemia, thrombocytopenia, sore tongue, progressive neuropathy, and impaired cognition, all of which are related to the dysfunction of the bone marrow.

4. **Discuss the specific relationship of thrombocytes (platelets) and vitamin B_{12} deficiency and nursing management.** In vitamin B_{12} deficiency anemia, thrombocytes may be decreased, increasing the risk for easy bruising or bleeding. After identifying platelet deficiency, the nurse should institute precautions to avoid bleeding. These precautions include instructing the client or significant others (S.O.) to avoid flossing or using hard toothbrushes when providing oral care, and to avoid being constipated by increasing intake of fluids and foods high in fiber. Nurses should avoid administering injections, and should use the smallest needle size possible if injections are mandatory. The use of an air mattress and frequent positioning of the client is needed, and persons drawing blood specimens should avoid prolonged use of tourniquets. Nursing attendants can be assigned to monitor the client's skin for signs of ecchymoses, petechiae, complaints of epistaxis, gingival bleeding, and hematuria. Licensed practical nurses can test stool for occult bleeding, measure and monitor changes in abdominal girth, and monitor signs of changes in level of consciousness. A current blood sample should be kept in the laboratory for crosshatching if needed in an emergency.

5. **Discuss common nursing diagnoses for vitamin B_{12} deficiency anemia.**

   - Imbalanced nutrition: less than body requirements R/T poor nutritional intake, anorexia, and treatment – The nurse needs to collaborate with the registered dietitian in planning a dietary regimen for the client, until the client can become involved in the decision-making process. The client should be taught about foods high in protein, iron, and calories, needed to increase essential nutrients for hematopoiesis development. The nurse should monitor the amount of food consumed during meal times and teach the client about the dietary content of the foods that are eaten. The nurse should teach the client the importance of eating small, frequent meals with snacks throughout the day upon discharge.
   - Ineffective therapeutic regimen management R/T lack of knowledge of disease process and essential nutrients to retard vitamin B_{12} deficiency

The following are prescribed:

- Cyanocobalamin (vitamin B_{12}) 2,000 mcg PO per day for two weeks, then 1,000 mcg PO per day
- Folic acid (Apo-Folic) 0.4 mg PO daily

6. **What are the purposes for the prescribed medications?** *Oral cyanocobalamin* replaces the lack of B_{12} in the body. *Oral vitamin B_{12}* has been shown to have an efficacy equal to that of injections in the treatment of pernicious anemia. It contains B complex vitamins that are essential for cell reproduction, maturation of RBCs, nucleoprotein synthesis, and maintenance of nervous system (myelin synthesis). *Folic acid* stimulates the

production of RBCs, white blood cells (WBCs), and platelets to improve symptoms directly related to vitamin B_{12} deficiency.

7. **What are the most common adverse reactions, drug-to-drug, drug-to-food/herbal interactions of cyanocobalamin (vitamin B_{12})?** The most common adverse reaction of *cyanocobalamin* is hypokalemia. Drug-to-drug interactions may occur with the simultaneous use of aminosalicylic acid, neomycin sulfate, anticonvulsants, extended-release potassium supplements, colchicine, and cimetidine, which may decrease absorption of oral *cyanocobalamin* and vitamin C. The simultaneous use with chloramphenicol may interfere with the therapeutic response of *cyanocobalamin*, and delay hematopoiesis growth. Drug-to-food/herbal interactions may occur with the simultaneous use of foods high in vitamin C, which may decrease oral absorption and effectiveness of vitamin B_{12}. Common adverse reactions of *folic acid* are not clinically established. Drug-to-drug interactions may occur with the simultaneous use of pyrimethamine; methotrexate, trimethoprim, and triamterene may prevent the activation of folic acid. The simultaneous use of sulfonamides, antacids, and cholestyramine may decrease folic acid absorption. *Folic acid* requirements are increased with the simultaneous use of estrogens, phenytoin, phenobarbital, primidone, carbamazepine, or corticosteroids. There are no clinically significant drug-to-food/herbal interactions established for **folic acid.**

8. **Discuss factors that may inhibit folic acid absorption.** Factors that may inhibit folic acid absorption are poor nutrition, especially a lack of leafy green vegetables (particularly spinach, asparagus, and broccoli), liver, citrus fruits, yeast, dried beans, nuts and grains, because all of these contain folic acid. Other factors include malabsorption syndromes, particular small bowel disorders that interfere with adequate intestinal absorption of essential vitamins such as folic acid, or inflammatory disorders, such as regional enteritis, ulcerative colitis, or alcoholism. Regional enteritis, ulcerative colitis, and alcoholism cause inflammation of the stomach, pancreas, and intestine, resulting in the interference of the normal processes of digestion and absorption. Alcohol also increases the body's requirements for B vitamins, which are needed to metabolize alcohol. Because alcoholism has a direct relationship with malnutrition by potentiating destructive effects on the liver, there are gastrointestinal changes that take place, with folic acid deficiency being the most responsible for the malabsorption caused by alcoholic malnutrition. Clients on hemodialysis have also the risk for folic deficiency because folic acid is lost during dialysis.

9. **Discuss client education for vitamin B_{12} deficiency anemia.** Vitamin B_{12} deficiency is treated by replacement of vitamin B_{12}. If the deficiency is due to defective absorption or absence of the IF, the client will need monthly intramuscular injections of the vitamin. To prevent development of complications in clients with pernicious anemia or an inability to absorb B_{12}, the client will need life-long injections of the vitamin. The client may eat foods that are rich sources of vitamin B_{12} such as nutrient-added breakfast cereals, fortified soy milk, organ meats, clams, oysters, egg yolk, crab, salmon, sardines, muscle meat, milk, and dairy products.

10. **Discuss nursing implications for clients with vitamin B_{12} deficiency.** The use of Schilling test for detection of pernicious anemia has been supplanted for the most part by serologic testing for parietal cell and intrinsic factor antibodies. Gastrectomy predisposes clients to the development of cobalamin deficiency. Because cobalamin plays an important role in DNA synthesis and neurologic function, deficiency can lead to a wide spectrum of hematologic and neuropsychiatric disorders. However, early diagnosis and prompt treatment can delay the progression of the disorder. Although the daily requirement of cobalamin is approximately 2 mcg, the initial oral replacement dosage consists of a single daily dose of 1,000 to 2,000 mcg. This high dose is required because of the variable absorption of oral vitamin B_{12} in doses of 500 mcg or less. Nurses need to be cognizant that even when anemia is severe in persons with pernicious anemia, RBC transfusions may not be used because the person's body has compensated over time by expanding the total blood volume. Therefore, administering transfusion to such persons, particularly those who are elderly and/or have cardiac dysfunction, can precipitate pulmonary edema. If transfusions are required for life-threatening conditions, the RBCs should be transfused slowly, with careful attention to signs and symptoms of overload.

References

Black, J.M. and Hawks, J.H (2005). *Medical-Surgical Nursing: Clinical Management for Positive Outcomes.* Philadelphia: W. B. Saunders.

Broyles, B.E. (2005). *Medical-Surgical Nursing Clinical Companion.* Durham, NC: Carolina Academic Press.

Corbet, J.V. (2004). *Laboratory Tests and Diagnostic Procedures with Nursing Diagnoses* (6th ed.). Upper Saddle River, NJ: Pearson Prentice Hall.

Gahart, B.L. and Nazareno, A.R. (2005). *2005 Intraveneous Medications.* St. Louis: Elsevier Mosby.

Green, R. (March 1996). "Screening for Vitamin B_{12} Deficiency: Caveat Emptor." *Annals of Internal Medicine* 124(5): 509–511. Available at http://annals.org/cgi/content/full/124/5/509

Huether, S.E. and McCance, K.L. (2004). *Understanding Pathophysiology* (3rd ed.). St. Louis: Mosby.

Ignatavicius, D.D. and Workman, M.L. (2006). *Medical-Surgical Nursing across the Health Care Continuum* (5th ed.). Philadelphia: W.B. Saunders.

Spratto, G.R. and Woods, A.L. (2005). *2005 Edition: PDR Nurse's Drug Handbook.* Clifton Park, NY: Thomson Delmar Learning.

CASE STUDY 2

Renal Calculi

GENDER
- M

AGE
- 34

SETTING
- Clinic

ETHNICITY/CULTURE
- Japanese/Asian

PREEXISTING CONDITIONS

COEXISTING CONDITIONS

LIFESTYLE
- Employed for the last four years as a computer analyst for a U.S. company

COMMUNICATION
- English as a second language

DISABILITY

SOCIOECONOMIC STATUS
- Upper

SPIRITUAL/RELIGIOUS
- Shinto

PHARMACOLOGIC
- Morphine sulfate (Duramorph)
- Oxybutynin chloride (Ditropan)
- Hydrochlorothiazide (HydroDIURIL)

PSYCHOSOCIAL
- Fear
- Pain
- Anxiety

LEGAL

ETHICAL

ALTERNATIVE THERAPY
- Imagery
- Relaxation techniques

PRIORITIZATION
- Pain management
- Prevent kidney damage

DELEGATION
- RN
- Client education

EASY

THE DIGESTIVE AND URINARY SYSTEMS

Level of difficulty: Easy

Overview: This case involves pain management as well as questioning the client about personal or family history of urologic stones, obtaining a diet history, including fluid intake patterns. If the client has a history of stone formation, it should be determined if chemical analysis of the stone(s) was performed in the past and what the preventive measures were.

Client Profile

Mr. J is a 34-year-old male who arrives at the emergency department (ED) of a busy urban hospital accompanied by his brother, who drove Mr. J from his office to the ED. Mr. J is 5'6" and weighs 134 pounds.

Case Study

On arrival, Mr. J reports an "unbearable" pain that is intermittent in nature. He describes the pain as more intense while he was walking to his brother's car. Mr. J also reports that the pain began insidiously, one day ago, and he noticed it while working at his desk. He said that, later that day, he felt nauseated and was diaphoretic. He tried to take some fluids but the nausea would not subside, which decreased his fluid intake. Later that night, he felt warm, but did not know what his temperature was. Upon awakening in the morning, the pain had decreased much. However, when he urinated, the amount was small, and the color was pink-red. He prepared and left for work, trying to avoid the discomfort. While preparing a report for presentation at a luncheon meeting, he felt a pain that radiated from his left side to his abdomen. The pain was severe for about one minute. He informed his brother, who works in an adjoining building, and the brother transported him to the ED. Mr. J denies previous episodes of this type of pain. He reports no past or current medication history. Social history includes racquetball on weekends, occasional games of tennis, and he enjoys drinking white wine with the evening meal, which usually includes rhubarb and wheat germ. He is triaged by a nurse. His vital signs are:

   Blood pressure: 130/82
   Pulse: 94 and regular
   Respirations: 18
   Temperature: 101.0° F

He is seen by the ED health care provider, who does a history and physical, then orders a stat dose of morphine sulfate 5 mg/SQ. An intravenous line with dextrose 5% and 0.45 sodium chloride at 100 mL/hr is initiated. A computed tomography (CT) scan is done and calcium oxalate stones are identified in the left kidney calyx. A urine dipstick test is positive for hematuria, and urinalysis reveals red blood cells (RBCs) in the urine. There is no turbidity or odor from the urine specimen. Mr. J's laboratory results are:

   Serum calcium: 10.5 mg/dL
   Serum phosphate: 5 mg/dL
   Serum uric acid: 9 mg/dL
   Urine uric acid: 800 mg/24 hr
   Urine calcium: 260 mg/24 hr
   Urine phosphate: 1.3 g/24 hr
   Urine specific gravity: 1.026

After the health care provider reviews the laboratory data and diagnostic results, a diagnosis of renal calculi is confirmed. Mr. J's pain has subsided and he denies feeling nauseated. He has voided 100 mL of dusky-colored urine with trace elements of blood. The urine is strained and there is one visible stone. A sample of the urine is sent to the lab for microscopic analysis. Mr. J's vital signs are:

   Blood pressure: 110/70
   Pulse: 78 and regular
   Respirations 14
   Temperature: 98.4° F

Mr. J will be discharged in the late evening. Mr. J is to return to his primary health care provider for follow-up care in two weeks.

Questions and Suggested Answers

1. **Discuss factors that contribute to urolithiasis.** *Metabolic abnormalities* result in increased urine levels of calcium, oxaluric acid, uric acid, or citric acid. *Warm climates* cause increased fluid loss, low urine volume, and increased solute concentration in urine. A *diet* with large intake of dietary proteins increases uric acid excretion. Excessive amounts of tea or fruit juices elevate urinary oxalate level. Large intake of calcium and oxalate, and low fluid intake increase urinary concentration.

2. **Discuss the most common types of kidney stones.** Calcium stones are the most common kidney stones, and are composed of calcium oxalate and/or calcium phosphate. *Calcium oxalate* are small stones that often get trapped in the ureter. Their predisposing factors include idiopathic hypercalciuria, hyperoxaluria, independent of urinary pH, and family history. *Calcium phosphate struvite* are mixed stones (typically) with struvite or oxalate stones. They are common in women, always in association with urinary tract infections, and are large staghorn types. The predisposing factors are alkaline urine, primary hyperparathyroidism, and urinary tract infections, usually Proteus organisms. *Uric acid stones* are predominant in men, with a high incidence in Jewish men. The predisposing factors include gout, acid urine, and heredity. *Cystine stones* are related to a genetic autosomal recessive defect, and defective absorption of cystine in the gastrointestinal (GI) tract and the kidney, with excess concentrations causing stone formation. The predisposing factor is acid urine.

3. **Discuss common manifestations of urolithiasis.** A common manifestation is sharp, severe pain with sudden onset. If the stone is in the renal calyces, the pain is referred to as renal colic and originates deep in the lumbar region. Pain radiates around the side and down toward the testicles in the male, and the bladder in the female. Pain that is referred to as ureteral colic pain radiates toward the genitalia and thigh. When the pain is severe, the client will usually exhibit nausea, vomiting, pallor, and diaphoresis, and be quite anxious, due to an autonomic response to the severity of the pain.

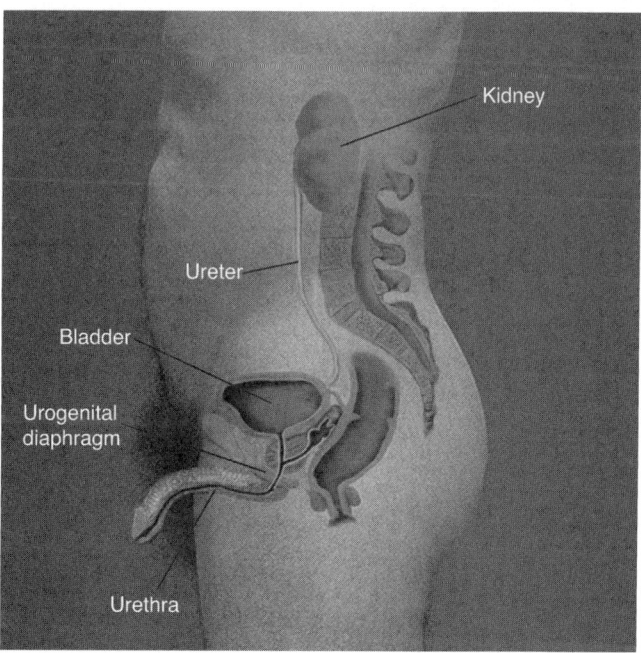

Male urinary tract

4. **Discuss common complications of urolithiasis.** *Urinary tract obstruction* is an interference with the flow of urine at any site along the urinary tract. An obstruction may be anatomic or functional, which impedes blood flow proximal to the blockage, dilates the urinary system, increases the risk for infection, and compromises renal function. *Hydronephrosis* occurs because of an obstruction resulting in dilation of the ureter and accumulation

of urine in the ureter, and dilation of the renal pelvis and calyces proximal to a blockage, resulting in enlargement of the renal pelvis and calyces (hydronephrosis). ***Hypertension*** may develop because, during acute renal obstruction, the renin-angiotensin-aldosterone process is activated; there is retention of sodium, water, and urea. ***Urinary tract infection*** occurs due to obstruction of the lower urinary tract because of incomplete bladder emptying and urethral turbulence. Infection that involves an obstructed kidney causes further damage to the renal parenchyma and may be difficult to eradicate because of urinary stasis. If the infection affects the renal pelvis, and causes scarring, this will increase the damage caused by the obstruction.

The following are prescribed:

- Morphine sulfate (Astromorph PF) 1–2 mg IV q1–2h
- Oxybutynin chloride (Ditropan) 5 mg PO two times per day, today only
- Hydrochlorothiazide (HydroDIURIL) 50 mg PO two times per day
- IV D 5.45% NS at 100 mL/hr until 5:00 PM today and encourage fluid intake of two to three liters today
- Accurate intake and output, and strain all urine
- Discharge after 5:00 PM with follow-up appointment in two weeks

5. **What are the purposes for the prescribed orders?** ***Morphine sulfate*** is a narcotic analgesic that helps to relieve moderate to severe pain. It helps to relief the pain of renal calculi by binding with receptors at the supraspinal level to produce analgesia. ***Oxybutynin chloride*** helps to control the pain of bladder spasms. It is a spasmolytic drug that acts within the spinal cord to suppress hyperactive reflexes involved in regulation of muscle movement. When the reflexes are suppressed, spasms are decreased or obliterated, and pain is relieved. ***HydroDIURIL*** promotes diuresis and helps to eliminate stones from the kidneys. It is a thiazide diuretic that promotes calcium resorption from the renal tubules back into the body, thereby reducing urine calcium loads and preventing formation of calcium stones. ***IV D 5.45% NS at 100 mL/hr*** and ***fluid intake*** of two to three liters per day help to dilute the urine and prevent dehydration and formation of calcium stones. ***Accurate intake*** and ***output*** provides information on how the kidneys are filtering and eliminating waste products. If there were a deficit in urinary output, it would be an indicator of possible urinary obstruction. Straining all urine will aid in identifying stones and will guide management. Follow-up care is important to re-evaluate the effectiveness of medication therapy.

6. **What are the most common adverse reactions, drug-to-drug, drug-to-food/herbal interactions of the prescribed medications?** The most common adverse reactions of ***oxybutynin chloride*** are drowsiness, blurred vision, dry mouth, constipation, pruritus at application site (if drug is patch), aggravation of benign prostatic hypertrophy, and glaucoma. Drug-to-drug interactions may occur with the simultaneous use of other anticholinergic agents, including amantadine, antidepressants, phenothiazines, and disopyramide. Additive central nervous system (CNS) depression may occur with alcohol, antihistamines, opioids, and sedative/hypnotics. The simultaneous use with nitrofurantoin may increase the serum levels of oxybutynin and cause toxicity. If used simultaneously with levodopa, oxybutynin chloride may decrease the effectiveness of levodopa. When used with atenolol, digoxin, or nitrofurantoin, it increases the absorption of these agents, increasing their effects. Simultaneous use with haloperidol may result in tardive dyskinesia, worsening of schizophrenia and decreased haloperidol levels. If used simultaneously with doxycycline and biphosphonates, it may exacerbate esophagitis, because doxycycline and biphosphonates cause esophagitis. There is increased anticholinergic action with jimsonweed and scopolia. The most common adverse reactions of ***hydroDIURIL*** are hypokalemia, hyperuricemia, and hyperglycemia. Drug-to-drug interactions may occur with the simultaneous use with other antihypertensives, resulting in additive hypotension. Additive hypokalemia may occur with the simultaneous use of corticosteroids, amphotericin B, mezlocillin, piperacillin, or ticarcillin. When used simultaneously with lithium, lithium excretion is decreased and the risk of toxicity develops. The use of cholestyramine or colestipol with hydroDIURIL decreases absorption of the drugs. There is no clinically significant drug-to-drug, drug-to-herb/food clinically established for hydroDIURIL.

7. **Discuss other diagnostic tests used to identify urolithiasis.** *Intravenous pyelogram (IVP)* also known as the excretory urogram (EUG) is most frequently performed to evaluate the calyces and pelvis of the kidneys, ureters, and urinary bladder when abnormalities of these organs are suspected. It can localize the degree and site of obstruction or confirm the presence of a radiolucent stone, such as a uric acid or cystine calculus. Because a contrast medium is used, the client is asked about allergies to iodine or iodinated contrast media, and if the client has history of allergies to these, or other types of allergies, an antihistamine such as diphenhydramine (Benadryl) or steroidal therapy is initiated before the contrast is administered. The status of the kidney's ability to excrete the dye is determined by the assessment of the blood urea nitrogen (BUN) and creatinine level. The normal BUN is 5-20 mg/dL, and the creatinine is 0.5 to 1.3 mg/dL (values may vary depending on the parameters of different agencies). *Renal ultrasonography* identifies radiopaque or radiolucent calculus in the renal pelvis, calyx, or proximal ureter. *Flat-plate X-ray (KUB)* identifies larger, radiopaque stones.

8. **Discuss endourologic procedures used to remove or crush urolithiasis.** *Cystolitholapaxy* is the use of a lithotrite (stone crusher) to crush large stones in the bladder. The bladder is then irrigated, and the stones washed out. The use of a nephroscope (*percutaneous nephrolithotomy*) requires general or spinal anesthesia. A probe is inserted through a sinus tract from the skin into the kidney pelvis, producing ultrasonic waves, which break the stones into sandlike particles, which are then removed and the pelvis irrigated. However, this procedure is only used for large stones and after other lithotripsy procedures have failed. The electrohydraulic lithotripsy uses a probe to break stones into fragments that are then removed by forceps or suction. The probe is placed directly on a stone, then crushes it. For this procedure, a continuous saline irrigation is implemented to flush out the stone particles, and the outflow drainage is strained and the particles analyzed. The calculi can also be removed by forceps or basket extraction. *Extracorporeal shock wave lithotripsy* is a non-invasive procedure. However, the client is anesthetized (spinal or general anesthesia) and placed in a water bath. The anesthesia is necessary to keep the client very still during the procedure. A fluoroscopy or ultrasound is used to guide or focus the lithotripter on the affected kidney, and a high-voltage spark generator produces high-energy acoustic shock waves that shatter the stone without damaging surrounding tissues. The stone is broken into fine sand, which is excreted into the client's urine within a few days after the procedure.

9. **Discuss the difference between a ureterolithotomy and a pyelolithotomy.** Surgical therapy is needed for some clients, such as the very obese or individuals with complex abnormalities in the calyces or at the point where the ureter crosses the iliac vessels, referred to as the UPJ. A ureterolithotomy is one of the surgical therapies that involve making of an incision in the affected ureter to remove a calculus. A pyelolithotomy is another surgical therapy that involves the making of an incision into and removal of a stone from the kidney pelvis.

10. **Discuss client education for urolithiasis.** The client should avoid foods that are high in calcium oxalate (the type of stone identified in the urine), such as spinach, black tea, and rhubarb, Swiss chard, coca, beets, wheat germ, pecans, okra, lime peel, and chocolate. The client must finish the entire prescription of medications to ensure that stones will be eliminated from the body. The client must drink at least three liters (3,000 mL) of fluid a day to dilute potential stone-forming crystals, prevent dehydration, and promote urine flow. Pain in the region of the kidneys or bladder may signal the beginning of an infection or the formation of another stone. If the client experiences this type of pain, the primary health care provider should be consulted. The client should keep follow-up appointments as scheduled.

References

Black, J.M. and Hawks, J.H (2005). *Medical-Surgical Nursing: Clinical Management for Positive Outcomes*. Philadelphia: W.B. Saunders.

Broyles, B.E. (2005). *Medical-Surgical Nursing Clinical Companion*. Durham, NC: Carolina Academic Press.

Gahart, B.L. and Nazareno, A.R. (2005). *2005 Intravenous Medications*. St. Louis: Mosby.

Huether, S.E. and McCance, K.L. (2004). *Understanding Pathophysiology* (3rd ed.). St. Louis: Mosby.

Ignatavicius, D.D. and Workman, M.L. (2006). *Medical-Surgical Nursing across the Health Care Continuum* (5th ed.). Philadelphia: W.B. Saunders.

Skidmore-Roth, L. (2006). *Mosby's Handbook of Herbs & Natural Supplements*. St. Louis: Mosby.

Spratto, G.R. and Woods, A.L. (2005). *2005 Edition: PDR Nurse's Drug Handbook.* Clifton Park, NY: Thomson Delmar Learning.

CASE STUDY 3

Stage IIC Cancer of the Prostate

GENDER
- M

AGE
- 52

SETTING
- Urology outpatient clinic of a medical center

ETHNICITY/CULTURE
- Mexican American

PREEXISTING CONDITIONS

COEXISTING CONDITIONS
- Strong familial predisposition; two brothers with colon cancer

LIFESTYLE
- Utility employee
- Worked with asbestos for 28 years

COMMUNICATION
- English as a second language

DISABILITY

SOCIOECONOMIC STATUS
- Middle

SPIRITUAL/RELIGIOUS
- Catholic

PHARMACOLOGIC

PSYCHOSOCIAL
- Anxiety
- Depression
- Fatigue

LEGAL
- Work-related factor may result in compensation

ETHICAL
- Possibility of early retirement

ALTERNATIVE THERAPY
- St. John's Wort

PRIORITIZATION
- Initial interview
- Questions about genitourinary history

DELEGATION
- RN
- Client education

THE DIGESTIVE AND URINARY SYSTEMS

Level of difficulty: Moderate

Overview: This case involves the use of the nursing process, systems assessment, and critical-thinking skills to provide optimum care while monitoring fluid and electrolyte status. Focus will be on family history, knowledge of the disease process, and the importance of compliance with treatment regimens.

Client Profile

Mr. G is a 52-year-old married male who is 5'10" and weighs 190 pounds. He is employed by a major utility gas company. Mr. G is scheduled for an office visit with his family health care provider due to results of prior laboratory and diagnostic tests.

Case Study

Mr. G reports frequency of urination with reduction in urinary stream, dysuria, nocturia, change in bowel habits (constipation and occasional diarrhea), and a feeling of incomplete bowel emptying. He is concerned about the symptoms because of his family history of colon cancer. He also reports having had a history of gastric ulcers for five years and a family history cancer in both of his brothers. When questioned about his dietary habits, Mr. G reports maintaining a diet low in fiber, and high in fat, protein, and refined carbohydrates. However, every year since he turned 40, he has undergone an annual physical exam with his primary health care provider that includes digital/rectal examination His most recent digital/rectal examination was "abnormal;" his stools have been negative guaiac annually. At age 50, he had a proctosigmoidoscopy because of unusual constipation. His vital signs are:

- Blood pressure: 140/78
- Pulse: 80
- Respirations: 18
- Temperature: 98.4° F

During a rectal assessment at the clinic, a colon mass is located and will be staged as needed after further examination. The health care provider does a complete history and physical examination, then the client is scheduled for the following diagnostic tests: colonoscopy, serum for prostatic-specific antigen, acid phosphatase, alkaline phosphatase, and a transurethral ultrasonography (TRUS). Mr. G returns to the medical center on different dates to have the tests done. The tests are done as scheduled, and the results are received and reviewed by an oncologist and the medical team. Mr. G's laboratory results are:

- Prostatic-specific antigen (PSA): 3.8 ng/mL
- Acid phosphatase: 0.53 I/L
- Serum alkaline phosphatase: 128 U/L

The TRUS reveals small tumors in the prostate gland. The oncologist, surgeon, and health care provider explain the results to Mr. G and make a diagnosis of prostate cancer Stage IIC. Plans for treatment are explained to the client and the decision is made for treatment. Mr. G remains in the Same Day Care oncology unit of the hospital for further instructions but will be sent home today.

Questions and Suggested Answers

1. **Discuss the risk factors and pathophysiology of prostate cancer.** Age, ethnicity, and family history are three nonmodifiable risk factors for prostate cancer. A high-fat diet is thought to be associated with an increased risk for prostate cancer. A family history of prostate cancer, especially first-degree relatives (fathers, brothers) is also associated with prostate cancer. Prostate cancer is usually slow growing. It can spread by three routes: direct extension, through the lymph system, or through the bloodstream. Spread by direct extension involves the seminal vesicles, urethral mucosa, bladder wall, and external sphincter. The cancer later spreads through the lymphatic system to the regional lymph nodes, and the veins from the prostate seem to be the mode of spread to the pelvic bones, head of the femur, lower lumbar spine, liver, and lungs. Once the tumor

has spread to distant sites, the major problem becomes the management of pain, with pain becoming severe, especially in the back and the legs, because of compression of the spinal cord and destruction of bone.

2. **Discuss clinical manifestations of prostate cancer.** Prostate cancer is usually asymptomatic in the early stages. Eventually the client may have symptoms of dysuria, hesitancy, dribbling, frequency, urgency, hematuria, nocturia, retention, interruption of urinary stream, and inability to urinate. Pain in the lumbosacral area that radiates down to the hips or legs, when coupled with urinary symptoms, may indicate metastasis.

3. **Discuss cultural and ethnic considerations for the male reproductive system.** Prostate cancer occurs twice as frequently among black American men as among white men. Black American men tend to be diagnosed with prostate cancer at an earlier age, have more advanced disease at the time of diagnosis, and have a higher mortality rate than do white men. Hispanic and Asian American men have a lower incidence of prostate cancer and lower mortality rates as compared with white American men. Testicular cancer occurs most frequently among white Americans compared with other ethnic groups and is rare in black Americans.

4. **Discuss diagnostic studies used to aid the confirmation of prostate cancer.** The two primary screening tools for prostate cancer are direct rectal examination (DRE) and the PSA. The normal level of PSA is 0 to 4 nanogram (ng)/mL to 4 microgram (μg)/Liter. The diagnosis of prostate cancer is confirmed by a histologic examination of tissue removed surgically by transurethral resection, open prostatectomy, transurethral needle biopsy. Fine-needle aspiration is a quick, painless method of obtaining prostate cells for cytologic examination. This procedure hel mg ps to determine the stage of the disease. TRUS studies are indicated for men who have elevated PSA levels and abnormal DRE findings.

The following are prescribed:

- External-beam irradiation with 175 rads × one week. Start first dose today then discharge to home.
- Oxybutynin chloride (Ditropan) 5 mg PO two times per day
- Return to Same Day Care oncology unit × six more days

5. **What are the purposes of the prescribed treatment and medication?** *External-beam irradiation* is prescribed for Mr. G because the tumors are confined to the prostate and do not require higher dose of irradiation. *Oxybutynin chloride* is prescribed because it decreases the urinary bladder spasms that may occur from external-beam radiation.

6. **What are common adverse reactions to the prescribed treatment and medication?** Common adverse reactions include radiation-induced cystitis, radiation-induced proctitis, and erectile dysfunction.

7. **Discuss other therapies that may be prescribed to treat prostate cancer.** *Interstitial irradiation* (implantation of radioactive seeds of iodine or palladium), also referred to as brachytherapy, is a procedure that allows higher radiation doses directly into the tissue while sparing surrounding tissue (rectum and bladder). The radioactive seeds are placed in the prostate gland with a needle through a grid template guided by transrectal ultrasound. The grid template and ultrasound ensure accurate placement of the seeds. Hormonal therapy is focused on reducing the levels of circulating androgens in order to reduce tumor growth. However, one of the biggest challenges with hormonal therapy is the development of hormone-refractory disease.

8. **Discuss surgical procedures used for Stage IIC prostate cancer.** A *suprapubic prostatectomy* is one of the surgical procedures used with prostate cancer. It requires a surgical approach through the bladder, permits exploration for cancerous lymph nodes, allows for more complete removal of obstructing gland, and permits treatment of associated bladder lesions. A *transurethral resection (TURP)* is used to remove prostatic tissue with the use of an instrument introduced through the urethra.

9. **Discuss postoperative complications of prostate surgeries.** Complications associated with a prostatectomy depend on the type of surgery and include hemorrhage, clot formation, catheter obstruction, and altered sexual dysfunctions. All prostatectomies carry a risk of impotence because of the potential damage to the pudendal nerves, through which most of the skeletal motor fibers are transmitted to the external bladder

sphincter, which aids in bladder emptying. If retrograde ejaculation occurs (during ejaculation, the seminal fluid goes into the bladder and is excreted into the urine) and is not corrected, the seminal fluid mixed with urine can spread from the prostatic urethra through the vas deferens into the epididymis, resulting in infection. If this is detected, a vasectomy may be performed to correct the abnormality.

10. **Discuss client education for prostate cancer.** Radiation-induced cystitis may develop. Signs of radiation-induced cystitis include discomfort with voiding, daytime voiding frequency, increased number of times awakened to void, and suprapubic discomfort. Signs of cystitis will subside within four to six weeks of the therapy. Radiation-induced proctitis may occur and is characterized by frequent defecation, bowel cramping or urgency. The defecation of blood and mucus also may occur, but will subside within four to six weeks. External-beam radiation therapy may irritate the perineal skin. Therefore, the perineal area should be cleansed daily with mild cleanser and lukewarm water, dried thoroughly and small amounts of cornstarch-based or talcum-based powder should be applied to the area. The client needs to rest during the day, because external-beam radiation causes fatigue. Significant others should be included in the discharge planning discussion, if they are available, and meal planning should be included in the discussion. Foods high in protein and carbohydrates should be identified at this time.

References

Abel, L., Dafoe-Lambie, J., Butler, W.M., and Merrick, G.S. (2003). "Treatment Outcomes and Quality-of-Life Issues for Patients Treated with Prostate Brachytherapy." *Clinical Journal of Oncology Nursing* 7(1): 48–54.

Black, J.M. and Hokanson-Hawks, J. (2005). *Medical-Surgical Nursing: Clinical Management for Positive Outcomes* (7th ed.). Philadelphia: W.B. Saunders.

Broyles, B.E. (2005). *Medical-Surgical Nursing Clinical Companion.* Durham, NC: Carolina Academic Press.

Claker-Tasker, V. (June 2003). "Socioeconomic Status and African Americans' Perceptions of Cancer." *Journal of National Black Nurses Association* 14(6): 13–19.

Corbet, J.V. (2004). *Laboratory Tests and Diagnostic Procedures with Nursing Diagnoses* (6th ed.). Upper Saddle River, NJ: Prentice Hall.

Gahart, B.L. and Nazareno, A.R. (2005). *2005 Intraveneous Medications.* St. Louis: Mosby.

Haughney, A. (2004). "Nausea and Vomiting in End-Stage Cancer." *American Journal of Nursing* 104(11): 40–48.

Huether, S.E. and McCance, K.L. (2004). *Understanding Pathophysiology* (3rd ed.). St. Louis: Mosby.

Ignatavicius, D.D. and Workman, M.L. (2006). *Medical-Surgical Nursing across the Health Care Continuum* (5th ed.). Philadelphia: W.B. Saunders.

Spratto, G.R. and Woods, A.L. (2005). *2005 Edition: PDR Nurse's Drug Handbook.* Clifton Park, NY: Thomson Delmar Learning.

Wickham, R. (2003). "Nausea and Vomiting: Palliative Care Issues across the Cancer Experience." *Oncology Supportive Care* 4(1): 44–54.

CASE STUDY 4

Ulcerative Colitis

GENDER
- F

AGE
- 35

SETTING
- Hospital

ETHNICITY/CULTURE
- White American

PREEXISTING CONDITIONS
- Stress

COEXISTING CONDITIONS
- Recurrent respiratory infection
- Emotional stress

LIFESTYLE
- Phlebotomy supervisor for a large private, nonprofit medical organization

COMMUNICATION

DISABILITY

SOCIOECONOMIC STATUS
- Middle

SPIRITUAL/RELIGIOUS
- Episcopalian

PHARMACOLOGIC
- Mesalamine (Asacol)
- Sulfasalazine (Azulfidine)
- Metronidazole (Flagyl)

PSYCHOSOCIAL
- Anxiety

LEGAL

ETHICAL
- Is the quality of life optimal for a 35-year-old client with ulcerative colitis disease?

ALTERNATIVE THERAPY
- Flaxseed
- Vitamin C
- Aloe vera

PRIORITIZATION
- Assess pain
- Maintain
- fluid and electrolyte balance

DELEGATION
- RN
- Client education

MODERATE

THE DIGESTIVE AND URINARY SYSTEMS

Level of difficulty: Moderate

Overview: This case involves accurate assessment of fluid loss, monitoring for signs of dehydration, and critical assessment of the abdomen for characteristics of bowel sounds, distention, and tenderness. It also involves prioritization in a triage situation to prevent serious complications.

Client Profile

Ms. V is a 35-year-old, unmarried phlebotomy supervisor for a large medical team. Ms. V is 5'10" and weighs 120 pounds. She has a two-year history of inflammatory bowel disease and has been hospitalized twice for exacerbations of intermittent diarrhea and colicky pain in the right lower quadrant. She appears anxious upon arrival at the emergency department (ED) and verbalizes frustration with the recurring problems. Ms. V also reports occasional periods of depression, which she relates to the disease.

Case Study

Ms. V's fiancé accompanies her to the ED. Her vital signs on admission are:

Blood pressure: 110/68
Pulse: 104 and regular
Respirations: 20
Temperature: 101.2° F

Ms. V experienced ten bloody bowel movements of moderate amounts accompanied by localized abdominal pain prior to arriving in the ED. An intravenous line with IV fluid of D_5LR at 150 cc/hr is initiated via a peripheral venous access. Ms. V is later seen by the ED health care provider and a gastroenterologist for initial assessment and data collection to help determine her diagnosis. Ms. V is placed on "nothing by mouth" (NPO) status, except ice chips. Plans to insert a nasogastric tube if she vomits are discussed with the health care provider and nurse. Serum labs prescribed prior to invasive diagnostic work-up include: hematocrit, hemoglobin, white blood cell count, erythrocyte sedimentation rate, serum sodium, serum potassium, serum chloride, albumin, stool for occult blood, ova, parasites, culture, and sensitivity. Results of the serum labs are:

White blood cell (WBC) count: $12,000/mm^3$
Erythrocyte sedimentation rate (ESR): 24 mm/hr
Hemoglobin (Hgb): 15.2 g/dL
Hematocrit (Hct): 30.5%
Potassium (K+): 2.6 mEq/L
Blood urea nitrogen (BUN): 18 mg/dL
Sodium (Na): 134 mEq/L
Chloride (Cl^-): 98 mEq/L
Creatinine: 0.09 mg/dL

A double-contrast barium enema with air contrast and colonoscopy with biopsies are discussed with Ms. V and will be scheduled for the next day if the vomiting and diarrhea subsides. The vomiting and diarrhea subside and the double-contrast barium enema and biopsies are done, which provide the definitive diagnosis of ulcerative colitis (UC). The results are reviewed by the radiologist, followed by discussion with the multidisciplinary team and the client, and the plan of care is initiated.

Questions and Suggested Answers

1. **What are common nursing diagnoses for the client with UC?**

   - Diarrhea R/T irritated bowel and intestinal hyperactivity
   - Anxiety R/T possible social embarrassment, unfamiliar environment, diagnostic tests and treatment

- Imbalanced nutrition: less than body requirements R/T decreased intake, decreased absorption, and increased nutrient loss through diarrhea
- Impaired skin integrity R/T diarrhea and altered nutritional status

2. **What are the expected findings of the barium enema with air contrast and endoscopy?** The barium enema with air contrast identifies changes in mucosal pattern and incomplete filling, which are indicative of UC. The barium enema differentiates between ulcerative colitis and Crohn's disease. Ms. V's enema revealed areas of granular inflammation with ulcerations. The colon was narrow and shortened in appearance, and pseudopolyps were present.

3. **What is the purpose of intestinal biopsies in diagnosing UC?** Intestinal biopsies provide a definitive diagnosis of ulcerative colitis, by identifying cryptitis and crypt abscesses both of which are the hallmark for ulcerative colitis.

4. **What type of psychotherapy would be most effective for Ms. V at this time?** Interpersonal psychotherapy would be most effective for Ms. V at this time, because it deals with interpersonal relationships and social support, and is effective in managing anxiety and depression that are not related to organic causes.

5. **Discuss a serious cardiac complication that may develop due to Ms. V's low serum potassium level.** Potassium is a neurotransmitter and, with sodium, controls the electrical potential across cell membranes and maintains fluid volume. In the presence of hypokalemia, the cardiac muscle lacks adequate stimulations resulting in tachy and brady dysrhythmias, including ventricular dysrhythmia such as premature ventricular contractions and bradycardia.

The following are prescribed:

- Mesalamine (Asacol) 800 mg PO three times per day
- Sulfasalazine (Azulfidine) 250 mg PO four times per day
- Metronidazole (Flagyl) 7.5 mg/kg IV q6h
- Loperamide (Imodium) 4 mg PO followed by 2 mg after each formed stool
- Potassium chloride (K-chloride) 10 mEq/100 mL IV × four doses, repeat serum potassium after last dose

6. **What are the purposes for the prescribed medications?** *Sulfasalazine* and *mesalamine* provide relief of the symptoms by decreasing the inflammation and diarrhea. Sulfasalazine is a sulfonamide antibiotic as well as an aminosalicylate. Mesalamine is an anti-inflammatory agent that also is an aminosalicylate. When these agents are administered orally, they are converted in the colon by intestinal microflora to sulfapryidine and 5-aminosalicylic acid. They then exert an anti-inflammatory effect by inhibiting prostaglandin in the bowel, which helps to decrease production of inflammation and diarrhea. If diarrhea were to be stimulated by prostaglandin, intestinal mucosal transport and absorption of fluids and electrolytes would be further compromised, resulting in additional complications. The combining of both drugs enhances the anti-inflammatory and immunomodulatory properties, and enhances and provides a more effective control of the clinical manifestations. Combining oral and rectal *mesalamine* enhances the expected outcome because the combined method ensures that the entire colon is covered. *Metronidazole* is an antibacterial and antiprotozoal that is active against anaerobic organisms. It works by first being taken up by cells and then converted into its active form, which then interacts with DNA to cause strand breakage and loss of structure. When the structure is lost, there is inhibition of nucleic acid synthesis and, ultimately, cell death. *Loperamide* is effective because it inhibits gastrointestinal peristalsis by direct action on circular and longitudinal intestinal muscles, and prolongs transit time of intestinal content. *Potassium chloride* is an electrolyte solution that treats potassium deficiency secondary to bouts of diarrhea.

7. **What are the most common adverse reactions, drug-to-drug, and drug-to-food/herbal interactions of the prescribed medications?** The most common adverse reactions of *mesalamine* are sulfite sensitivity, headache, dizziness, fatigue, abdominal pain, cramps, or discomfort. Drug-to-drug interactions include a risk of neutropenia and increase in 6-thioguanine nucleotide levels in clients with Crohn's disease when mesalamine is used with azathioprine or mercaptopurine. There are no clinically significant drug-to-food/herbal interactions

established. The most common adverse reactions of ***sulfasalazine*** are headache, nausea, vomiting, anorexia, and allergic reactions. Drug-to-drug interaction may occur with the simultaneous administration of drugs containing iron or with antibiotics, which may alter the absorption of sulfasalazine. Use with digoxin decreases digoxin absorption and decreases folic acid absorption. There is a high rate of neutropenia when used with mercaptopurine or mercaptopurine. There are no clinically significant drug-to-food/herbal interactions established. The most common adverse reactions of ***metronidazole*** are abdominal cramping, anorexia, constipation, decreased libido, diarrhea, dizziness, mucous membrane dryness, and nausea. Drug-to-drug interactions may occur with simultaneous use of ritinavir, lopinavir/ritonavir, nitroglycerin, and phenobarbital, which may increase the metabolism of metronidazole. Alcohol and alcohol-containing products can cause toxic reactions. Cimetidine may increase serum metronidazole levels. Metronidazole potentiates hydantions and may decrease the metabolism of warfarin and increase its anticoagulant effects. Neurotoxicity is increased when used concurrently with other neurotoxic agents, such as ciprofloxacin, cyclosporine, and immipenem-cilastatin. There are no clinically significant drug-to-food/herbal interaction established. The most common adverse reactions of ***loperamide*** are drowsiness, constipation, dry mouth, and dizziness. Drug-to-drug interactions may occur with the simultaneous use of central nervous system (CNS) depressants, opioid analgesics, sedative or hypnotics. Drug-to-food/herbal interactions are seen with the simultaneous use of kava, valerian, skullcap, or chamomile, which can increase CNS depression. The most common adverse reactions of ***potassium chloride*** are nausea, vomiting, and hyperkalemia. Drug-to-drug interactions may occur with the simultaneous use of potassium-sparing diuretics resulting in hyperkalemia, and with angiotensin-converting enzyme (ACE) inhibitors causing potentiation of the potassium chloride and increasing the risk of hyperkalemia. There are no clinically significant drug-to-food/herbal interactions.

8. **Identify complementary and alternative therapies for clients with UC.** Alternative therapies for clients with ulcerative colitis include biofeedback, hypnosis, yoga, and acupuncture. Biofeedback is a technique used especially for stress-related conditions. It is a tool for empowering the mind by training it to take control of certain conscious and autonomic processes. It is an excellent tool for teaching relaxation. Biofeedback uses various monitoring devices to help clients become more aware of and able to control their own physiologic responses.

9. **Discuss specific nursing intervention activities for clients receiving intravenous potassium replacement for hypokalemia.**
    - Determine current serum potassium level prior to administering the prescribed dose, to avoid hyperkalemia.
    - Determine that the client is voiding at least 30 mL of urine per hour before administering intravenous K+ supplement. If kidney function is altered, supplemental potassium elimination will be delayed, and acute renal failure may develop.
    - Monitor intravenous site for infiltration during infusion therapy, because potassium is an irritating drug that could cause irritation to the tissues if infiltrated.
    - Do not administer more than 10 mEq/hr in any given amount of infusion fluid, to avoid development of cardiac dysrhythmias.
    - Monitor serum potassium level after supplemental doses to determine the need for modification.

10. **Discuss community-based nursing care for clients with risk for hypokalemia being discharged to home.**
    - The nurse should discuss common symptoms of hypokalemia with the client.
    - The symptoms should be listed on a card for the client to take home upon discharge.
    - Foods high in potassium and the importance of including them in the diet should be discussed.
    - The client and significant other, if applicable, should be taught to take the radial pulse and peripheral pulses, and the necessary action to take if the pulses are difficult to locate. The importance of checking them properly should be emphasized.
    - The importance of keeping clinic appointments and having serum potassium lab data monitored should be stressed during the client education and discharge discussion.

References

Broyles, B.E. (2005). *Medical-Surgical Nursing Clinical Companion.* Durham, NC: Carolina Academic Press

Corbet, J.V. (2004). *Laboratory Tests and Diagnostic Procedures with Nursing Diagnoses* (6th ed.). Upper Saddle River, NJ: Prentice Hall.

Gahart, B.L. and Nazareno, A.R. (2005). *2005 Intravenous Medications.* St. Louis: Mosby.

Huether, S.E. and McCance, K.L. (2004). *Understanding Pathophysiology* (3rd ed.). St. Louis: Mosby.

Ignatavicius, D.D. and Workman, M.L. (2006). *Medical-Surgical Nursing across the Health Care Continuum* (5th ed.). Philadelphia: W.B. Saunders.

Lehne, R.A. (2004). *Pharmacology for Nursing Care* (5th ed.). Philadelphia: W.B. Saunders.

LeMone, P. and Burke, K.M. (2004). *Medical-Surgical Nursing: Critical Thinking in Client Care* (3rd ed.). Upper Saddle River, NJ: Prentice Hall.

Lewis, S.M., Heitkemper, M.M., and Dirksen, S.R. (2004). *Medical-Surgical Nursing* (6th ed.). St. Louis: Mosby.

Phipps, W.J., Monahan, F.D., Sands, J.K., Marek, J.E., and Neighbors, M. (2003). *Medical-Surgical Nursing: Health and Illness Perspectives* (7th ed.). St. Louis: Mosby.

Spratto, G.R. and Woods, A.L. (2005). *2005 Edition: PDR Nurse's Drug Handbook.* Clifton Park, NY: Thomson Delmar Learning.

CASE STUDY 5

Acute Renal Failure

GENDER
- F

AGE
- 60

SETTING
- Hospital

ETHNICITY/CULTURE
- Black American

PREEXISTING CONDITIONS
- Hypertension
- Diabetes mellitus type 2

COEXISTING CONDITIONS
- Diabetes
- Hypertension

LIFESTYLE
- Housewife

COMMUNICATION
- Spanish and English

DISABILITY
- Yes

SOCIOECONOMIC STATUS
- Low

SPIRITUAL/RELIGIOUS
- Catholic

PHARMACOLOGIC
- Dopamine HcL
- Lantus (Insuline glargine)
- Human regular insulin (Humulin R)
- Nifedipine (Procardia)
- Furosemide (Lasix)
- Calcium carbonate (Os-cal)
- Digoxin (Lanoxin)
- Sodium polystyrene sulfonate (Kayexelate)

PSYCHOSOCIAL
- Depression

LEGAL

ETHICAL
- Is there an ethical dilemma of randomizing clients with ARF to a certain dialysis modality?

ALTERNATIVE THERAPY
- Prayer

PRIORITIZATION
- Determine risk factors for ARF
- Assess fluid balance
- Monitor serum potassium levels

DELEGATION
- RN
- Client education

MODERATE

THE DIGESTIVE AND URINARY SYSTEMS

Level of difficulty: Moderate

Overview: This case involves critical assessment of the client. The nurse must question the client about decrease in urinary output; history of hypertension; use of prescribed medications/herbals taken independently; history of constipation or diarrhea, anorexia, nausea or vomiting, and unusual fatigue. The case involves prioritization in a triage situation with other clients experiencing acute onset of other diseases. The nurse must use critical thinking in triaging clients in order of highest priority to avoid or manage complications that could develop. The nurse must be knowledgeable about sites of drug metabolism and must constantly monitor for unintended effects of prescribed drugs.

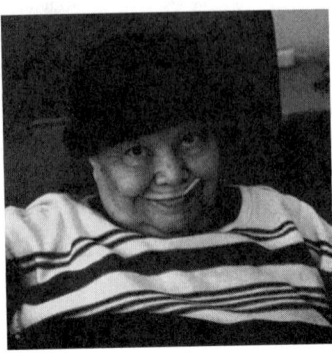

Client Profile

Ms. D is a 60-year-old client who lives in an apartment building in a "comfortable" two-bedroom apartment. Her significant others include her parents, who are alive and reside in a nursing home; and four younger brothers and one sister, all of whom are alive and well and have frequent contact with Ms. D. Her family history includes both parents having hypertension and a younger brother having type I diabetes for five years. Ms. D is 5'5" and weighs 190 pounds.

Case Study

Ms. D is admitted to the hospital with complaints of increased fatigue, lethargy, and occasional confusion. After the initial interview, history, and physical examination by a registered nurse (RN) and a physician's assistant (PA), Ms. D is transferred from the triage area to a medical care unit. Vital signs in the emergency department (ED) are:

Blood pressure: 160/98
Pulse: 78
Respirations: 16
Temperature: 98.5° F

Ms. D informs the receiving nurse in the medical unit that she is on lantus (Insulin glargine) ten units daily at bedtime, and does fingerstick glucose monitoring every four hours during the day. She admits being anxious because during the past two weeks she has experienced unusual dryness of the skin, which requires scratching. Ms. D decided to come to the hospital and goes to the ED because she believes she will get attention faster. When Ms. D is asked about the amount of urine voided since she awoke, she informs the receiving nurse and PA that since she has awakened, she has urinated a smaller amount within a seven-hour period when compared to other times. However, Ms. D believes the decrease in urinary output is related to her decrease in appetite, including fluids. Ms. D is currently taking furosemide 40 mg PO daily, captopril 50 mg PO two times per day for high blood pressure, and ibuprofen or naproxen occasionally for joint pains. She is also taking insulin for diabetes and ibuprofen PRN joint pain prescribed by her primary health care provider. Ms. D also reports a noted decrease in urinary output and unusual irritation frequently. She is admitted to the unit and placed on a cardiac monitor. A peripheral intravenous line is inserted, and IV fluid of NaCL 0.45% at 75 mL/hr is initiated. The nurse continues with the physical assessment and auscultation of her heart sounds. There is S_3 gallop and bilateral rales over lung fields, especially at the bases, and +1 pedal edema at the ankles. Ms. D is placed in a semi-Fowler's position, and the nurse assigns a certified nursing assistant to remain with Ms. D, while she documents her findings. A chest X-ray is done and signs of congested heart failure are evident. Furosemide 40 mg IV is administered stat. Ms. D is seen by a health care provider and a history and physical examination are done, the history and assessment done by the nurse are reviewed, and the following diagnostic and laboratory tests are ordered: X-ray of the kidneys, ureters, and bladder (KUB); renal ultrasonography; and a cystoscopy. Ms. D's laboratory values are:

Blood urea nitrogen (BUN): 25 mg/dL

Creatinine: 2.8 mg/dL

Sodium (Na): 130 mEq/L

Potassium (K+): 6.8 mEq/L

Calcium: 8 mg/dL

Magnesium: 3 mEq/L

Phosphorous: 6 mg/dL

Glucose: 118 mg/dL

Urine specific gravity: 1.002

Urine sodium concentration: 48 mEq/L

A consent is signed for a cystoscopy and central venous pressure catheter insertion. The catheter is inserted and an X-ray is negative for malposition of the catheter. Intravenous fluid is changed to Lactated Ringers at 75 mL/hr, and a foley catheter is inserted and attached to a urometer collecting bag. The results of the diagnostic and labs tests are received and reviewed by the health care provider: the KUB is negative for stones obstructing the renal pelvis, ureters or bladder; the renal ultrasonography is negative for urinary obstruction, but the renal calyces and collecting ducts are dilated, and tissue perfusion is impaired. The cystoscopy is negative for obstruction of the lower urinary tract. The medical doctor, the PA, the RN, an endocrinologist, and a cardiologist review the results of the diagnostic studies. A primary diagnosis of ARF is made, and secondary diagnosis of congested heart failure. The health care provider discusses the plan of care, including hemodialysis, with Ms. D. She is transferred to the medical intensive care unit (MICU), an electrocardiogram (EKG) is done, and the client is placed on continuous telemetry to monitor for life-threatening arrhythmias. Because of the current elevated serum potassium level, the EKG reveals tall, peaked T waves, widening of the QRS complex, and ST segment depression. Dopamine HcL (Intropin) infusion 2 microgram/kg is initiated.

Questions and Suggested Answers

1. **Discuss your understanding of the medical diagnosis of ARF, considering all of the information provided in the case study, and the pathophysiology of ARF.** Ms. D's history of hypertension has accelerated the progression of diabetic neuropathy diabetes mellitus. Hypertension is a leading cause of end-stage renal disease (ESRD), especially among black Americans. It is also the most common cardiovascular abnormality, which usually exists pre-end stage renal disease. Common complications of hypertension include peripheral vascular disease and renal failure. Some degree of renal dysfunction is usually present in the hypertensive client, even a person with a minimally elevated blood pressure. Renal dysfunction is the direct result of ischemia caused by the narrowed lumen of the intra-renal blood vessels. Gradual narrowing of the arteries and arterioles leads to atrophy of the nephrons, which often leads to renal failure. In congested heart failure, there is decreased tissue perfusion to major organs such as the kidneys, and the long-term effects of diuretic therapy such as diuresis, gradually affects the renal system. A history of diabetes mellitus eventually results in diabetic nephropathy, a microvascular complication associated with damage to the small blood vessels that supply the glomeruli of the kidneys, resulting in the development of renal dysfunction. Ms. D's serum potassium is 6.8 mEq/L on admission. It is the most serious electrolyte associated with kidney disease, usually a result of decreased excretion by the kidneys, the breakdown of cellular protein, bleeding, or metabolic acidosis. A review of the elevated potassium, serum BUN, and creatinine indicates that the kidney function is altered. A normal serum potassium is 3.5–5.0 mEq/L. Even small changes in the level can have profound effects on cardiac muscle. Although potassium can be lost in the gastrointestinal (GI) drainage, the kidneys excrete almost all the potassium. Therefore, an elevated potassium level is an indicator of altered renal

function. A normal BUN level is 5–20 mg/dL in adults, but may be slightly higher in the elderly. Although urea diffuses freely into both the extracellular and intracellular fluid, it is ultimately excreted by the kidneys. Therefore, elevated levels are an indication of altered renal function, unless the client is dehydrated, which would cause the urea to be elevated. A normal serum creatinine level is 0.6–1.3 mg/dL for men and 0.5–1.0 mg/dL for women. Ms. D's creatinine is 2.8 mg/dL. In the absence of disorders affecting muscle mass, elevated creatinine levels indicate decreased renal function. If the urea nitrogen is elevated and the creatinine is normal, this finding usually indicates a nonrenal cause for the excessive urea. However, when both values are elevated in addition to the other disease entities, renal failure is usually a primary cause. Because the renal ultrasonography shows renal calyces, dilated collecting ducts, impaired tissue perfusion, and alteration of the renal labs, there is strong evidence of renal failure. Ms. D is in the oliguric phase of acute renal failure, and the manifestations of this phase are changes in urinary output, fluid and electrolyte abnormalities, and uremia (the presence of excessive amounts of urea and other nitrogenous waste products in the blood).

2. **Discuss some of the common causes of ARF.** ARF is a clinical syndrome characterized by a rapid loss of renal function with progressive azotemia, which is the accumulation of nitrogenous waste products such as BUN and increasing levels of creatinine. There are three phases of acute renal failure (pre-renal, intra-renal, and post-renal). The *pre-renal factors* that cause ARF are those external to the kidneys that reduce renal blood flow, and lead to decreased glomerular perfusion and filtration. A critical factor in the pre-renal phase is decreased circulating volume of the blood, which may be related to hypovolemia, decreased cardiac output, decreased peripheral vascular resistance, and vascular obstruction. *Intra-renal* factors include conditions that cause direct damage to the renal tissue, resulting in impaired nephron function. Some of these factors include nephrotoxic drugs (e.g. aminoglycoside antibiotics, contrast media). Nephrotoxins can cause obstruction of intra-renal structures by crystallization or actual damage to the epithelial cells of the tubules. *Intra-renal* causes may also be related to the release of hemoglobin from hemolyzed red blood cells (RBCs) or myoglobin released from necrotic muscle cells. Acute tubular necrosis (ATN) is a type of intra-renal ARF caused by ischemia, nephrotoxins, or pigments, and both nephrotoxic ATN and ischemia are responsible for 90% of intra-renal ARF cases. *Intra-renal* causes account for approximately 35% to 40% of all causes of ARF. *Post-renal causes* include mechanical obstruction of urinary outflow. The common causes are benign prostatic hyperplasia, prostate cancer, calculi, trauma, and extrarenal tumors. However, the two most common causes of ARF are prolonged renal ischemia and nephrotoxic drugs.

3. **Discuss the phases that ARF progresses through.** Acute renal failure may progress through four phases. The *initial phase* begins at the time of the insult and continues until the signs and symptoms become apparent, and can last for hours or days. The *oliguric phase* is caused by a reduction in the glomerular filtration rate (GFR), with oliguria being less than 400 mL of urine in 24 hours. This phase usually occurs within one to seven days of the causative event. If the cause is ischemia, oliguria may occur within 24 hours. Elevated potassium (hyperkalemia) is the leading cause of death in the oliguric phase of ARF. It is the most critical factor to cause death in this phase because in the oliguric phase there is a reduction in GFR, and potassium is eliminated by the kidneys. If the GFR is reduced, potassium accumulates. Accumulation of potassium results in lethal arrhythmias and impairment of neuromuscular function, including muscle weakness, flaccid paralysis, absence of deep tendon reflexes and cardiac conduction abnormalities, and eventually fatality. In the *diuretic phase* there is a gradual increase in the daily urine output to one to three liters per day, but it may reach three to five liters or more per day. However, although urine output is increasing, the nephrons are still not fully functional. Instead, the high urine volume is caused by osmotic diuresis from the high urea concentration in the glomerular filtrate and the inability of the tubules to concentrate the urine. In this phase, the kidneys have recovered their ability to excrete wastes, but not to concentrate the urine. In this phase, hypovolemia and hypotension can occur from the massive fluid losses. Although there is massive diuresis, uremia may still be severe, which will be reflected by low creatinine clearances, elevated serum creatinine and blood urea nitrogen, and persistent signs and symptoms. In this phase, the client is monitored for hyponatremia, hypokalemia and dehydration. The diuretic phase may last for one to three weeks, and it is at this time that the client's acid-base, electrolyte, blood urea nitrogen, and creatinine values begin to

normalize. The *recovery phase,* the fourth phase of ARF begins when the GFR increases, which allows the BUN and serum creatinine levels to plateau and then decrease. The major improvements occur in the first one to two weeks of this phase, but renal function may take up to 12 months to stabilize.

4. **What are the primary strategies of treatment for ARF?** The primary strategies for treating ARF are to eliminate the cause with prescribed medications such as potassium resins, or to conduct short-term hemodialysis to remove excess potassium from the body. Another strategy is to educate the client about foods and drugs that may cause ARF, and about being knowledgeable of the early signs and symptoms of ARF and the appropriate interventions that should be applied to alleviate these signs and symptoms. It is also important to prevent complications such as hyperkalemia by monitoring serum potassium levels and urinary output, and reporting and documenting the levels. Effectively educate the client with acute renal failure about foods to avoid that will increase serum potassium levels, prescribed medications that may cause elevated serum potassium, and the importance of follow-up care with the primary healthcare provider.

5. **What are common nursing diagnoses for ARF?**

    - Excess fluid volume R/T renal failure and fluid retention
    - Risk for infection R/T invasive lines and altered immune responses
    - Imbalanced nutrition: less than body requirements R/T altered metabolic state and dietary restrictions
    - Disturbed thought process R/T effects of uremic toxins on central nervous system
    - Fatigue R/T anemia, metabolic acidosis, and uremic toxins
    - Anxiety R/T disease process, therapeutic interventions, and uncertainty of prognosis
    - Potential complication: arrhythmias R/T electrolyte imbalances
    - Potential complication: metabolic acidosis R/T inability to excrete H+, impaired
    - Sodium bicarbonate reabsorption, and decreased synthesis of ammonia

6. **Briefly discuss the types and purpose of hemodialysis use to eliminate toxic factors from the blood to prevent fatal complications.** The kidneys are the primary excretory organs for urea, an end product of protein metabolism, and creatinine, an end product of endogenous muscle metabolism. The best serum indicator of renal failure is creatinine because it is not significantly altered by other factors. The serum potassium levels increase in renal failure because the normal ability of the kidneys to excrete 80% to 90% of the body's potassium is impaired. When potassium levels exceed 6 mEq/L or arrhythmias are identified, treatment must be initiated immediately because hyperkalemia is one of the most serious complications in ARF. There are two options available for dialysis. One is hemodialysis (HD) and the other is peritoneal dialysis (PD). HD is the method of choice when rapid changes are required in a short time, but it is technically more complicated than PD because specialized staff, equipment, and vascular access are required. The process of HD requires anticoagulation therapy to prevent blood from clotting when blood contacts the foreign membrane material in the dialysis blood circuit. Other reasons why HD is more complicated than PD involve the complications that could occur during or after HD, such as hypotension from the rapid removal of vascular volume (fluid shifting) during HD. If hypotension occurs during HD, the usual treatment is to decrease the volume of fluid being removed and infuse 0.9% normal saline solution (remembering that those clients with heart failure will require slower infusion and less volume of normal saline). Painful muscle cramps may occur due to rapid removal of sodium and water, or from neuromuscular hypersensitivity. The treatment includes reduction of the ultrainfiltration rate and the infusion of hypertonic saline solution 3.0% slowly to replace sodium loss, while avoiding intravascular volume overload and pulmonary edema. Hepatitis is another complication that may occur with HD. The preventive measure is to maintain infection control measures as designed by the Centers for Disease Control (CDC), and the agency protocol. Sepsis may occur and is often related to infections of vascular access sites. The preventive measure is to use aseptic technique and to monitor clients for signs and symptoms of sepsis, such as fever, hypotension, and elevated WBC count. Disequilibrium syndrome occurs because of the rapid changes in the composition of the extracellular fluid. This results in the shift of fluid into the brain, causing cerebral edema, and manifestations of confusion and restlessness. The treatment consists

of slowing or stopping the dialysis and infusing hypertonic saline solution, albumin, or mannitol to draw fluid from the brain cells back into the systemic circulation.

The following are prescribed:

- Furosemide (Lasix) 40 mg IV q6h × 24 hours
- Nifedipine (Procardia) 20 mg PO three times per day
- Lantus (Insulin gargline) 10 units SC at bedtime
- Human regular insulin (Humulin R): Fingerstick sliding scale (FSS) q4h PRN for:
  Glucose less than 100 mg/dL, no insulin coverage; 100–140, two units SC; 141–180, four units SC; 181–220, six units SC; 221–260, eight units SC; 261–300, ten units SC; 301–340, twelve units SC; greater than 341, call the MD.
- Calcium carbonate (Os-cal) 4 g PO with meals
- Digoxin (Lanoxin) 125 mg PO every morning
- Sodium polystyrene sulfonate (Kayexalate) 15 g PO daily for potassium level greater than 5 mEq/L
- Monitor serum creatinine, BUN, serum sodium, potassium, glucose, hematocrit and hemoglobin, urine protein, and urine specific gravity daily.
- Dietary consultation, strict intake and output, record daily weight

7. **Including dopamine HcL, which was administered in the MICU, what are the purposes for the prescribed orders?** *Dopamine HcL* is an inotropic cardiac stimulant and vasopressor. With continuous intravenous infusion, it enhances renal perfusion by its direct action on alpha- and beta-adrenergic receptors and on specific dopaminergic receptors in mesenteric and renal vascular beds. In the dose prescribed, it increases cardiac output with minimal increase in myocardial oxygen consumption and dilates the renal and mesenteric blood vessels. However, in higher doses, it will increase the blood pressure. *Furosemide* is a loop diuretic that enhances the effects of the bolus fluid and increases urinary output by action on the proximal and distal ends of the tubule and the ascending limb of Henle's loop, blocking reabsorption of sodium and chloride. When these are blocked, passive reabsorption is prevented and the kidneys eliminate the excess urine. *Nifedipine* is a calcium channel-blocking agent that effectively treats the hypertension associated with ARF by decreasing peripheral vascular resistance through vasodilation. Further, it increases tissue perfusion to the kidneys. *Insulin glargine* is a long-acting recombinant human insulin analog that "differs from human insulin in that the amino acid asparagines at position A21 is replaced by glycine and two arginines are added to the C terminus of the B-chain." (Spratto and Woods, 622). After subcutaneous injection, it forms microprecipitates that gradually release the insulin for long-acting action. Further, it stimulates peripheral glucose uptake especially in muscle and fat tissue. When administered at bedtime, *insulin glargine* maintains glycemic levels by achieving blood levels that are relatively stable, and there is less risk for hypoglycemia or hyperglycemia during sleep. *Human regular insulin* is a rapid acting insulin that lowers and stabilizes elevated glucose levels by increasing peripheral glucose uptake especially by skeletal muscle and fat tissue. Further, it inhibits the liver from converting glycogen to glucose. It is the preferred agent for *sliding scale* use. *Calcium carbonate* is a calcium salt used to increase calcium levels, which simultaneously decreases the elevated phosphate levels occurring in ARF. This results from the inverse relationship between calcium and phosphate serum levels. *Digoxin* is a positive inotropic cardiac glycoside used to treat tachydysrythmias by slowing and strengthening the myocardial contractions, improving stroke volume and cardiac output. *Sodium polystyrene sulfonate (Kayexalate)* is a potassium-removing resin used to treat the hyperkalemia characteristic of ARF. It increases excretion of potassium through the large intestine. Monitoring of *serum creatinine* is significant in renal failure because the kidneys normally filter out large amounts of creatinine on a daily basis. However, when kidney filtration is altered, creatinine levels rise, requiring immediate interventions. Since *creatinine* is excreted only by the kidneys, its elevation is a significant indicator of damage to the nephrons. The BUN determines how effectively the kidneys are clearing waste product from the blood. Therefore, if the kidneys are not functioning properly, there will be excess urea in the bloodstream. *Serum sodium* determines if the client is retaining sodium, because clients in renal failure retain sodium. Monitoring *serum potassium* level is important because potassium level is elevated in renal failure and

the increase in serum potassium will result in renal failure if not corrected. Elevated *serum potassium* also affects the cardiac system and the musculoskeletal system in a significant manner, which could result in complications if not detected and corrected. Monitoring of *serum glucose* levels is important because the diabetic client in acute renal failure may experience changes in insulin requirements due to the decrease in glucose levels, and because diuretics adversely affect sodium and potassium levels by enhancing the excretion of urine, which causes an increase in excretion of both electrolytes and the increase of glucose levels. Monitoring the *hematocrit* and *hemoglobin levels* helps determine if anemia is present. *Hematocrit and hemoglobin* are decreased in persons with acute renal failure probably due to diminished erythropoietin production, which would require intervention to retard the development of anemia. Monitoring *urine protein* is important because blood proteins do not pass through the kidneys into the urine because they are too large. When kidney function is altered, protein may pass into the urine, and protein in the urine may be a sign of permanent kidney damage, or failure. *Urine specific gravity* helps in the diagnosis of acute renal failure, because the urine specific gravity is usually decreased and fixed, reflecting the inability of the tubules to produce a concentrated or diluted urine in response to changes in plasma osmolarity. *Dietary consultation* is required by a registered dietitian to calculate the client's daily dietary requirements. The dietitian is then prepared to work with the client, the medical doctor, the urologist, and the endocrinologist in developing a diet with specific levels of protein, sodium, potassium, and calories to compensate for the hypercatabolic state. Clients with ARF often have a high rate of metabolism. This hypercatabolic state causes a breakdown of muscle protein, which will lead to increase in azotemia if aggressive nutritional management is not in place. *Strict intake* and *output* provides information on the client's physiological response to fluid and the kidney's functioning status. When the kidneys are not functioning properly, as in ARF, accurate assessment of intake and output is paramount to management of fluid and electrolyte imbalance. *Daily weight* determines water retention and the effectiveness of medical interventions used to improve the client's state of health, such as furosemide.

8. **What are the most common adverse reactions to the prescribed medications?** The most common adverse reactions to *dopamine HcL* are hypotension, bradycardia, headache, hypertension, palpitations, tachycardia, vomiting, and arrhythmias. The most common adverse reactions to *furosemide* are hypokalemia, hypotension, hyponatremia, hypochloremia, hypomagnesemia, hypovolemia, metabolic alkalosis, and dehydration. The most common adverse effects associated with *nifedipine* are marked hypotension, peripheral and pulmonary edema, tachycardia, nausea, diarrhea, dizziness, lightheadedness, and disturbances in equilibrium. The most common adverse reaction to *insulin glargine* is hypoglycemia and its manifestations, including diaphoresis, nausea, nervousness, palpitations, and weakness. The most common adverse reaction to *human regular insulin* is hypoglycemia and its manifestations as noted above. The most common adverse reaction to *calcium carbonate* is constipation, anorexia, nausea and vomiting, diarrhea, and rebound hyperacidity may occur. The most common adverse effects of *digoxin* are bradycardia (most common) and hypotension and those associated with digoxin toxicity (diarrhea, anorexia, nausea and vomiting, headache, blurred vision and halo effects, disorientation, restlessness, confusion, dysrrythmias, and AV heart block). The most common adverse effects of *sodium polystyrene sulfonate* include hypocalcemia, hypokalemia, hypomagnesemia, hypernatremia, constipation, nausea, vomiting, and gastric irritation.

9. **Discuss the drug-to-drug, drug-to-food/herbal interactions for the prescribed medications.** Drug-to-drug interactions may occur with the simultaneous use of *dopamine HcL* and phenytoin, which will cause severe bradycardia and hypotension. Halothane and cyclopropane, when used concurrently with *dopamine HcL,* increase the risk of hypertension and ventricular arrhythmias. The simultaneous use with monoamine oxidase (MAO) inhibitors, ergot alkaloids (ergotamine), doxapram, guanethidine, guanadrel, and some antidepressants may result in severe hypertension. Dopamine may be antagonized by alpha- or beta-blocking agents. The vasopressor response may be decreased in the presence of tricyclic antidepressants, requiring higher doses of dopamine (Gahart and Nazareno, 426). There are no clinically significant drug-to-food/herbal interactions established. With intravenous *furosemide,* drug-to-drug interactions may occur with the simultaneous use of thiazide diuretics or corticosteroids and may increase the risk of hypokalemia. Furosemide potentiates antihypertensive agents including nitroglycerin and nitroprusside sodium.

Aminoglycosides, cisplatin, and amphotericin B increase the risk of ototoxicity and amphotericin B also increases the risk of nephrotoxicity. Furosemide may increase the activity of warfarin sodium, heparin, streptokinase, beta-blocking agents, lithium (may cause lithium toxicity), and nonpolarizing muscle relaxants. The simultaneous use with digoxin or amiodarone may cause dysrrythmias, and increased risk of cardiotoxicity if used concurrently with pimozide or sparfloxacin. When used with insulin or sulfonylureas, dopamine may cause hyperglycemia by decreasing glucose tolerance. Dopamine effects may be inhibited by phenytoin, ACE inhibitors, nonsteroidal anti-inflammatory agents (NSAIDs), probenecid, or salicylates (if used in clients with liver cirrhosis or ascites). (Gahart and Nazareno, 570). Smoking may increase the secretion of antidiuretic hormone, decreasing the diuresis and cardiac output effects of furosemide. There are no clinically significant drug-to-food/herbal interactions with intravenous furosemide established. Drug-to-drug interactions are numerous with concurrent use with *nifedipine.* Simultaneous use of rifampin, quinupristin/dalfopristin, itroconazole, and diltiazem increases the effects of nifedipine. Barbiturates, nafcillin, cimetidine, and ranitidine decrease the serum levels of nifedipine. Nifedipine increases the effects of anticoagulants, cyclosporine, digoxin, diltiazem, magnesium sulfate, tacolimus, theophylline, and vincristine with higher risk of toxicity of these agents. When quinidine is used concurrently with nifedipine, quinidine's effects are decreased and there is an increased risk of hypotension, bradycardia, pulmonary edema, atrioventricular block, and ventricular tachycardia. Grapefruit juice increases nifedipine serum levels and St. John's Wort and melatonin decrease nifedipine effects. Drug-to-drug interactions with the simultaneous use of *insulin glargine* and other agents either increase or decrease the glucose-lowering effects of insulin glargine. Those agents that increase the insulin's effects include ACE inhibitors, dispyramide, fluoxetine, MAO inhibitors, octreotide, phopoxyphene, salicylates, and sulfonamides. Those that decrease its glucose-lowering effects are danazol, diuretics, isoniazid, niacin, and somatropine. Clonidine and lithium salts may potentiate or decrease insulin's effects. Although drug-to-food/herbal interactions technically may not occur, eating foods high in simple sugars or other carbohydrates will decrease the effectiveness of insulin glargine by increasing serum glucose levels, requiring an increase in the dose of insulin. The only drug-to-drug interaction associated with *regular insulin* is that the use of oral hypoglycemics will increase the effects of regular insulin and, because this type of insulin is rapid acting, the concurrent use would greatly increase the risk of hypoglycemia. As with all insulins, the increased intake of simple sugars and carbohydrates will require increasing the dose of regular insulin. Drug-to-herbal interactions may occur with the simultaneous use of garlic and ginseng, which may potentiate hypoglycemic effects. Drug-to-drug interactions may occur with the simultaneous use of *calcium carbonate* and quinidine or amphetamines, increasing the effects of these agents. Decreased levels of salicylates, calcium channel blocking agents, ketoconazole, tetracyclines, and iron salts are seen with concurrent use of calcium carbonate. Drug-to-food/herbal interactions include increased action and adverse effects when used with lily of the valley, pheasant's eye, and squill. Drug-to-drug interactions may occur with the simultaneous use of oral diazepam and thiazides, loop diuretics, barbiturates, CNS depressants, alcohol, SSKIs, cimetidine, and muscle relaxants by potentiating their effects. Fluoxetine and isoniazid increase the half-life of diazepam, ranitidine decreases GI absorption of diazepam, and oral contraceptives, valporic acid, disulfiram, isoniazid, and propranolol cause decreased metabolism of diazepam. Kava increases the action of diazepam. Numerous drug-to-drug interactions are associated with the use of *digoxin.* Amiodarone, anticholinergics, atorvastatin, benzodiazepines, captopril, diltiazem, dipyridamole, erythromycin, esmolol, flecainide, fluoxetine, hypoglycemic agents, levothyroxine, hydroxychloroquine, ibuprofen, indomethacin, itraconazole, methimazole, nifedipine, propranalol, quinidine, quinine, telmisartan, tetracyclines, tolbutamide, and verapamil increase digoxin levels, increasing the risk of digoxin toxicity. Albuterol increases digoxin binding to skeletal muscle and amphotericin B increases potassium depletion, thus increasing the risk of digoxin toxicity. The following agents decrease digoxin effects: amilaride, aminoglycosides, aminosalicylic acid, antacids, cholestyramine, colestipol, diopyramide, metoclopramide, spirolactone, sulfasalazine, and thyroid. Beta-blocking agents pose an increased risk of complete heart block. Parenteral calcium preparations cause cardiac dysrrhythmias and large volume glucose infusions increase potassium loss and increase the risk of digoxin toxicity. Chlorthalidone, ethacrynic acid, furosemide, and thiazides increase potassium and magnesium loss resulting in an increased risk of digoxin toxicity. Ephedra, ephedrine, and epinephrine increase the chance of cardiac dysrhythmias. Aloe, buckthorn bark/berry, cascara sagrada bark, German chamaomile flower, ginseng, hawthorn, Iceland moss, Indian snakeroot, ivy leaf, licorice, marshmallow root, rhubarb root, sarsaparilla root, castor bean oil, may apple root, yellow dock root, oleander, purple foxglove, squill, and senna pod/leaf must be used with extreme caution because they increase the effects of digoxin. St. John's Wort decreases digoxin's action. Drug-to-drug interactions may occur with the simultaneous use of *sodium polystyrene sulfonate* and antacids or laxatives that will decrease the effects of sodium polystyrene sulfonate. No clinically significant drug-to-food/herbals have been established.

10. **Discuss the gerontologic considerations of ARF.** The older adult is more susceptible than the younger adult to ARF as the number of functioning nephrons decrease with age. Impaired function of other organ systems (e.g. cardiovascular disease, impaired pancreas function) can increase the risk of developing ARF. The aging kidneys are less able to compensate for changes in fluid volume, solute load, and cardiac output. The prognosis after an episode of ARF is generally worse in the older adult than in the younger person. The mortality rate of ARF is 5% to 25% higher in the older adult than in the younger adult, and death is usually caused by infection, gastrointestinal hemorrhage, or myocardial infarction.

11. **Discuss client education for ARF.** The client should be taught to avoid exposure to nephrotoxins, particularly those in the over-the-counter products, prevent infection and other major stressors that can slow healing, and to monitor weight, blood pressure, and pulse daily. Also advise the client to maintain dietary restriction as planned with the registered dietitian and the health care provider or nurse practitioner. The importance of follow-up care should also be discussed.

References

Black, J.M. and Hawks, J.H. (2005). *Medical-Surgical Nursing: Clinical Management for Positive Outcomes.* Philadelphia: W.B. Saunders.

Broyles, B.E. (2005). *Medical-Surgical Nursing Clinical Companion.* Durham, NC: Carolina Academic Press.

Cavanaugh, B.M. (2003). *Nurse's Manual of Laboratory Diagnostic Tests.* Philadelphia: F.A. Davis.

Corbet, J.V. (2004). *Laboratory Tests and Diagnostic Procedures with Nursing Diagnoses* (6th ed.). Upper Saddle River, NJ: Prentice Hall.

Gahart, B.L. and Nazareno, A. R. (2005). *2005 Intravenous Medications.* St. Louis: Mosby.

Heitz, U. and Horne, M.M. (2005). *Mosby's Pocket Guide Series: Fluid, Electrolyte and Acid-Base Balance* (5th ed.). St. Louis: Mosby.

Huether, S.E. and McCance, K.L. (2004). *Understanding Pathophysiology* (3rd ed.). St. Louis: Mosby.

Ignatavicius, D.D. and Workman, M.L. (2006). *Medical-Surgical Nursing across the Health Care Continuum* (5th ed.). Philadelphia: W.B. Saunders.

Spratto, G.R. and Woods, A.L. (2005). *2005 Edition: PDR Nurse's Drug Handbook.* Clifton Park, NY: Thomson Delmar Learning.

CASE STUDY 6

Appendicitis

GENDER
- M

AGE
- 38

SETTING
- Hospital

ETHNICITY/CULTURE
- Black American/West Indian

PREEXISTING CONDITIONS

COEXISTING CONDITIONS

LIFESTYLE
- RN specializing in psychiatry

COMMUNICATION

DISABILITY

SOCIOECONOMIC STATUS
- Middle

SPIRITUAL/RELIGIOUS
- Anglican

PHARMACOLOGIC
- Ampicillin sodium/sulbactam sodium (Unasyn)
- Gentamicin sulfate (Garamycin)
- Metoclopramide HcL (Reglan)
- Metronidazole (Flagyl)
- Morphine sulfate (Duramorph)

PSYCHOSOCIAL
- Anxiety

LEGAL

ETHICAL

ALTERNATIVE THERAPY

PRIORITIZATION
- Assess and manage pain
- Prepare for surgery

DELEGATION
- RN

MODERATE

THE DIGESTIVE AND URINARY SYSTEMS

Level of difficulty: Moderate

Overview: This case involves critical thinking and focused assessment skills to prioritize care for a client with appendicitis with peritonitis. It involves accurate assessment of pain with specific identification of location of pain and thorough assessment and auscultation of the chest to rule out lower lobe pneumonia. The triage nurse should be skilled at detecting signs of septic shock that could occur with the client with ruptured appendix.

Client Profile

Mr. W is a 38-year-old registered nurse who has specialized in psychiatric nursing. He is 5′4″ and weighs 210 pounds. Mr. W is brought by a neighbor to the emergency department (ED), accompanied by his wife. The mode of transportation is a car.

Case Study

Mr. W denies past medical or surgical history. He reports that while preparing to leave for his place of employment, he had an unusually sharp pain in his abdomen. He tells the triage nurse that he had been having "on and off" pain in the abdominal area and that, at times, the pain was continuous. He said today he felt "unusually cool" but thought it was due to the weather. However, when the pain shifted to his right lower quadrant and remained localized at the area halfway between the umbilicus and the right iliac crest (McBurney's point), he informed his wife of the need to go the ED. On arrival at the ED, Mr. W is complaining of nausea, and begins vomiting. He is assisted to a stretcher, and immediately positions himself on his side with his right leg flexed. The ED health care provider is notified and the triage nurse continues to gather the history by focusing on Mr. W's description of the origin of the pain, intensity, and duration. Upon completion of the pain assessment, the nurse proceeds to perform a physical examination, using the system's approach, then examines the most tender quadrant of the abdomen last. The lungs are clear on auscultation and normal breath sounds are present, ruling out any relationship with the abdominal pain and lower lobe pneumonia. The ED nursing technician monitors the vital signs and reports:

- Blood pressure: 110/70
- Pulse: 80
- Respirations: 18
- Temperature: 100.0° F

The ED health care provider sees Mr. W and history and assessment examination are completed. Mr. W is transferred to a medical surgical unit in preparation for further evaluation and probable emergency surgery. He is given morphine sulfate 4 mg IM. He is on NPO ("nothing by mouth") status but has intravenous fluid 0.9% sodium chloride at 125 mL/hr. Electrocardiogram (EKG) and chest X-ray results are normal. Results from serum labs drawn on arrival to the ED reveal:

- White blood cell (WBC) count: 20,000/mm^3
- Hematocrit (Hct): 30%
- Hemoglobin (Hgb): 15 mg/dL

Urinalysis reveals hematuria, albuminuria, and pyuria. Blood culture reveals gram-negative anaerobic bacilli. Ultrasound study shows the presence of appendicitis. Diagnostic tests and lab results done in the ED are reviewed, and a diagnosis of appendicitis is confirmed. Mr. W is informed of the need for surgery, an order for type and cross match for two units of packed red blood cells (PRBCs) is placed, an informed consent is signed, and the operating room staff is notified. Ampicillin sodium/sulbactam sodium (Unasyn) 1 g IV is administered stat, and the client is waiting "on call" to the operating room for an appendectomy.

Questions and Suggested Answers

1. **Define appendicitis.** Appendicitis is an inflammation of the appendix, which is a narrow blind tube that extends from the inferior part of the cecum.

2. **Discuss the etiology and pathophysiology of appendicitis.** The most common causes of appendicitis are obstruction of the lumen by a fecalith (accumulation of feces), foreign bodies, tumor of the cecum or appendix.

Obstruction results in distention, venous engorgement, and the accumulation of mucus and bacteria, which can lead to gangrene and perforation.

3. **Discuss the classic manifestations of appendicitis and some diseases that mimic appendicitis.** The classic manifestations begin with periumbilical pain, followed by anorexia, nausea, and vomiting. The pain is persistent and continuous, eventually shifting to the right lower quadrant and localizing at McBurney's point (located halfway between the umbilicus and the right iliac crest). Further assessment of the client reveals localized tenderness, rebound tenderness, and muscle guarding. The client usually prefers to lie still, often with the right leg flexed. Low-grade fever may or may not be present, and coughing aggravates pain. Rovsing's sign may be elicited by palpating of the left lower quadrant, causing pain to be felt in the right lower quadrant.

4. **Discuss the complications associated with acute appendicitis.** *Perforation* of the appendix occurs when the appendix becomes obstructed and intraluminal pressure increases, leading to decreased venous drainage, thrombosis, edema, and bacterial invasion of the bowel wall. If the obstruction continues, perforation will result. An abrupt change in the character of the pain as described by the client and a high fever are indicators of perforation. If the pain becomes generalized throughout the abdomen and the abdomen is rigid and boardlike, rupture may have occurred. If a ruptured (perforated) appendix is suspected, the symptoms should be reported to the health care provider immediately so that the client can be prepared for surgery. The nurse can initiate an intravenous line with the use of a Hep-lock, and anticipate that IV antibiotics will be initiated to decrease the infection. *Peritonitis* is another complication that may develop, and refers to inflammation of the peritoneum. It is usually caused by enteric bacteria entering the peritoneal cavity, such as seen with a perforated appendix. The enteric bacteria cause contamination, resulting in the development of generalized inflammation of the peritoneal cavity. This is due to a shift of fluid into the peritoneal space (third spacing), and circulating blood volume is depleted, leading to hypovolemia. The manifestations of peritonitis depend on the severity and extent of the infection, as well as the age and general health of the client. Classic symptoms include an acute abdomen, an abrupt onset of diffuse, severe abdominal pain. The pain may localize and intensify near the areas of infection, and movement may intensify the pain. The entire abdomen is tender, with guarding or rigidity of abdominal muscles, and the abdomen is boardlike. There is rebound tenderness over the area of inflammation, and paralytic ileus may be present because peritoneal inflammation inhibits peristalsis. Until the infecting organism has been identified, a broad-spectrum antibiotic effective against organisms commonly implicated in peritonitis is prescribed. If perforation is the cause of the peritonitis, a laparotomy is done to close the perforation or remove the damaged, inflamed tissue. If surgery is done, the client returns from surgery with gastric tubes, intravenous fluids, and orders for bedrest in Fowler's position to help localize the infection and promote lung ventilation. Oxygen is usually ordered to facilitate cellular metabolism and healing. *Abscess formation* may develop as a complication of appendicitis. Treatment involves broad-spectrum antibiotic before surgery, surgical draining of the abscess depending on its location, and administration of a broad-spectrum antibiotic after surgery.

5. **Discuss the collaborative management for appendicitis.** Examination of the client with a complete history and physical done by a health care provider or nurse practitioner, with focus on palpation of the abdomen. A differential WBC test should be done to look for both the total WBC count and the number of immature WBCs that are usually present with appendicitis. A *urinalysis* is done to rule out (R/O) genitourinary conditions that mimic the manifestations of appendicitis. *Abdominal X-rays* may be done with the client in the flat and upright positions. A fecalith or calculus may be noted in the right upper quadrant, or a localized ileus. An *abdominal ultrasound* is done and is currently the most effective test for diagnosing acute appendicitis. It is effective because it allows high-frequency sound waves to reflect back to a doppler device to create a computer-generated image. The test also takes less than 30 minutes, is non-invasive, and is particularly useful if symptoms are atypical. An intravenous pyelogram (IVP) may be used to differentiate appendicitis from possible urinary tract disease.

6. **What are common nursing diagnoses for appendicitis?**
   - Acute pain R/T nerve irritation from inflammation
   - Deficient fluid volume R/T NPO status and vomiting

- High risk for infection R/T rupture of appendix
- Deficient knowledge R/T condition, treatment, and health maintenance

7. **If the client starts to vomit, what interventions should be carried out by the nurse, in order of priority?** Position the client on the side to prevent aspiration, and provide an emesis basin in close proximity. Prepare for insertion of nasogastric tube (NGT), start intravenous fluid as prescribed, and maintain intake and output record. The NGT is needed for this client due to the risk for vomiting, and a NGT aids in the prevention of vomiting.

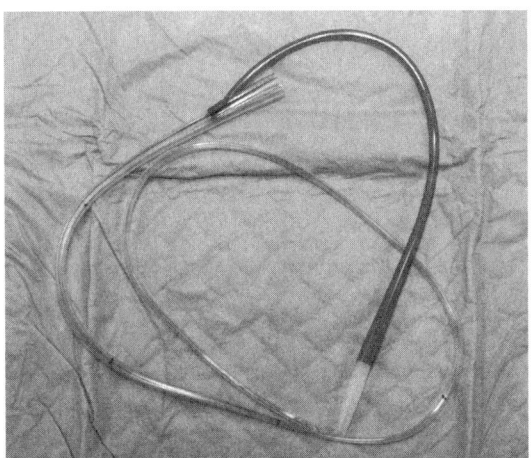

Nasogastric tube

After getting a request from a health care provider or nurse practitioner, send the request to the X-ray department or keep it on the unit, but notify X-ray department that an X-ray will be needed after the insertion of an NGT. The nurse delegates to a certified nursing attendant the role of gathering all equipment needed, but it is the nurse who checks to ensure that the suction apparatus is working. Inform the client of the need for the tube and give clear instructions on what will be done. Place the client in an upright position (high Fowler's) that enhances the ability to swallow as the tube is being passed into the stomach. If this position is contraindicated, the client is placed in a recumbent position. The nurse determines which of the client's nostrils is most open and proceeds to occlude one of the nostrils, while listening for the client's breathing through the other nostril. Inspect the nasal septum for deviation, and ask the client about past problems with intubation. Mark the length of the tube to be passed, then lubricate the final three inches at the top of the tube. Have the client position the head in a neutral position, insert the tube through the client's most patent nostril and pass it through the nasopharynx. Tape the tube to the nose using only one side of a split piece of tape, so that position of the tube can be maintained. Verification of the tube is done by X-ray and, after verification, the nurse attaches the tube to suction as per protocol or as ordered. The nurse documents the reason for the NGT, and monitors the client's abdomen and auscultates bowel sounds, amount and character of drainage if the tube is attached to suction. If the tube is attached to suction and the drainage exceeds 100 mL/hr, notify the health care provider. If the tube stops draining, first assess the equipment for proper functioning. If the tube needs irrigating, consult with the health care provider, nurse practitioner, or institution protocol. Normal saline is the only acceptable irrigating solution because its isotonicity will not further compromise the client's fluid and electrolyte status.

The following are prescribed:

- NPO, start IV fluid D %.45% NaCL at 125 mL per hour
- Metoclopramide HcL (Reglan) 10 mg IV q6h PRN. Dilute in 50 mL normal saline and infuse over 30 minutes.
- Morphine sulfate (Duramorph) 8 mg q4h PRN pain
- Ampicillin sodium/sulbactam sodium (Unasyn) 1.5 g IV × one before surgery

- Gentamicin sulfate (Garamycin) 80 mg loading dose IV × one before surgery
- Metronidazole (Flagyl) 15 mg/kg IV before surgery

8. **What are the purposes for the prescribed medications?** *Metoclopramide HcL* is a gastric stimulant and increases gastric emptying. It is a dopamine antagonist that acts by increasing sensitivity to acetylcholine and results in greater motility of the upper gastrointestinal (GI) tract, increasing gastric emptying time, and relaxation of the pyloric sphincter and duodenal bulb (Spratto and Woods, 782). *Morphine sulfate* is an opiate analgesic that alters processes affecting pain perception and emotional response to pain. It alters these processes by binding to opioid receptors in the brain and spinal cord and activating endogenous analgesia system. *Ampicillin sodium/sulbactam sodium* is a penicillin and beta-lactamase inhibitor that is effective against gram-positive and gram-negative bacteria. *Gentamicin* is a broad-spectrum aminoglycoside antibiotic action and is used for serious infections of the GI tract. *Metronidazole* is an antifungal agent active against gram-negative anaerobic bacilli. It is effective against serious intra-abdominal infections.

9. **What are the most common adverse reactions to the prescribed medications?** The most common adverse reactions to *metoclopramide HcL* are headache, transient hypertension, mild sedation, fatigue, restlessness, drowsiness, and diarrhea. The most common adverse reactions to *ampicillin sodium/sulbactam sodium* are the full scope of hypersensitivity reactions (rash), diarrhea, nausea, and burning and pain at injection site, especially if infused too rapidly through a peripheral IV access. The most common adverse reactions to *gentamicin sulfate* are anorexia, muscle twitching, roaring in the ears, tinnitus, nausea, vomiting, and decreased creatinine clearance. If used in high doses, gentamicin is ototoxic as well as nephrotoxic. The most common adverse reactions to *metronidazole* are anorexia, constipation, cystitis, diarrhea, dryness of the mucous membranes (mouth, vagina, vulva), fever, peripheral neuropathy, dizziness, headache, abdominal pain, overgrowth of candida, and nausea. The simultaneous use of oral anticoagulants may potentiate hypoprothrombinemia.

10. **Discuss the drug-to-drug and drug-to-food/herbal interactions for the prescribed medications.** Drug-to-drug interactions may occur with the simultaneous use of *metoclopramide* and alcohol, or and other central nervous system depressants, which may increase sedating effects, and opioid analgesics decrease metoclopramide's effects. Concurrent use with acetaminophen, cyclosporine, ethanol, levodopa, succinylcholine, and tetracycline increases the absorption and effects of these agents. It decreases the effects of cimetidine and digoxin if used simultaneously. If used with monoamine oxidase (MAO) inhibitors, there is increased release of catecholamines and greater risk of toxicity. Metoclopramide used in conjunction with sertraline or venlafaxine can result in possible serotonin syndrome. There are no clinically significant drug-to-food/herbal interactions established. Drug-to-drug interactions may occur with the simultaneous use of *ampicillin sodium/sulbactam sodium* with allopurinol, which increases incidence of rash. The simultaneous use with aminoglycosides (i.e., gentamicin sulfate) may be impaired in clients with severe end stage renal failure and, although frequently used concomitantly, should never be mixed in the same infusion and preferably should be administered a minimum of one hour apart if using the same IV access site. Streptomycin potentiates its bacteriocidal effects against enterococci. Concurrent use with beta-adrenergic blocking agents (propranolol) may increase the risk of anaphylaxis (Gahart and Nazareno, 106). The simultaneous use of probenicid decreases renal excretion and increases the blood levels of ampicillin sodium/sulbactam sodium. It may decrease the clearance, thus increasing the risk of toxicity of methotrexate. The simultaneous use of chloramphenicol, erythromycin, and tetracycline may antagonize the bactericidal effects of ampicillin sodium/sulbactam sodium. There are no clinically significant drug-to-food/herbal interactions established. With *gentamicin sulfate,* drug-to-drug interactions may occur with the simultaneous use of other aminoglycosides, vancomycin, and amphotericin B, which may increase the risk of ototoxicity. Gentamicin is synergistic when used in combination with beta-lactase antibiotics including sulbactam sodium, clavulanate potassium, cephalosporins, and penicillins, as well as vancomycin. Neuromuscular blocking agents are potentiated by aminoglycoside and apnea may occur. Gentamicin may be antagonized by bacteriostatic agents, such as chloramphenicol, erythromycin, and tetracyclines and potentiated by anticholinesterases and antineoplastics, such as cisplatin and nitrogen mustard. Dangerous additive effects may occur with the concurrent use of

gentamicin and enflurane, kanamycin, streptomycin, cephalosporins, furosemide, vancomycin, and many other agents so drug interactions should be closely checked if administering other agents with gentamicin. There is no clinically significant drug-to-food/herbal interactions established. Drug-to-drug interactions may occur with the simultaneous use of **metronidazole HcL** and alcohol, oral solutions of citaloprim, ritinavir, lopinavir, and IV formulations of sulfamethoxazole may elicit disulfiram effects and cause acute psychosis. Simultaneous use with fluorouracil or azathioprine increases the risk of leukopenia. Barbiturates, chloramphenicol, erythromycin, and tetracyclines may negate bacteriocidal effects of metronidazole. Cimetidine may increase metronidazole serum levels and neurotoxicity may increase with the concurrent use of ciprofloxacin, cyclosporine, and imipenum-cilastatin. Metronidazole increases lithium levels, creating an increased risk of lithium toxicity, and potentiates phenytoin and warfarin (Gahart and Nazareno, 797). There are no clinically significant drug-to-food/herbal interactions established.

References

Black, J.M. and Hawks, J.H. (2005). *Medical-Surgical Nursing: Clinical Management for Positive Outcomes.* Philadelphia: W.B. Saunders.

Broyles, B.E. (2005). *Medical-Surgical Nursing Clinical Companion.* Durham, NC: Carolina Academic Press.

Corbet, J.V. (2004). *Laboratory Tests and Diagnostic Procedures with Nursing Diagnoses* (6th ed.). Upper Saddle River, NJ: Prentice Hall.

Deglin, J.H. and Vallerand, A.H. (2005). *Davis's Drug Guide for Nurses* (9th ed.). Philadelphia: F.A. Davis.

Gahart, B.L. and Nazareno, A.R. (2005). *2005 Intravenous Medications.* St. Louis: Mosby.

Huether, S.E. and McCance, K.L. (2004). *Understanding Pathophysiology* (3rd ed.). St. Louis: Mosby.

Ignatavicius, D.D. and Workman, M.L. (2006). *Medical-Surgical Nursing across the Health Care Continuum* (5th ed.). Philadelphia: W. B. Saunders.

Lewis, S.M., Heitkemper, M.M., and Dirksen, S.R. (2004). *Medical-Surgical Nursing* (6th ed.). St. Louis: Mosby.

Spratto, G.R. and Woods, A.L. (2005). *2005 Edition: PDR Nurse's Drug Handbook.* Clifton Park, NY: Thomson Delmar Learning.

CASE STUDY 7

Lower Gastrointestinal Bleeding

GENDER
- M

AGE
- 70

SETTING
- Hospital

ETHNICITY/CULTURE
- Black American

PREEXISTING CONDITIONS

COEXISTING CONDITIONS

LIFESTYLE
- Professional painter

COMMUNICATION

DISABILITY

SOCIOECONOMIC STATUS
- Middle

SPIRITUAL/RELIGIOUS
- Episcopalian

PHARMACOLOGIC
- Aluminum hydroxide (Amphogel)
- Misoprostol (Cytotec)
- Ferrous sulfate (Feosol)

PSYCHOSOCIAL
- Anxiety

LEGAL

ETHICAL

ALTERNATIVE THERAPY

PRIORITIZATION
- Stop the bleeding
- Increase tissue perfusion
- Prevent shock

DELEGATION
- RN
- Client education

MODERATE

THE DIGESTIVE AND URINARY SYSTEMS

Level of difficulty: Moderate

Overview: This case involves a thorough account of the current problem, symptoms, and any treatments related to the current problem; exploration of characteristics associated with reported or overt symptoms and factors that may be the cause of symptoms; assessment for pain, a common problem with gastrointestinal (GI) tract disorders. Observation of the skin for discoloration, jaundice, or ecchymosis should be included in the assessment.

Client Profile

Mr. G is a 70-year-old male who travelled with his wife for a family reunion but upon arrival at the city of destination, he was taken from the airport to the emergency department (ED) of a city hospital because he had fainted in the parking lot of the airport after clearing customs. Mr. G is 5'9" and weighs 204 pounds.

Case Study

Mr. G is brought from the airport by emergency medical services (EMS) to the ED, accompanied by his wife. On arrival, Mr. G is alert, and oriented to all stimuli. His vital signs are:

Blood pressure: 110/78
Pulse: 108
Respirations: 16
Temperature: 98.4° F

A nurse practitioner (NP) initiates the assessment. The sclera of both eyes are almost white, but his skin is dry and warm. His wife reports that he has not been eating as he usually does and he has slept much more than usual for the past three weeks. She also reports that his steps have been much slower than normal and he has not been as "jovial" as he usually is. Mr. G reports loss of appetite and a decrease in bowel movement, with only one bowel movement every other day (his usual is daily). He denies past medical or surgical history but informs the nurse that he has noticed that his bowel movement has been black and tarry, but he did not think anything about it. He reports taking "aspirin" for arthritic pain during the past six months. His heart sounds are normal, bilateral breath sounds are clear, and respirations are normal. His abdomen is soft and nontender to the touch, and bowel sounds are hyperactive. On rectal exam, there is dark-colored blood and tarry stool. Stool for guaiac is done and is positive for occult blood. There are no other abnormalities on rectal examination. Specimen is drawn and sent to the lab for hematocrit, hemoglobin, red blood cell count, partial thromboplastin time, activated partial thromboplastin time, serum iron, transferrin, and blood for type and cross match. A 12-lead electrocardiogram (EKG) is done and reveals normal sinus rhythm. A health care provider continues with the assessment after discussing the initial findings with the NP. An 18-gauge intravenous catheter is inserted and 0.9% NaCL is initiated at 100 mL per hour. A nasogastric tube (NGT) is inserted, and aspirate is analyzed for bleeding but is negative for the presence of blood. Results of the labs reveal:

Hematocrit (Hct): 24%
Hemoglobin (Hgb): 10 mg/dL
Red blood cell (RBC) count: $4.5/mm^3$
Partial thromboplastin time (PTT): 48 seconds
Activated partial thromboplastin time (aPTT): 48 seconds
Serum iron: 50 mg/dL
Transferrin: 230 mg/dL

Mr. G is transferred to the surgical unit where he receives two units of packed red blood cells (PRBCs). Mr. G is prepared for a virtual colonoscopy by receiving two cleansing enemas before the procedure. After the transfusion, Mr. G. reports "feeling much better." The colonoscopy is done and reveals hemorrhoids and small gastric ulcers in the area of the lower GI tract. The multidisciplinary team discusses the findings of the diagnostic studies with Mr. G and plans to do a proctosigmoidoscopy at a later time, depending on his length of stay, since he is from "out of town." Post-transfusion labs reveal:

Hct: 26%
Hgb: 12 mg/dL

Post-transfusion vital signs are:

> Blood pressure: 110/74
> Pulse: 98
> Respirations: 18
> Temperature: 98.4° F

Because Mr. G is not from the state where he is hospitalized, he is discharged to home with referral to his primary health care provider for a proctosigmoidoscopy, further evaluation to rule out diverticular diseases and benign anorectal diseases, and to reevaluate hematologic and GI status. A diagnosis of lower GI bleeding is confirmed by clinical symptoms and the colonoscopy.

Questions and Suggested Answers

1. **Discuss common causes for lower GI bleeding in adults.** Some common causes are diverticulosis/diverticulitis of the small intestine; diverticulosis/diverticulitis of the colon, Crohn's disease of the small bowel or the colon, ulcerative colitis, noninfectious gastroenteritis and colitis, hemorrhoids, anal fissure, and fistula-in-ano. Active lower GI bleeding may be from an unknown cause.

2. **Discuss the purpose of the NGT inserted on admission and nursing implications for persons with NGTs.** The NGT is inserted because the bleeding could also be from the upper GI tract, and the NGT helps to prevent aspiration of secretions, which could result in aspiration or chemical pneumonia, and prolonged hospitalization.

3. **Discuss the potentially severe transfusion-related complications and the nursing implications.** One potential complication is *febrile, nonhemolytic reaction* that is caused by antibodies to donor white blood cells (WBCs) that are still present in the unit of blood or blood component. The signs and symptoms of a febrile, nonhemolytic transfusion reaction are chills (absent to severe) followed by fever (more than 1° Celsius elevation). The fever typically begins within two hours after the transfusion is begun. Muscle stiffness is present and can be frightening. To diminish this type of reaction, the use of a leukocyte reduction filter is suggested. *Acute hemolytic reaction* occurs when the donor blood is incompatible with that of the recipient, because antibodies already present in the recipient's plasma rapidly combine with antigens on donor RBCs, and the RBCs are hemolyzed (destroyed) in the circulation (intravascular hemolysis). Symptoms consist of fever, chills, low back pain, nausea, chest tightness, dyspnea, and anxiety. The transfusion must be discontinued immediately, and blood and urine specimens must be obtained and analyzed for evidence of hemolysis. Prevention of acute hemolytic reaction requires detail in labeling the blood samples, blood components, and identifying the recipient before initiating the transfusion. *Allergic reaction* is believed to occur from sensitivity to a plasma protein within the blood component being transfused. The symptoms of allergic reaction are urticaria, itching, and flushing. The reactions are usually mild and respond well to antihistamines (Benadryl). Severe reactions such as bronchospasm, laryngeal edema, and shock are managed with epinephrine, corticosteroids, and pressor support.

4. **What are common nursing diagnoses directly related to Mr. G's situation?**

   - Ineffective tissue perfusion R/T blood loss
   - Anxiety R/T treatment regimen and unfamiliar environment
   - Imbalanced nutrition: less than body requirements R/T decreased intake
   - Risk for injury R/T blood transfusion reactions
   - Deficient knowledge R/T condition, treatment, and health maintenance

The following are prescribed on discharge:

- Aluminum hydroxide (Amphogel) 60 mL one to three hours after meals
- Ferrous sulfate (Feosol) 325 mg PO three times per day
- Misoprostol (Cytotec) 200 mcg/50 mg

5. **What are the purposes for the prescribed orders?** *Aluminum hydroxide* buffers and neutralizes acid in the GI tract by raising the pH of gastric acid, which neutralizes the stomach acid content. *Ferrous gluconate* corrects erythropoietic abnormalities induced by iron deficiency, and helps to reduce gastric tissue changes caused by decrease in iron. The mechanism by which it corrects iron abnormalities is not clear. *Misoprostol* is a synthetic prostaglandin that protects the gastric mucosa from ulcerogenic agents such as aspirin by inhibiting basal and nocturnal gastric acid secretion and acid secretion in response to a variety of stimuli.

6. **What are the most common adverse reactions, drug-to-drug, drug-to-food interactions of the prescribed medications?** The most common adverse reaction to *aluminum hydroxide* is constipation. Drug-to-drug interactions may occur with the simultaneous use of tetracyclines, allopurinol, corticosteroid, diflunisal, histamine-2 antagonists, penicillamine, thyroid hormones, ticlopidine, anticholinergics, phenothiazines, isoniazid, quinidine, phenytoin, digoxin, iron salts, warfarin, detoconazole, and ciprofloxacin, which will decrease their absorption, and administration should be separated by at least two hours. There are no clinically significant drug-to-food/herbal interactions established. The most common adverse reactions of *ferrous gluconate* are nausea, heartburn, constipation, and black stools. Drug-to-drug interactions may occur with the simultaneous use of antacids, cimetidine, and cholestyramine, which will decrease the absorption. Ferrous gluconate decreases the serum levels of fluoroquinolones, levodopa, levothyroxine, methyldopa, mycophenalate mafetil, penicillamine, and tetracycline by decreasing their absorption. Drug-to-food interaction is seen with a decrease in iron absorption with vitamin E, and vitamin C if taken with iron, increases its absorption. St. John's Wort decreases iron absorption. The most common adverse reactions of *misoprostol* are diarrhea, nausea, abdominal cramps, dyspepsia, and abdominal pain. Drug-to-drug interactions may occur with the simultaneous use of magnesium-containing antacids, which may increase diarrhea. No clinically significant drug-to-food/herbal interactions have been established.

7. **Discuss other diagnostic tests the health care provider could have ordered to locate the source of bleeding.** *Enteroscopy* is the visualization of the small intestine. There are different types of enteroscopies, such as the capsule endoscopy referred to as M2A, which is a small bowel enteroscopy that visualizes the entire small bowel, including the distal ileum. It is also used to evaluate and locate the source of GI bleeding. *Invasive colonoscopy* is the insertion of a probe to view to view the entire large bowel. Tissue biopsy specimens or the removal of polyps can be done through the colonoscope. *Proctosigmoidoscopy* is an endoscopic examination that allows for the direct visualization of the mucosa of the anal canal, the rectum and the distal sigmoid colon using a flexible or rigid scope. The purpose is to screen for colon cancer, investigate the source of bleeding, or diagnose or monitor inflammatory bowel disease. An *esophagogastroduodenoscopy* (EGD) is the direct visualization of the mucosa of the upper gastrointestinal tract, which includes the esophagus, stomach, and upper duodenum, using a flexible fiber-optic endoscope.

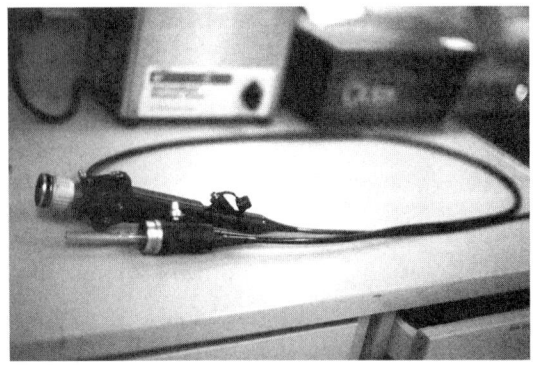

Endoscope

8. **Discuss the similarity and differences between invasive colonoscopy and virtual colonoscopy.** Both the invasive (endoscopic) colonoscopy and the virtual colonoscopy procedure need a bowel preparation. *Invasive colonoscopy* allows for the direct visualization of the mucosa of the entire colon and terminal ileum by means of a flexible fiber-optic colonoscope. Fluoroscopy can be used to assist in guiding the advancement of the scope. A *virtual colonoscopy* is a noninvasive procedure that uses a scanner to view the colon.

9. **Discuss the nursing responsibilities for the client experiencing a proctosigmoidoscopy.** A signed consent is required if tissue is to be removed or if required by the protocol of the agency. The nurse assures that the consent is updated. The nurse reviews the prescribed bowel preparation that is needed before the procedure and explains that the preparation is to clear the rectum and sigmoid colon of feces to enhance visualization. Tell the client that a light meal the evening before and liquids the morning of the procedure are allowed. Inform the client that when the scope is inserted, the urge to defecate may be experienced and that he or she will be asked to take slow, deep breaths through the mouth to help alleviate the urge to defecate. Inform the client that he or she will be placed on the left side in the knee-chest position or on a special table in the proctoscopic position. The endoscope is lubricated and inserted into the anus to the required depth for visualization. Inform the client that slight rectal bleeding might be experienced after the procedure if polyps or tissue are excised but that it should not persist for longer than two days.

10. **Discuss client education for lower GI bleeding.** The client should comply with follow-up care. The client should avoid stress and nonprescribed medications that can cause gastric irritation. The client should avoid foods that are irritating to the stomach, such as caffeine, coffee, and hot spicy foods. The client should monitor bowel movements daily.

References

Black, J.M. and Hawks, J.H. (2005). *Medical-Surgical Nursing: Clinical Management for Positive Outcomes.* Philadelphia: W.B. Saunders.

Broyles, B.E. (2005). *Medical-Surgical Nursing Clinical Companion.* Durham, NC: Carolina Academic Press.

Corbet, J.V. (2004). *Laboratory Tests and Diagnostic Procedures with Nursing Diagnoses* (6th ed.). Upper Saddle River, NJ: Prentice Hall.

Gahart, B.L. and Nazareno, A.R. (2005). *2005 Intravenous Medications.* St. Louis: Mosby.

Huether, S.E. and McCance, K.L. (2004). *Understanding Pathophysiology* (3rd ed.). St. Louis: Mosby.

Ignatavicius, D.D. and Workman, M.L. (2006). *Medical-Surgical Nursing across the Health Care Continuum* (5th ed.). Philadelphia: W. B. Saunders.

Spratto, G.R. and Woods, A.L. (2005). *2005 Edition: PDR Nurse's Drug Handbook.* Clifton Park, NY: Thomson Delmar Learning.

CASE STUDY 8

Chronic Renal Failure (End-Stage Renal Disease)

GENDER
- F

AGE
- 64

SETTING
- Hospital

ETHNICITY/CULTURE
- White American

PREEXISTING CONDITIONS

COEXISTING CONDITIONS

LIFESTYLE
- Retired interior decorator

COMMUNICATION

DISABILITY

SOCIOECONOMIC STATUS
- Middle

SPIRITUAL/RELIGIOUS
- Presbyterian

PHARMACOLOGIC
- Epoetin alfa recombinant (Epogen)
- Calcium carbonate (Os-cal)
- Aluminum hydroxide (Amphogel)
- Nifedipine (Procardia)
- Folic acid (Apo-Folic)
- Ferrous sulfate (Feosol)
- Ducosate sodium (Colace)
- Furosemide (Lasix)

PSYCHOSOCIAL
- Anxiety

LEGAL

ETHICAL
- Do all clients with renal failure have an unconditional right to dialysis, given the cost of dialysis and the relative few who benefit from it?

ALTERNATIVE THERAPY

PRIORITIZATION
- Complete history, including nutritional habits and current medications
- Discuss urinary elimination in detail

DELEGATION
- RN
- CNA
- Client education

THE DIGESTIVE AND URINARY SYSTEMS

Level of difficulty: Difficult

Overview: This case involves a thorough assessment of the client's condition, including current medications as well as careful systems assessment to prioritize care and prevent further complications and maintain kidney function and homeostasis for as long as possible. Accurate monitoring of blood pressure and serum potassium are critical since hypertension and hyperkalemia are common complications of end-stage renal disease (ESRD). Critical assessment of fluid status to identify imbalance is needed.

Client Profile

Mr. P, a 64-year-old retiree, is 4'10" and weighs 170 pounds. He shares a private home with his younger brother, who transported him to the emergency department (ED) of the hospital. On arrival, he complains of having had a headache for the past two hours. His vital signs are:

Blood pressure: 200/150

Pulse: 110

Respirations: 30

Temperature: 98.6° F

He is alert and oriented but is slow to respond to questions. He denies chest pain but reports nausea and feels he will vomit at anytime.

Case Study

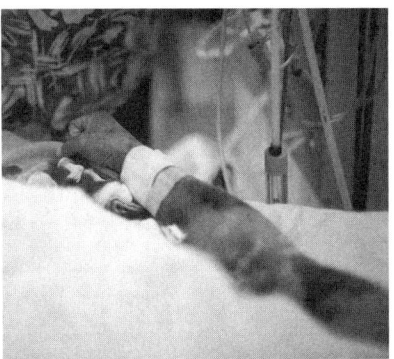

Double-lumen nasogastric tube

Mr. P was diagnosed a year ago with end-stage renal failure secondary to hypertension, requiring treatment with hemodialysis. He is dialyzed at the clinic three times per week and is restricted to 1000 mL of fluid each day. He has a primary arteriovenous (AV) fistula in his left forearm (he is right handed). He reports current medications as:

Folic acid: 0.1 mg PO daily

Ferrous sulfate: 325 mg three times per day

Aluminum hydroxide: gel 500 mg PO twice

Erythropoietin alpha: self medicates with 50 units SC three times per week

Nifedipine: 30 mg PO three times per day

Mr. P reports not feeling his usual self, feeling tired on awakening this morning, and having difficulty getting out of bed. He is triaged and transferred to the medical intensive care (MICU), where an electrocardiogram (EKG) is done and shows sinus tachycardia and occasional unifocal premature ventricular contractions. Physical assessment reveals rales at the bases of the lungs and pitting edema of the lower extremities. Serum laboratory reports reveal:

Creatinine: 12 mg/dL

Blood urea nitrogen (BUN): 40 mg/dL

Sodium (Na): 150 mEq/L

Chloride: 100 mEq/L

Potassium (K+): 7.8 mEq/L

Phosphorous: 6.5 mg/dL

Calcium: 6 mg/dL

Hemoglobin (Hgb): 19 g/dL

Hematocrit (Hct): 28%

Glucose: 98 mg/dL

Arterial blood gas (ABG):
    pH: 7.32
    $PaCO_2$: 18 mm Hg
    HCO_3: 8 mEq/L
    PaO_2: 54

Mr. P is transferred to the dialysis unit soon after being transferred to the MICU and is dialyzed. A multidisciplinary team will participate in the overall plan of care, and the social worker, dietitian, and case manager will plan and coordinate home-care management.

Questions and Suggested Answers

1. **Discuss the pathophysiology of chronic renal failure, or ESRD.** Chronic renal failure, or ESRD, is a progressive, irreversible deterioration in renal function in which the body's ability to maintain metabolic fluid and electrolyte balance fails, resulting in uremia or azotemia (retention of urea and other nitrogenous wastes in the blood). As renal function declines, the end products of protein metabolism (which are normally excreted in urine) accumulate in the blood. Uremia develops and adversely affects every system in the body. The greater the buildup of waste products, the more severe the symptoms. Many of the symptoms of uremia are reversible. In ESRD, there are decreased glomerular filtration rates (GFR). As GFR decreases due to the nonfunctioning glomeruli, the creatinine clearance will decrease and the serum creatinine level will rise. In addition, the BUN level is elevated. The BUN is affected not only by renal disease, but also by protein intake in the diet, catabolism (tissue and red blood cell [RBC] breakdown), and medications such as steroids. Because the kidney is unable to concentrate or dilute the urine normally in ESRD, appropriate responses by the kidney to changes in daily intake of water and electrolytes do not occur. The client often retains sodium and water, increasing the risk of edema formation, congestive heart failure, and hypertension. *Acidosis* develops with advanced renal disease; metabolic acidosis occurs as the kidney is unable to excrete increased loads of acid (H+). Decreased acid secretion primarily results from inability of the kidney tubules to secrete ammonia (NH_3^-) and to reabsorb sodium bicarbonate (HCO_3^-). There is also decreased excretion of phosphates and other organic acids. *Anemia* develops as a result of inadequate erythropoietin production, the shortened life span of the RBCs, nutritional deficiencies, and the uremic client's tendency to bleed, particularly from the gastrointestinal (GI) tract. Erythropoietin is a substance normally produced by the kidney that functions to stimulate bone marrow to produce RBCs. In renal failure, erythropoietin production decreases and profound anemia results, producing fatigue, angina, and shortness of breath. *Metabolic changes* occur because clients with ESRD exhibit glucose intolerance, which is due to insulin resistance, as evident by reduced sensitivity to the hypoglycemic action of insulin. Elevated triglycerides related to increased production of lipids by the liver in response to the elevated blood glucose and insulin levels. *Pericarditis* develops due to accumulation of uremic toxins. *Hematologic changes* with normochromic, normocytic anemia, and platelet deficiencies occur due to the interference of uremic toxins with platelet adhesiveness. *GI changes* occur, with constipation being a common problem due to phosphate-binding agents, restriction of fluids, high-fiber foods, and decreased activity. *Immunologic changes* include depression of humoral antibody formation, increasing the risk for infection. *Changes in medication metabolism* occur due to a high level of the medication due to low serum albumin, which decreases the protein binding sites, impaired renal excretion, or impaired hepatic metabolism of the

medications. ***Cardiovascular changes*** result, with hypertension being the most frequent clinical manifestation due to the mechanisms of volume overload, stimulation of the renin-angiotensin system, sympathetically mediated vasoconstriction, and the absence of prostaglandins. ***Respiratory changes*** occur, with pleuritis being a frequent occurrence. ***Musculoskeletal changes*** occur with hypercalcemia, and the presence of renal osteodystrophy, which develops slowly in several forms such as in osteomalacia, osteitis fibrosis, osteoporosis, or osteosclerosis. ***Integumentary changes*** result, with severe and intractable pruritus developing secondary to hyperparathyrodism and calcium deposits on the skin. ***Neurologic changes*** develop, with the presence of peripheral neuropathy resulting in "restless legs syndrome", and reduction of deep tendon reflexes and vibratory sense. ***Reproductive changes*** manifest with decreased libido in both sexes. ***Endocrine changes*** manifest hypothyroidism because of the thyroid-stimulating hormone demonstrating a blunted response to thyrotropin-releasing hormone.

2. **Discuss the incidence, prevalence, and etiologies of ESRD in the United States.** The incidence of ESRD has increased by almost 8% per year for the past five years and, according to the National Kidney Foundation, more than 378,000 Americans need dialysis to stay alive. In addition, more than 50,000 clients are waiting for renal transplants, but only about 14,000 will actually receive transplants annually because of the shortage of suitable organs. ESRD occurs more often in men than in women, and the greatest increase in ESRD is in clients 65 years and older. Also, according to the National Kidney Foundation, diabetes mellitus is the leading cause of chronic renal failure, accounting for 44% of the new cases diagnosed annually in the United States. Uncontrolled or poorly controlled hypertension is the second leading cause. The prolonged hyperglycemia in diabetes mellitus results in diabetic nephropathy, in which the glomeruli are injured by protein denaturation due to the high glucose levels, which causes hyperfiltration, and intraglomerular hypertension exacerbated by systemic hypertension. Progressive changes include glomerular enlargement, glomerular basement membrane thickening with proliferation of cells and matrix of the kidneys. The overall result is diffuse intercapillary glomerulosclerosis and decreased blood flow. Eventually, there is microalbuminuria as the first manifestation of renal dysfunction. Later, hypoproteinemia, reduction in plasma oncotic pressure, fluid overload, anasarca (generalized body edema) and hypertension may occur. Cardiovascular disease is the predominant cause of death in clients with ESRD. In chronic hemodialysis clients, approximately 45% of the overall mortality is attributable to cardiac disease. The most common cardiovascular abnormality is hypertension, which usually precedes ESRD and is worsened by sodium retention sand increased extracellular fluid volume. Hypertension accelerates atherosclerotic vascular disease, produces intrarenal arterial spasm, and eventually leads to left ventricular hypertrophy and congestive heart failure.

3. **Discuss why Mr. P was dialyzed soon after he was transferred to the MICU.** He was dialyzed in an effort to correct electrolytes imbalances, remove metabolic waste products that the kidneys were not capable of performing, and regain as much normalcy of fluid, electrolyte, and metabolic balance as possible.

4. **Discuss Mr. P's AV fistula and the purpose for it.** An AV fistula is an anastomosis between an artery and a vein that allows arterial blood to flow into the vein, causing venous engorgement and enlargement. The vein is then used as an access to the bloodstream for hemodialysis. Patency of the access must be assessed frequently each day, which can be determined by palpating for a buzzing sensation (a thrill) or by auscultating with a stethoscope for a bruit (buzzing sound). Signs of infections such as redness, pain, or swelling along the fistula area must be reported promptly. Infection should be treated before dialysis or it could become systemic, resulting in complications. No blood pressure, drawing of blood samples or intravenous lines should be performed in this hand. A sign over the client's bed is a helpful reminder.

5. **Discuss why the client is in metabolic acidosis.** The client is in metabolic acidosis because of the kidney's inability to excrete hydrogen ions as a result of decreased reabsorption of sodium bicarbonate and decreased formation of dihydrogen phosphate and ammonia. This condition accentuates hyperkalemia and the reabsorption of calcium from the bones.

6. **What is the relationship between calcium, phosphorous, and chronic renal failure?** Another major abnormality seen in chronic renal failure is a disorder in calcium and phosphorous metabolism. The body's serum calcium and phosphate levels have a reciprocal relationship in the body; as one rises, the other decreases. Due to decreased filtration through the kidney's glomerulus, there is an increase in the serum phosphate level and a reciprocal or corresponding decrease in the serum calcium level. The decreased calcium level causes increased secretion of parathormone from the parathyroid glands. However, in renal failure, the body does not respond normally to the increased secretion of parathormone and, as a result, calcium leaves the bone, often producing bone changes and bone disease. There is uremic bone disease, often called osteodystrophy, that develops from the complex changes in calcium, phosphate, and parathormone balance. Plasma calcium decreases in response to the hyperphosphatemia, and in the presence of the chronicity of the kidneys, conversion of vitamin D in its active metabolite phase is severely impaired, resulting in reduction of calcium absorption from the GI tract and impaired calcium mobilization from the bone, worsening hypocalcemia.

7. **What are common nursing diagnoses for clients with ESRD?**

   - Excess fluid volume R/T inability of kidneys to excrete fluid, inadequate dialysis, and excessive fluid intake
   - Impaired skin integrity R/T decrease in oil and sweat gland activity, hyperphosphatemia, deposition of calcium-phosphate precipitates, capillary fragility, excess fluid, and neuropathy
   - Risk for injury (fracture) R/T alterations in the absorption of calcium and excretion of phosphate, altered vitamin D metabolism
   - Activity intolerance R/T anemia and neuropathy
   - Imbalanced nutrition: less than body requirements R/T restricted intake of nutrients (especially protein), nausea, vomiting, anorexia, and stomatitis
   - Risk for infection R/T suppressed immune system, access sites, and malnutrition secondary to dialysis and uremia
   - Anticipatory grieving R/T loss of kidney function
   - Knowledge deficit R/T condition, treatment, and home care upon discharge

8. **Discuss hemodialysis (HD) versus peritoneal dialysis and the reason Mr. P was given hemodialysis instead of peritoneal dialysis.** HD was preferred at this time because it is a faster acting procedure when critical results are needed to maintain homeostasis and prevent complications. In HD, an artificial membrane (usually made of cellulose-based or synthetic materials) is used as the semipermeable membrane which is in contact with the client's blood. Dialysis is begun when the client's uremia can no longer be adequately managed conservatively. It is initiated when the GFR (or creatinine clearance) is less than 15 mL per minute. Peritoneal dialysis is used to treat clients with acute and chronic renal failure in the hospital or at home. The process is easily taught to clients, and clients can dialyze themselves at any location without machinery. Peritoneal dialysis involves instilling dialyzing fluid into the peritoneal cavity. The peritoneum serves as a dialyzing membrane, and access to the peritoneum is gained through the introduction of a catheter into the peritoneal space. Because introduction of a catheter presents a continuous portal of entry for organisms into the peritoneum, each client must be thoroughly instructed in the care of the catheter and the signs and symptoms of local or peritoneal infection, which must be reported to the health care provider. If the procedure is temporary, the catheter is removed and the incision is covered with a dry, sterile dressing and will heal in few days. Advantages of peritoneal dialysis include maintaining a balanced state of blood chemistry values. This type of dialysis also provides clients with more control over daily life. Disadvantages are minimal and relate mostly to infection if the catheter becomes contaminated. The advantages of HD are rapid removal of fluid, urea, and creatinine. It effectively removes potassium with minimal loss of protein. Home dialysis can be done and temporary access can be placed at the bedside. The disadvantages of HD include vascular access problems, therefore, heparinization may be necessary. Other disadvantages are the need for dietary and fluid restrictions, the loss of blood during dialysis (which could result in the development of anemia), the development of hypotension, the need for permanent access by surgical approach, and the self-image problems some clients may develop due to the need for the permanent access device.

The following are prescribed after the dialysis is completed:

- Folic acid (Apo-Folic) 0.1 mg PO daily
- Ferrous sulfate (Feosol) 325 mg PO three times per day
- Epoetin alfa (Epogen) 100 units/kg/dose SC three times per week
- Aluminum hydroxide gel (Amphogel) 500 mg PO four times per day
- Nifedipine (Procardia) 30mg PO three times per day
- Docusate sodium (Colace) 300 mg PO three times per day
- Calcium carbonate (Os-cal) 500 mg PO three times per day
- Furosemide (Lasix) 40 mg IV now and again in 4 hours

9. **What are the purposes for the prescribed medications?** *Folic acid* is a vitamin B complex supplement that replenishes the depletion that usually occurs with ESRD because of nutritional deficit. It is needed for the final maturation of the RBCs, and accomplishes this by synthesizing DNA which, when synthesized, results in the formation of thymidine triphosphate, one of the essential building blocks of DNA. *Ferrous sulfate* is an iron supplement that improves the anemic state of the client. It corrects erythropoietic abnormalities without stimulating erythropoiesis. Normal iron stores are needed for epoetin alfa to effectively correct the client's anemia. *Epoetin alfa* is an amino acid glycoprotein manufactured by recombinant DNA that stimulates the bone marrow to produce RBCs to increase the hematocrit, and oxygen-carrying capacity, decrease anemia, and reduce the need for blood transfusion. *Aluminum hydroxide* is an aluminum-based antacid that lowers phosphate by binding dietary phosphopate and forming insoluble aluminum phosphate in the GI tract, where it then is excreted in the feces. *Nifedipine* is a calcium channel-blocking agent that lowers blood pressure by vasodilating both coronary and peripheral vessels. It also prevents the influx of calcium into the kidney cells, helping to preserve cell integrity by improving GFR. *Docusate sodium* is a stool softener that prevents constipation caused by fluid restriction, iron supplement, and phosphate binding drugs and calcium channel blockers. It does this by lowering surface tension, which permits water and fats to penetrate and soften stools for easier passage. *Calcium carbonate* increases calcium levels to treat the hypocalcemia characteristic of ESRD. Because of the inverse relationship between calcium and phosphorous, by increasing the calcium level, the phosphorous level will decrease. *Furosemide* is a loop diuretic that is indicated here because of the client's pulmonary edema and hypertension. It acts on the proximal and distal ends of the renal tubule and the ascending loop of Henle to increase water and sodium excretion.

10. **What are the most common adverse reactions of the prescribed medications?** The most common adverse reactions of *folic acid* include allergic reactions, nausea, anorexia, and altered sleep patterns. The most common adverse reactions of *ferrous sulfate* are nausea, heartburn, constipation, black stools, hypotension, epigastric pain, and skin staining at intramuscular (IM) site. The most common adverse reactions of *epoetin alfa* are hypertension, headache, iron deficiency, and clotting of AV fistula. The most common adverse reaction of *aluminum hydroxide gel* is constipation. The most common adverse reactions of *nifedipine* are hypotension, tachycardia, headache, peripheral edema, and flushing. The most common adverse reaction of *docusate sodium* is diarrhea. The most common adverse effect of *calcium carbonate* is constipation. The most common adverse effects of *furosemide* include hypokalemia, hyponatremia, anorexia, hyperglycemia, leg cramps, and mental confusion.

11. **Discuss the drug-to-drug and drug-to-food/herbal interactions for the prescribed medications.** With *folic acid,* drug-to-drug interactions may be seen with the simultaneous use of pyrimethamine, methotrexate, trimethoprim, and triamterene, which may prevent the activation of folic acid. The concurrent use with sulfonamides, sulfasalazine, antacids, and cholesytramine decrease the absorption of folic acid. The simultaneous use of estrogens, phenytoin, phenobarbital, primidone, carbamazepine, or corticosteroids increases the requirements of folic acid. There are no clinically significant drug-to-food/herbal interactions established. With *ferrous sulfate* drug-to-drug interactions may occur with the simultaneous use of tetracycline and antacids decrease the absorption of iron. The simultaneous use of fluoroquinolones and penicillamine should be avoided, because it severely alters the effects of fluoroquinolones and decreases the serum levels

of both of these agents, The concurrent use with levodopa, methyldopa, mucophenolate mofetil, and levothyroxine because the ferrous sulfate decreases the absorption of these agents. Ascorbic acid 200 mg or more is needed to increase iron absorption; vitamin E decreases the effectiveness to ferrous sulfate; and St. John's Wort may decrease ferrous sulfate's GI absorption. Drug-to-drug interactions may occur with the simultaneous use of *epoetin alfa* and heparin, which may increase the requirement of heparin during hemodialysis. There are no clinically significant drug-to-food/herbal interactions established. With *aluminum hydroxide,* drug-to-drug interactions may occur with the simultaneous use of allopurinol, corticosteroids, diflunisal, histamine-2 antagonists, penicillamine, thyroid hormones, ticlopidine anticholinergics, phenothiazines, quinidine, phenytoin, warfarin, ciprofloxacin, tetracyclines, chlorpromazine, iron salts, isoniazid, digoxin, or fluoroquinolones, which may decrease the absorption of these drugs. Administration should be separated by at least two hours. There are no clinically established drug-to-food/herbal interactions established. With *nifedipine* drug-to-drug interactions may occur with the simultaneous use of fentanyl, antihypertensives, nitrates, alcohol, or quinidine, which may cause additive hypotension. The concurrent use with digoxin may increase serum digoxin levels and toxicity. Concurrent use with beta blockers, disopyramide, or phenytoin may result in bradycardia, conduction defects, or congestive heart failure (CHF). The concurrent use with cimetidine, diltiazem, itraconazole, quinupristin/dalfopristin, ranitidine, rifampin, and propranolol may decrease the metabolism and increase risk for nifedipine toxicity. Use with barbiturates decreases nifedipine's effects. Use with warfarin, cyclosporine, magnesium sulfate, tacolimus, theophylline, and vincristine increases the effects of these agents. Grapefruit juice increases serum levels and effect, and St. John's Wort increases the metabolism of nifedipine, thus decreasing its serum levels. Drug-to-drug interactions are seen with the concurrent use of *docusate sodium* and mineral oil, which will increase systemic absorption. There are no clinically significant drug-to-food/herbal interactions established. With *calcium carbonate* drug-to-drug interactions may occur with the simultaneous use of quinidine and amphetamines by increasing their plasma levels. Further, it decreases the levels of salicylates, calcium channel blocking agents, ketoconazole, tetracyclines and iron salts. Increased effects and adverse effects of lily of the valley, pheasant's eye, and squill are seen with concurrent use with calcium carbonate. Drug-to-drug interactions occur with the concurrent use of *furosemide* and corticosteroids, thiazide diuretics, and amphotericin B, resulting in increased risk of hypokalemia. It potentiates the effects of antihypertensive agents and may increase the potential for ototoxicity if used simultaneously with gentamycin, cisplatin, and amphotericin B. Increased risk of nephrotoxicity occurs with the use of amphotericin B, acyclovir, aminoglycosides, cyclosporine, and vancomycin. Furosemide may increase the serum levels of insulin, sulfonylureas, warfarin, heparin, streptokinase, propranolol, and lithium. Risk of cardiotoxicity increases if used with pimozide and sparfloxacin. Furosemide is inhibited by angiotensin-converting enzyme (ACE) inhibitors, nonsteroidal anti-inflammatory agents (NSAIDs), probenecid, phenytoin, and in clients with cirrhosis and ascites who also are taking salicylates. Smoking increases the secretion of the body's antidiuretic hormone resulting in decreases furosemide-induced diuresis.

12. **Discuss client education for ESRD.** Explanation of dietary intake (protein, sodium, potassium, phosphate) and fluid restrictions, and the need to modify diet and fluid intake is stressed. Teach alternative ways of reducing thirst, such as sucking on ice cubes, lemons, or hard candy. The client with ESRD and a vascular access should be provided with the following information: Avoid tight clothing around the access that may decrease the blood flow and cause clotting. The access site should be checked at least two times daily for the "buzz" that indicates adequate blood flow. If it becomes difficult to palpate or does not "buzz," the primary health care provider should be notified promptly, since this may indicate that the access has clotted. Discuss specific care of the AV fistula, and signs and symptoms to look for indicating the developing of infection (redness, heat, swelling or drainage at the fistula site), and the importance of reporting these findings to the primary health care provider immediately. If for any reason the access site starts to bleed, apply firm pressure and call for help immediately, since much blood loss can occur from the access site. Do not allow anyone to take blood pressure or withdraw blood from the extremity that has the access, and do not sleep with pressure on the extremity with the access. Avoid the use of creams or lotions over the access site. Stress the

adherence to medication prescription (phosphate binding drugs should be taken with meals, iron supplements should be taken between meals), and the importance of follow-up care with the primary health care provider (a nephrologist). Inform the client about the significance of reporting weight gain greater than two pounds in a week, increasing blood pressure, edema, shortness of breath or weakness, since these are indications of the need for re-dialysis.

References

Black, J.M. and Hawks, J.H. (2005). *Medical-Surgical Nursing: Clinical Management for Positive Outcomes.* Philadelphia: W.B. Saunders.

Broyles, B.E. (2005). *Medical-Surgical Nursing Clinical Companion.* Durham, NC: Carolina Academic Press.

Corbet, J.V. (2004). *Laboratory Tests and Diagnostic Procedures with Nursing Diagnoses* (6th ed.). Upper Saddle River, NJ: Prentice Hall.

Gahart, B.L. and Nazareno, A.R. (2005). *2005 Intravenous Medications.* St. Louis: Mosby.

Guyton, A.C. and Hall, J.E. (2006). *Textbook of Medical Physiology* (11th ed.). Philadelphia: W.B. Saunders.

Huether, S.E. and McCance, K.L. (2004). *Understanding Pathophysiology* (3rd ed.). St. Louis: Mosby.

Ignatavicius, D.D. and Workman, M.L. (2006). *Medical-Surgical Nursing across the Health Care Continuum* (5th ed.). Philadelphia: W.B. Saunders.

National Kidney Foundation. (2004). www.kidney.org.

Spratto, G.R. and Woods, A.L. (2005). *2005 Edition: PDR Nurse's Drug Handbook.* Clifton Park, NY: Thomson Delmar Learning.

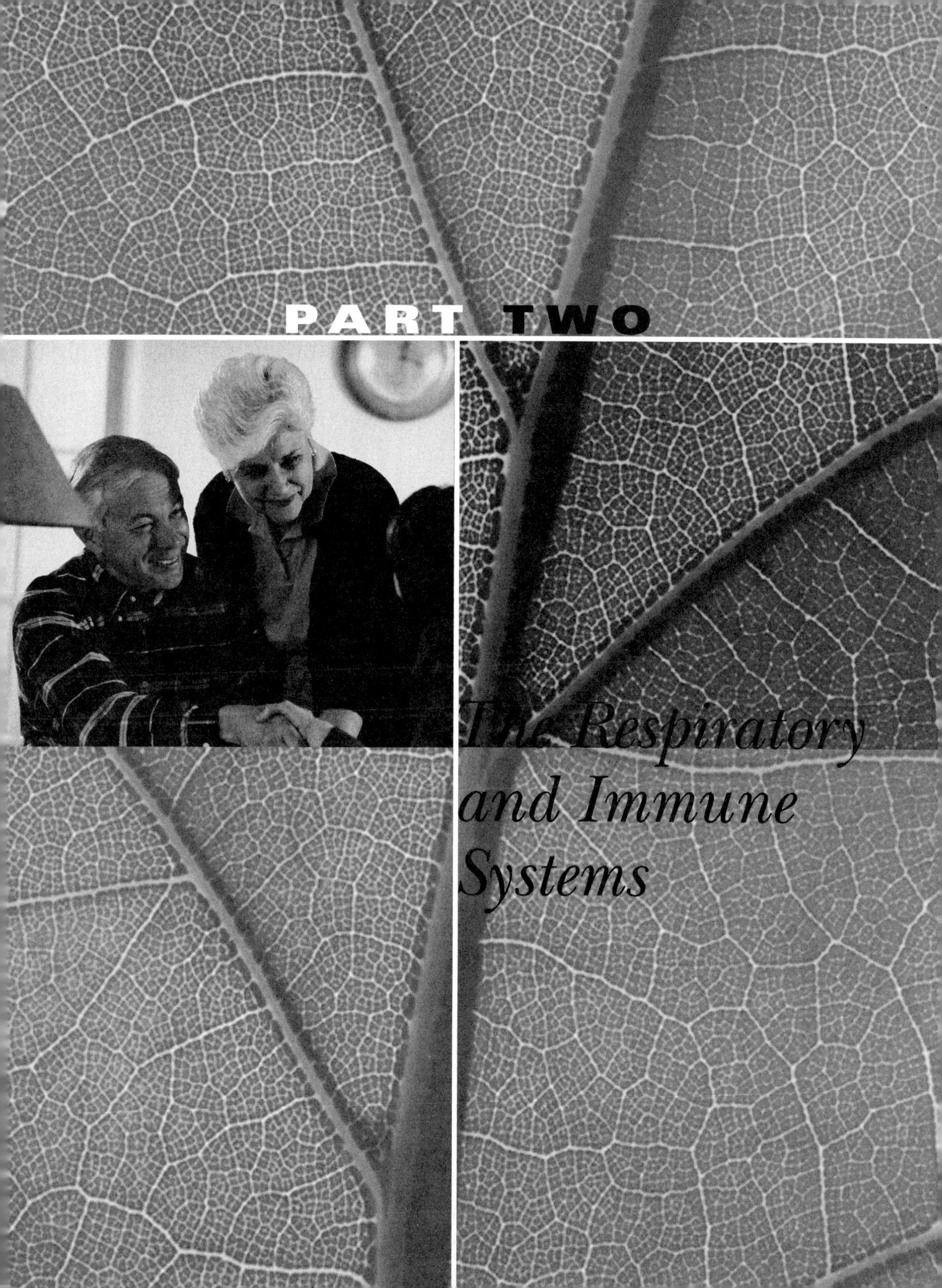

PART TWO

The Respiratory and Immune Systems

CASE STUDY 1

Chronic Bronchitis

GENDER
- M

AGE
- 76

SETTING
- Skilled nursing facility

ETHNICITY/CULTURE
- White American

PREEXISTING CONDITIONS

COEXISTING CONDITIONS
- Viral infection
- Bacterial infection

LIFESTYLE
- Apartment building supervisor

COMMUNICATION

DISABILITY
- Decreased exercise tolerance

SOCIOECONOMIC STATUS
- Middle

SPIRITUAL/RELIGIOUS
- Protestant

PHARMACOLOGIC
- Albuterol (Proventil)
- Guaifenesin (Robitussin)
- Amoxicillin (Amoxil)
- Cefepime HcL (Maxipime)
- Ipratropium bromide (Atrovent)
- Acetaminophen (Tylenol)

PSYCHOSOCIAL
- Anxiety
- Depression

LEGAL

ETHICAL

ALTERNATIVE THERAPY

PRIORITIZATION
- Maintain patent airway

DELEGATION
- RN
- Client education

THE RESPIRATORY AND IMMUNE SYSTEMS

Level of difficulty: Easy

Overview: This case involves prioritization of care to identify client's immediate needs and effective planning to have these needs met. The case also involves competence in identifying subtlety of grave changes with the client, such as absence of wheezing.

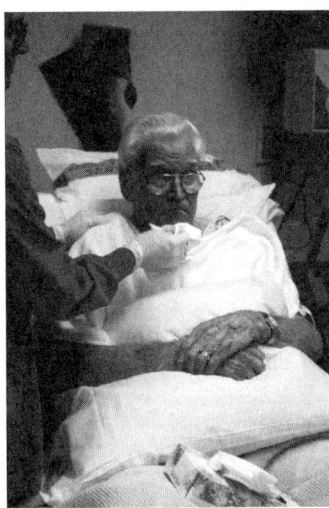

Client Profile

Mr. K, a 76-year-old male, is readmitted to the hospital's emergency department (ED) from a skilled nursing facility via an ambulette. On arrival, Mr. K shows signs of respiratory compromise as manifested by use of accessory muscles of the neck. The report from the nursing facility indicates that prior to this episode of respiratory impairment, Mr. K had been capable of carrying out basic activities of daily living such as combing his hair, mouth care, and dressing himself with only minimal assistance.

Case Study

During the past two weeks, Mr. K has been complaining of "stuffy" nose and has gradually begun to expectorate moderate amounts of respiratory secretions. The facility's health care provider is called because Mr. K has a temperature of 101° F and complains of chills even though the window of his room is closed and the air conditioning is off. His vital signs are:

Blood pressure: 124/86
Pulse: 80 and regular
Respirations: 20
Temperature: 101.0° F

Mr. K has a long history of cigarette smoking. On admission, he has thick, productive cough. The licensed practical nurse accompanying him informs the triage nurse that the cough has been unusually productive for more than one month, and Mr. K has had elevation of temperature of 101° F in the past that responded to Tylenol suppository. On auscultation, the ED nurse elicits loud rhonchi and wheezes. A complete history and physical is done, with physical findings that include clubbing of the fingers but no cyanosis or peripheral edema. A chest X-ray done on arrival to the ED reveals increased pulmonary congestion in the right lower lobe but no filtration or pleural effusion. Spirometry reveals airflow limitation with forced expiratory volume and forced vital capacity (FEV_1/FVC) 80%. Arterial blood gas (ABG) test reveals:

pH: 7.35
PO_2: 80
PCO_2: 47
HCO_3: 27

Mr. K is placed on two liters of oxygen via nasal cannula and is transferred to a respiratory unit of the hospital. On arrival at the unit, he continues to cough and, at times, coughs up blood-tinged sputum. A lab specimen is ordered, and results reveal sputum for culture and gram stain positive for Staphylococcus aureus and gram negative bacilli, white blood cell (WBC) with differential: WBC 14,000/mm^3 and eosinophils 600/mm^3. After the physical and laboratory data are reviewed, an admitting diagnosis of chronic bronchitis is confirmed.

Questions and Suggested Answers

1. **Discuss the cultural considerations for clients with chronic bronchitis related to history of cigarette smoking.** The prevalence of smoking remains higher among black Americans, blue-collar workers, and less educated people than in the overall population of the United States. Smoking prevalence is highest among Northern Plains American Indians/Native Americans and Alaskan Natives. The overall prevalence of smoking for both men and women has decreased over the past two decades, but the decrease for women has been less than for men. Development of culturally appropriate smoking cessation programs, as well as research examining barriers to cessation in these populations, may help reduce this disparity.

2. **Discuss specific criteria used to diagnose chronic bronchitis.** In order to diagnose chronic bronchitis, inflammation of the bronchi must continue for three months of the year and for two consecutive years in a client in whom other causes for cough have been excluded. Specific criteria to diagnose chronic bronchitis include complete history, occupation, number of packs per day of cigarettes smoked to determine smoking habits, chest X-ray, pulmonary function studies such as vital capacity and forced expiratory volume (both of which will be decreased), and an increased residual volume.

3. **Discuss the classic findings of clients with chronic bronchitis.**
   - Increased mucus production and chronic cough due to inflammation of the bronchi; an increased number of goblet cells, which also secrete mucus, and impaired ciliary function, which reduces mucus clearance
   - Pursed-lip breathing, when the small and large airways become involved and the thick mucus and inflamed bronchi obstruct the airway, especially during expiration
   - Reduced alveolar ventilation due to collapse of the airways and trapping of air in the distal portion of the lung
   - Abnormal ventilation-perfusion (V/Q) ratio due to a fall in PaO$_2$ and an increase in PaCO$_2$
   - Slight gynecomastia R/T the side effect of corticosteroid therapy used to counteract the inflammatory process that is usually present
   - Raised shoulders due to shortness of breath and increased work of breathing

4. **What are common nursing diagnoses for clients with chronic bronchitis?**
   - Impaired gas exchange R/T decreased ventilation
   - Ineffective airway clearance R/T excessive secretions and ineffective cough
   - Ineffective breathing pattern R/T fatigue and decreased energy
   - Activity intolerance R/T inadequate oxygenation and dyspnea
   - Sleep pattern disturbance R/T dyspnea and external stimuli
   - Risk for infection R/T increase mucus secretions and ineffective cough
   - Imbalanced nutrition: less than body requirements R/T dyspnea on exertion, anorexia

5. **What are the key features of cor pulmonale (right-sided heart failure), a complication of chronic bronchitis?**
   Key features of cor pulmonale are hypoxia and hypoxemia, increasing dyspnea, fatigue, weakness, enlarged, tender liver, warm, cyanotic extremities with bounding pulses, cyanotic lips, distended neck veins, right ventricular enlargement (hypertrophy), lower sternal or epigastric pulsations, gastrointestinal disturbances, such as nausea or anorexia, dependent edema, metabolic and respiratory acidosis, and pulmonary hypertension. Pulmonary hypertension occurs because the client's PaO$_2$ is depressed, which causes pulmonary

vasoconstriction, resulting in an increase in pulmonary blood pressure (pulmonary hypertension). Because the pressure in the right ventricle must increase to eject blood into the narrowed pulmonary vessels, but is too high for normal ejection, the increased pressure eventually leads to right-sided heart failure, also called pulmonary heart disease or cor pulmonale.

6. **Discuss the breathing patterns commonly seen in clients with respiratory muscle fatigue.**
   - Abdominal paradox, in which the diaphragm is nonfunctional; inspiration is accomplished by the intercostal and abdominal accessory muscles.
   - Respiratory alternans, in which diaphragmatic breathing alternates with abdominal paradox, may serve to rest the diaphragm.
   - Asynchronous breathing, in which the chest wall motion is unorganized, reflecting the uncoordinated activity of fatigued muscles.

The following are prescribed:

- Albuterol (Proventil) 2 puffs q4h and Ipratropium bromide (Atrovent) Soln, Inhl, 2.5 mL nebulization q4h
- Acetaminophen (Tylenol) 650 mg PO PRN temp greater than 100°
- Cefepime HcL (Maxipime) 1.5 g IV q12h
- Guaifenesin (Robitussin) 200 mg PRN q4h for cough
- D 5.45% NS IV infusion at 125 mL per hour

7. **What are the purposes for the prescribed orders?** *Albuterol* is a bronchodilator administered to enhance and prolong bronchodilation. *Albuterol* promotes bronchodilation by acting primarily on the smooth muscles of the bronchi, which enhances the airway diameter, and promotes better ventilation. *Acetaminophen* is a nonopioid analgesic and effective antipyretic that lowers the elevated temperature by its direct action on the hypothalamus heat-regulating center with consequent peripheral vasodilation, sweating, and dissipation of heat. *Cefepime HcL* is a fourth-generation cephalosporin that is bacteriocidal to both gram positive and gram negative pathogens including many strains that have developed a resistance to aminoglycosides and third-generation cephalosporins. This agent is prescribed to treat the client's respiratory infection. *Guaifenesin* is an expectorant that liquefies secretions, making them easier to clear out of the respiratory passages. Because of its expectorant property, the *intravenous infusion* replenishes electrolyte and water loss due to the insensible loss. *Dextrose in the IV solution* helps provide energy and rehydration, which is usually depleted during times of elevated fever.

8. **What are the most common adverse reactions of the prescribed medications?** The most common adverse drug reactions of *albuterol* are tachycardia, nervousness, restlessness, tremor, chest pain, and palpitation. A common adverse reaction seen with acetaminophen is *hepatotoxicity* in persons who are alcoholics. The most common adverse effects of *cefepime HcL* include a full range of allergic reactions, bone marrow suppression, and superinfections. There are no clinically significant common adverse drug reactions established for *guiafenesin*.

9. **Discuss the drug-to-drug and drug-to-food/herbal interactions for the prescribed medications.** With *albuterol*, drug-to-drug interaction may occur with the simultaneous use of epinephrine, which may increase adrenergic side effects. The simultaneous use with monoamine oxidase (MAO) inhibitors may lead to hypertensive crisis, and beta blockers may negate the therapeutic effect. Risk for hypokalemia is seen with the simultaneous use of potassium-losing diuretics, which would increase the risk of digoxin. There are no clinically significant drug-to-food interactions established, but drug-to-herbal interactions are seen with the simultaneous use of cola nut, guarana, tea, and coffee, which may increase stimulant effects. Drug-to-drug interactions may occur with the simultaneous use of *acetaminophen* and cholestyramine or activated charcoal, which may decrease acetaminophen absorption and delay effects of acetaminophen. Barbiturates, alcohol, carbamazepine, hydantoins, and isoniazid, if taken simultaneously with acetaminophen, increase the risk of

hepatotoxicity. The simultaneous use with warfarin increases the risk of bleeding, and if taken with loop diuretics, it may decrease their therapeutic effects. There are no clinically significant drug-to-food/herbal interactions established. Risk of nephrotoxicity increases with the simultaneous use of **cefepime HcL** and aminoglycosides, loop diuretics, and other potentially nephrotoxic agents. Cefepime HcL may be antagonized by chloramphenicol, erythromycin, and tetracyclines. When used with agents that affect platelet aggregation or are gastrointestinal ulceragenics, the risk of bleeding may increase. There are no clinically significant drug-food/herbal interactions. With **guaifenesin,** drug-to-drug interactions may occur with the simultaneous use of agents that affect platelet aggregation, increasing the risk of bleeding. There are no clinically significant drug-to-food/herbal interaction established.

10. **Discuss the key elements of stepped therapy for clients with chronic bronchitis.** The key elements are:

    - Drug therapy: Step I/Stage I includes the use of ipratropium by metered dose inhaler (MDI) with a spacer. Beta$_2$ agonist for rescue as needed by MDI with spacer. Step 2/Stage II includes adding a short-acting beta$_2$ agonist by metered dose inhaler. Step 3/Stage III includes adding long-acting theophylline for a therapeutic blood level of 8–12 microgram (mcg)/mL, and Step 4/Stage IV includes adding prednisone and, if the client improves, tapering the dose to the lowest dose that manages the symptoms. For the lowest prednisone dose, consider the use of an inhaled steroid.
    - Monitoring the client: Assessing at least every two hours, providing oxygen as needed, assessing and documenting the client's response to treatment.
    - Control of environmental irritants and allergens: Includes educating clients about the avoidance of factors that may trigger respiratory discomfort, such as tightening of the chest, and staying away from known allergens. Emphasizing the importance of complying with medication regimen.

11. **What are the complementary and alternative therapies that help clients control dyspneic episodes?** The complementary and alternative therapies are progressive relaxation, hypnosis, and biofeedback. Progressive relaxation includes self-teaching or instructor-directed exercise that involves learning to contract and relax muscles in a systematic way, beginning with the face and ending with the feet. The exercise may be combined with breathing exercises. Hypnosis places the client in a state of restful alertness, allowing the client to become more aware of his or her surroundings so that behavior can be changed and more healthful practices developed. Biofeedback is a therapeutic modality that enables individuals to monitor skin temperature, muscle tension, heart rate, brain waves, and/or skin conductance to learn to control these physiologic responses to stressful or challenging exercises. During biofeedback training, people use information (e.g., electroencephalogram, electrocardiogram, electromyogram, galvanic skin responses, skin temperature) to recognize normal or desirable physiologic states and then use techniques such as imagery or relaxation training to achieve these states.

References

Broyles, B.E. (2005). *Medical-Surgical Nursing Clinical Companion.* Durham, NC: Carolina Academic Press.
Corbet, J.V. (2004). *Laboratory Tests and Diagnostic Procedures with Nursing Diagnoses* (6th ed.). Upper Saddle River, NJ: Prentice Hall.
Gahart, B.L. and Nazareno, A.R. (2005). *2005 Intravenous Medications.* St. Louis: Mosby.
Huether, S.E. and McCance, K.L. (2004). *Understanding Pathophysiology* (3rd ed.). St. Louis: Mosby.
Ignatavicius, D.D. and Workman, M.L. (2006). *Medical-Surgical Nursing across the Health Care Continuum* (5th ed.). Philadelphia: W.B. Saunders.
LeMone, P. and Burke, K.M. (2004). *Medical-Surgical Nursing: Critical Thinking in Client Care* (3rd ed.). Upper Saddle River, NJ: Prentice Hall.
Spratto, G.R. and Woods, A.L. (2005). *2005 Edition: PDR Nurse's Drug Handbook.* Clifton Park, NY: Thomson Delmar Learning.

CASE STUDY 2

Human Immunodeficiency Virus Infection (CDC Category A)

GENDER
- F

AGE
- 32

SETTING
- Community clinic, a tertiary care center of a medical center

ETHNICITY/CULTURE
- Black South African

PREEXISTING CONDITIONS

COEXISTING CONDITIONS

LIFESTYLE
- Elementary school teacher

COMMUNICATION
- Xhosa and English as a second language

DISABILITY

SOCIOECONOMIC STATUS
- Middle

SPIRITUAL/RELIGIOUS
- Catholic

PHARMACOLOGIC
- Abacavir sulfate (Ziagen)
- Ritonavir (Norvir)
- Lamivudine/Zidovudine (Combivir)

PSYCHOSOCIAL
- Anxiety

LEGAL
- Client does not have the right not to release the names of those who may have contracted the disease from her.

ETHICAL
- Confidentiality—HIV is a reportable disease that carries a stigma.

ALTERNATIVE THERAPY
- Prayer
- Herbal medicines

PRIORITIZATION
- Maintain confidentiality
- Prepare for diagnostic tests

DELEGATION
- RN
- Client education

EASY

THE RESPIRATORY AND IMMUNE SYSTEMS

Level of difficulty: Easy

Overview: This case involves a thorough psychosocial and systems assessment and the use of optimum therapeutic communication to develop a sense of trust between client and health care providers. Room assignment is important due to the stigma of human immunodeficiency virus (HIV) and the client's lack of awareness of varying cultural views of the disease.

Client Profile

Ms. J is a 32-year-old female from Johannesburg, South Africa. She is vacationing with relatives who have resided in the United States for the past 40 years. Ms. J is accompanied by a cousin, a registered nurse, to the community center of a major city.

Case Study

On arrival at the clinic, Ms. J is restless as she waits for the next available nurse. During the initial interview, Ms. J informs the nurse that she is sexually active, practicing unprotected sex because she has been dating only her high-school sweetheart for years. Her reasons for seeking medical assistance are related to recent flu-like symptoms, including headache, fatigue, and occasional night sweats. Her report of unprotected sex and country of origin suggests the possibility of an early stage of human immunodeficiency virus (HIV). Her vital signs are:

Blood pressure: 150/98
Pulse: 120
Respirations: 22 and shallow
Temperature: 98.4° F

Ms. A is initially seen in the triage area of the ED by a nurse practitioner (NP), who notifies the ED physician of Ms. A's arrival and presenting symptoms. After the NP completes the history and physical, it is determined that Ms. J will need to return to the hospital for further evaluation. The NP, in collaboration with the clinic physician, assigns a tentative diagnosis of HIV to Ms. J, who is seen by a counselor and will return to the clinic in three weeks for a follow-up report on lab tests, then will see the primary health care provider at the hospital for a conclusive diagnosis. Lab results reveal CD4+/CD8 cell count 400 CD4+ cells/mm^3 of blood. Enzyme linked immunosorbent assay (ELISA) and Western Blot tests are positive for HIV, chest X-ray reveals normal lung field, and structures within the thorax are normal. Purified protein derivative (PPD) injection is administered, is read in 72 hours, and is negative for tuberculosis. The health care provider and NP review the diagnostic reports and the laboratory data and confirm the diagnosis of HIV. The findings are discussed with the client, after which the health care provider and NP spend much time listening to the client and allowing verbalization of feelings about the diagnosis. Request for consultation with a psychiatrist and social worker is submitted. The HIPPA (Health Insurance Portability and Accountability Act of 1996) form is discussed with and signed by the client. A copy of the form is given to the client.

Questions and Suggested Answers

1. **Discuss the pathophysiology of the HIV infection.** HIV is a ribonucleic acid (RNA) virus that replicates in a "backward" manner by going from RNA to deoxyribonucleic acid (DNA). It has to go into the cell before replication can take place and needs a living cell to perform its function. Once it enters the cell, it binds itself to the specific CD4 receptor sites on the cell's surface, and once bound, viral genetic material enters the cell. In the cell, viral RNA is transcribed into a single strand of viral DNA with assistance of reverse transcriptase, an enzyme made by HIV and other retroviruses. This strand copies itself, becoming double-stranded viral DNA. The initial infection with HIV results in viremia (large amounts of virus in the blood).

    Once infected, activated cells support viral replication and assist in spreading infection throughout the body. Over a period of time, HIV causes significant damage to the lymph system, allowing the virus to spill over into the blood, causing significant impairment of the immune system. The HIV destroys the CD4+ T cells in three different ways. One is through viral replication, which includes a process called *budding*. Budding leaves small holes in the cell's membrane, allowing leakage of the contents of the cells, which then results in cell death. A second method of destruction involves infected cells that can also fuse with other cells. The fusion continues until many cells, some of which are not infected, combine into a mass called a *syncytium* that destroys all affected cells. The third process of destruction is initiated by the infected person's immune system and the antibodies that are produced against HIV. These antibodies bind to the surface of infected cells and activate the complement system, ultimately destroying the infected cells.

2. **Discuss the modes of transmission that have remained constant throughout the course of the HIV pandemic.** The virus is spread through certain sexual practices, through exposure to blood, and through perinatal transmission. An important lesson that health care professionals have learned from the HIV epidemic is that sexual practices, not sexual preferences, place people at risk for sexually transmitted diseases such as HIV. The infection is preventable, and education and behavior change have shown to be the most effective prevention tools. However, educational messages should be specific to the client's need, culturally sensitive, language appropriate, and age specific.

3. **Discuss the protozoal infections detected in persons with HIV.** *Pneumocystis carinii pneumonia (PCP)* is the most common opportunistic infection in persons with HIV. The person with PCP has dyspnea on exertion, tachypnea, and a persistent dry cough, and fever may be observed. The client is fatigued and loses weight. On auscultation of the lung, crackles, or rales will be heard. *Toxoplasmosis encephalitis* caused by Toxoplasma gondii is acquired through contact with contaminated cat feces or by ingesting infected undercooked meat. The client may have subtle changes in mental status, neurologic deficits, headaches, and fever. Another protozoal infection is *cryptosporidiosis*, an intestinal infection caused by Cryptosporidium organisms. When HIV progresses to acquired immunodeficiency syndrome (AIDS), this illness ranges from mild diarrhea to a severe wasting with electrolyte imbalance. The diarrhea may result in fluid loss of up to 15–20 liters per day.

4. **Discuss how HIV is classified.** The Centers for Disease Control and Prevention (CDC) classifies HIV infection by combining clinical conditions that occur with HIV infection and three ranges of CD4 cell counts. The classification begins with acute HIV infection (clinical category A) and spans a continuum that ends with AIDS, clinical category C. The classifications are further divided into 1, 2, and 3 based on the client's CD4 cell count. *Clinical category A* refers to a person that is HIV positive, although the person might not have symptoms at this stage, but may have persistently enlarged lymph nodes (lymphadenopathy), or may have acute but temporary "flu-like" symptoms as the only disease manifestations. *Clinical category B* refers to a person with one or more symptoms (e.g., bacterial endocarditis, oropharyngeal candidiasis, herpes zoster, pulmonary mycobacterium tuberculosis infection) caused by HIV infection. *Clinical category C* refers to a person who has HIV and has progressed to AIDS if the person has any of the following: esophageal candidiasis, invasive cervical cancer, HIV-related encephalopathy, Kaposi's sarcoma, PCP, or wasting syndrome.

5. **Discuss the clinical manifestations of HIV and how the infection is diagnosed.** The ELISA test is accurate for HIV. However, the test can be false-positive if testing is done during the "window period." When the ELISA test is positive, confirmation is done with the Western Blot analysis, because the test detects serum antibodies to four specific major HIV antigens. The positive result of the Western Blot analysis is based on the presence of antibodies to at least two of the major HIV antigens. The interdisciplinary team and the client decide to initiate a medication regimen and to have the client return to the HIV clinic for follow-up care, including monitoring of serum lab values.

6. **List common nursing diagnoses for clients with HIV infection diseases.**

   - Risk for infection R/T immunodeficiency
   - Impaired gas exchange R/T anemia, respiratory infections, pulmonary Kaposi's sarcoma (KS), fatigue, or pain
   - Acute pain or chronic pain R/T neuropathy, myelopathy, malignancy, or infection
   - Imbalanced nutrition: less than body requirements R/T high metabolic need, nausea and vomiting, diarrhea, difficulty chewing or swallowing, or anorexia
   - Diarrhea R/T infection, food tolerance, or drugs

- Impaired skin integrity R/T KS, infection, altered nutritional state, incontinence, immobility, hyperthermia, or malignancy
- Disturbed thought processes R/T AIDS dementia complex (ADC), central nervous system infection, or malignancy
- Chronic low self-esteem R/T changes in body image, decreased self-esteem, or helplessness
- Deficient knowledge R/T condition, treatment, and health maintenance

The following are prescribed:

- Abacavir sulfate (Ziagen) 300 mg PO two times per day
- Ritonavir (Norvir) 600 mg PO two times per day
- Lamivudine/zidovudine (Combivir) one combination tablet (150 mg lamivudine/300 mg zidovudine) PO two times per day
- Epzicom (Abacavir) 300 mg PO two times per day

7. **Discuss highly active antiretroviral therapy (HAART) and whether the prescribed medications meet its criteria.** HAART is a combination of therapy regimens established for the treatment of HIV/AIDS that consists of multiple drugs used together in regimens popularly called "cocktails." These regimens consist of combinations of different types of antiretroviral agents, and are showing good results as measured by reduced viral load and improved CD4+ lymphocyte counts. A regimen may be a combination of two protease inhibitors and one non-nucleoside reverse transcriptase inhibitor or two protease inhibitors and one other antiretroviral agent.

8. **What are the purposes for the prescribed medications?** *Epzicom* is a nucleoside analog reverse transcriptase inhibitor that converts to carbovir transphosphate intracellularly to block the HIV-1 reverse transcriptase necessary for viral DNA replication and growth (Broyles, 26). *Ritonavir* is a protease inhibitor that acts by blocking the HIV protease enzyme necessary for viral replication. *Lamivudine/zidovudine* is a combination containing two nucleoside analog reverse transcriptase inhibitor acting by converting the virally infected cell into a "counterfeit" form of a nucleotide for placement in DNA to suppress production of reverse transcriptase and inhibit viral DNA synthesis and replication, thereby slowing the progression of the disease.

9. **What are the most common adverse reactions of the prescribed medications?** The most common adverse reactions of *epzicom* are hypersensitivity responses: myalgia, arthralgia, mouth ulcerations, headache, fever, chills, nausea, and diarrhea. Life-threatening hypotension, liver failure, renal failure, and anaphylaxis may occur. The most common adverse effects of *ritonavir* include nausea and vomiting, diarrhea, taste perversion, anorexia, constipation, anxiety, syncope, and hypotension. Serious allergic reactions have occurred with ritonavir's use. The most common adverse effects of *lamivudine/zidovudine* include lactic acidosis, hepatomegaly, nausea, vomiting, diarrhea, anorexia, abdominal pain, and stomatitis.

10. **Discuss the drug-to-drug and drug-to-food/herbal interactions for the prescribed medications.** Drug-to-drug interactions may occur with the simultaneous use of *abacavir* and ethanol, may decrease the excretion of abacavir and increase its serum level, resulting in toxicity. Concurrent use with methadone may increase methadone clearance, requiring increases in the dose to achieve desired effects. There is no clinically significant drug-to-drug/drug-to-food/herbal interactions established. Zidovudine, which may increase the maximum level of zidovudine and cause toxicity. The simultaneous use of zidovudine and clarithromycin may cause a decrease in the serum concentration of zidovudine. The simultaneous use of trimethoprim-sulfamethoxazole and *lamivudine* increases the serum level, which could increase the risk of lactic acidosis. There are no clinically significant drug-to-food/herbal interactions established. With *ritonavir* drug-to-drug interactions may occur with the simultaneous use of many different agents. It increases large increases in the plasma levels of amiodarone, atorvastatin, bepridil, bupropion, carbamazepine, cerivastatin, clonazepam, clozapine, desipramine, clarithromycin, indinavir, loperamide, cyclosporine, dexamethasone, dihydroergotamine, diltiazem, disopyramide, dronabinol, ergotamine, ethosuximide, fentanyl, flecainide, lidocaine, loperamide, daquinavir, sildenafil, lovastatin, methamnefazodone, nifedipine, perphenasone, propafenone,

propoxyphene, quinidine, quinine, risperidone, sildenafil, trazodone, selective serotonin reuptake inhibitors, simvastatin, tacrolimus, thioridazine, timolol, tramadol, tricyclic antidepressants, and verapamil leading to cardiac dysrhythmias, blood dyscrasias, and other serious adverse effects. Ritonavir decreases the plasma levels of dedanosine, ethynyl estradiol, atovaquone, clofibrate, daunorubicin, diphenoxylate, divalproex, ethinyl estrodiol, pravastatin, meperidine, lamotrigine, methadone, metoclopramide, phenytoin, pravastatin, sedative/hypnotics, theophylline, and warfarin requiring increased doses of these agents to achieve therapeutic effects. Azole antifungals and interleukins increase ritonavir serum levels while rifampin and rifabutin decrease its levels. No specific drug-to-food interactions have been established, however, St. John's Wort increases the action of ritonavir. Drug-to-drug interactions with the use of **lamivudine/zidovudine** include trimethoprim/sulfamethoxazole that significantly increases lamivudine levels, and zalcitabine that interacts with the lamivudine component, canceling the effects of both agents. The zidovudine component of this combination agent has many more interactions. Atovaquone, cytotoxic drugs, fluconazole, interferon beta 1b methadone, trimethoprim, and valproic acid increase the action of zidovudine. Increased risk of cytotoxicity occurs with the simultaneous use of zidovudine and acetaminophen, adriamycin, dapsone, flucytosine, gancicovir, interferon alfa, vinblastine, and vincristine. Rifampin and ritonavir decrease zidovudine levels. Doxurubicin and zidovudine antagonize each other and should not be used together. No specific drug-to-food/herbal interactions have been established.

11. **Discuss the importance of the client seeing an HIV social worker before leaving the clinic.** The social worker focuses on assessment and evaluation of the client's social situation. A comprehensive psychosocial history will be completed by the social worker to determine the client's financial needs. The social worker will also contact agencies for help as appropriate. Another important role of a social worker is to provide clients with referrals for links to community resources and recommendation to appropriate facilities if needed.

12. **Discuss dietary management for the person with HIV.** The immune system needs protein, carbohydrates, fat, and minerals in sufficient quantity to maintain optimal functioning. Therefore, nutrition is an essential component of the management of clients with HIV infection. Nurses caring for clients with HIV need to perform a complete nutritional assessment on these clients because it is key to improving their general nutritional status. Routine dental care is a part of the nutritional assessment, because clients with HIV have progressive gingival disease, which affects taste. Dietary guidelines need to include foods that take into account the cultural and economic status of the client.

References

Broyles, B.E. (2005). *Medical-Surgical Nursing Clinical Companion*. Durham, NC: Carolina Academic Press.
Centers for Disease Control and Prevention (2004). www.cdc.gov.
Corbet, J.V. (2004). *Laboratory Tests and Diagnostic Procedures with Nursing Diagnoses* (6th ed.). Upper Saddle River, NJ: Prentice Hall.
Deglin, J.H. and Vallerand, A.H. (2005). *Davis's Drug Guide for Nurses* (9th ed.). Philadelphia: F.A. Davis.
Gahart, B.L. and Nazareno, A.R. (2005). *2005 Intravenous Medications*. St. Louis: Mosby.
Huether, S.E. and McCance, K.L. (2004). *Understanding Pathophysiology* (3rd ed.). St. Louis: Mosby.
LeMone, P. and Burke, K.M. (2004). *Medical-Surgical Nursing: Critical Thinking in Client Care* (3rd ed.). Upper Saddle River, NJ: Prentice Hall.
Lewis, S.M., Heitkemper, M.M., and Dirksen, S.R. (2004). *Medical-Surgical Nursing: Assessment Management of Clinical Problems* (6th ed.). Philadelphia: Mosby.
Libster, M. (2002). *Delmar's Integrative Herb Guide for Nurses*. Albany, NY: Thomson Delmar Learning.
Spratto, G.R. and Woods, A.L. (2005). *2005 Edition: PDR Nurse's Drug Handbook*. Clifton Park, NY: Thomson Delmar Learning.
Swihart, D., Sprehe, J., and Page, M.C. (2003). "The HIV/AIDS Pandemic in 2003." *Advances for Nurses*. Available at https://nursing.advanceweb.com/Common/CE/Content.aspx?CourseID=174&CreditID=1&CC=19088&sid=825.

CASE STUDY 3

Pulmonary Tuberculosis

GENDER
- M

AGE
- 50

SETTING
- Hospital

ETHNICITY/CULTURE
- White American

PREEXISTING CONDITIONS

COEXISTING CONDITIONS

LIFESTYLE
- Unemployed for five years
- Consumes beer or vodka daily

COMMUNICATION

DISABILITY

SOCIOECONOMIC STATUS
- Low

SPIRITUAL/RELIGIOUS
- Catholic

PHARMACOLOGIC
- Isoniazid (Nydrazid)
- Pyridoxine HcL (Aminoxin)
- Pyrazinamide (Tebrazid)
- Rifampin (Rifadin)
- Streptomycin sulfate (Streptomycin)
- Megestrol acetate (Megace)

PSYCHOSOCIAL
- Anxiety

LEGAL
- The client does not have the right to refuse providing names of persons who may have contracted the disease.

ETHICAL
- Cases of TB must be reported.
- Client's concern for confidentiality must still be addressed appropriately.

ALTERNATIVE THERAPY

PRIORITIZATION
- Private room
- Respiratory isolation
- Arrest TB process

DELEGATION
- RN
- Client education

THE RESPIRATORY AND IMMUNE SYSTEMS

Level of difficulty: Easy

Overview: This case involves a thorough assessment of the client's respiratory status, including social history and past exposure to tuberculosis (TB); the client's native country; and travel to foreign countries prior to migrating to the United States.

Client Profile

Mr. B is a 50-year-old male who is brought to the hospital emergency department (ED) by emergency medical service (EMS) from a community clinic after having bouts of vomiting while waiting to be seen by a health care provider.

Case Study

Mr. B's vital signs on arrival to the ED are:

Blood pressure: 130/78
Pulse: 78
Respirations: 20
Temperature: 99.0° F

He is known at the hospital; he frequently comes to the hospital's ED in a state of stupor or is taken by EMS because he has fallen while walking in the street. Today, he is coherent, responding to questions appropriately. Mr. B is 5'8" and weighs 110 pounds. Social history reveals he is a high school graduate who worked as a bookkeeper for a trucking company. He has been unemployed for the past five years. His social history reveals cigarette smoking for 40 years; he has smoked two packs per day for 20 years. He is an undiagnosed alcoholic, a former cocaine and marijuana user, and was "detoxed" from the cocaine six years ago. He denies having used marijuana during the past eight years. Mr. B also reports infrequent feelings of depression and noted weight loss for the past two months. He has never been married but has a son whom he has not seen for several years. Mr. B is currently taking Megestrol acetate 200 mg PO every six hours as prescribed by a health care provider at the clinic he attends and reports compliance with the medication. The health care provider in the ED continues with the history and physical examination and gathers from Mr. B that he has been experiencing a dry cough and occasional night sweats. Mr. B is transferred from the ED to the respiratory unit, with written orders to place him on respiratory isolation. On arrival at the unit, he is placed in a single room, and respiratory precaution signs are initiated on the outside of the door that leads to his room. The pulmonologist meets with Mr. B on the unit and, after further gathering of data, orders: sputum for acid fast bacilli (AFB) × three sputum culture, Mantoux test with 0.1 ml of PPD intradermally, and chest X-ray. The results for the diagnostic tests are positive for the mycobacterium bacillus, and the diagnosis of pulmonary tuberculosis is confirmed.

Questions and Suggested Answers

1. **Discuss the incidence and prevalence of pulmonary TB.** TB is seen disproportionately in the poor, the underserved, and minorities. Individuals at risk for TB include homeless persons, residents of inner-city neighborhoods, foreign-born persons, older adults, those in institutions (long-term care facilities, prisons), injection drug users, the socioeconomically disadvantaged, medically underserved of all races, and people with immunosuppression from any etiology (e.g., HIV infections, malignancies). The prevalence of TB is high in a few areas of the United States where there is a large population of Native Americans, such as Arizona, New Mexico, and in counties near the Mexican border. Health care workers with increased exposure to TB are also at high risk.

2. **Discuss the etiology and pathophysiology of TB.** The primary infectious agent is the mycobacterium tuberculosis, gram positive AFB aerobic rod organism that usually spreads from person to person via airborne droplets, which are produced when the infected individual with pulmonary or laryngeal TB coughs, sneezes, speaks, or sings. Once the organisms are released into the air, they are dispersed and can be inhaled. However, brief exposure to a few tubercle bacilli rarely causes an infection. Instead, it is more commonly spread to the

individual who has had repeated close contact with an infected person. The disease cannot be spread by hands, books, glasses, dishes, or other fomites, since it requires a host in which to reside. Once the bacilli are inhaled, they pass down the bronchial system and implant themselves on the respiratory bronchioles or alveoli. The lower parts of the lungs are usually the site of initial bacterial implantation. After implantation, the bacilli multiply with no initial resistance from the host. The organisms are then engulfed by phagocytes (initially neutrophils and later macrophages) and may continue to multiply within the phagocytes. The organisms may spread through the lymphatic channels to regional lymph nodes and via the thoracic duct to the circulating blood, resulting in spread throughout the body. The organisms can spread throughout the body before sufficient activation of the cell-mediated immune response is available to bring the infection under control. The organisms find favorable environment for growth primarily in the upper lobes of the lungs, kidneys, epiphysis of the bone, cerebral cortex, and adrenal glands. Eventually the cellular immunity limits further multiplication and spread of the infection, and a characteristic reaction called an *epithelioid cell granuloma* results after the cellular immune system is activated. Dormant but viable organisms persist for years. Therefore, reactivation of TB can occur if the host's defense mechanisms become impaired.

3. **What are the risk factors for TB?** Risk factors include close contact with someone who has active TB, immunocompromised status, and preexisting medical conditions. Those who are suffering from substance abuse; are institutionalized; live in overcrowded, substandard housing; or do not have access to adequate health care are also at risk, as are those who emigrate from countries with a high prevalence of TB. Another risk factor is being a health care worker performing high-risk activities that exposure the worker to the inhalation of the organism.

4. **Discuss the Centers for Disease Control (CDC) recommendations for preventing transmission of TB in health care settings.** Many infectious agents can be prevented by the adherence by health care personnel to infection control practices and guidelines and practices related to the control and prevention of infections within the hospital settings. The CDC is a federal agency of the United States Public Health Service that focuses on epidemiology, prevention, control, and treatment of communicable diseases. Isolation procedures and other infection-control recommendations come from the CDC. In regards to TB, the CDC recommends early identification and treatment of persons with active TB, prevention of spread of infectious droplet nuclei by source control methods and by reduction of microbial contamination of indoor air, and surveillance for TB transmission such as droplet precautions and airborne precautions.

5. **Discuss the common clinical manifestations of clients with TB and how they reflect the pathophysiology of TB.** The common clinical manifestations are systemic in nature and include low-grade fever related to the infectious agent. Cough is a common symptom of respiratory disease and could be a reflexive action in response to an irritant such as infection irritating the airway or, if the irritant passes the bronchi, bronchioles, and alveoli, which are particularly sensitive to chemical stimulation, resulting in the triggering of a cough. Night sweats may occur in response to the low-grade fever, and fatigue may be due to imbalanced nutrition, because the client with TB may be anorexic from the effects of the disease process resulting in low hematocrit and low hemoglobin, and therefore weight loss related to decreased appetite and lack of sleep and rest.

6. **Discuss the gerontologic considerations for TB.** TB may have atypical manifestations in elderly clients whose symptoms may include unusual behavior and altered mental status, fever, anorexia, and weight loss. Many elderly clients may have no reaction (loss of immunologic memory) or delayed reactivity for up to a week (recall phenomenon). A second skin test is usually performed in one to two weeks.

7. **Discuss the specific diagnostic studies used to confirm TB.** The tuberculin skin test uses a purified protein derivative (PPD) of the tubercle bacillus administered by intradermal injection (Mantoux) test or multipuncture technique (Tine) to determine sensitization to the tuberculosis bacillus from a previous exposure, not the presence of the disease. The AFB smear is a staining method used primarily to identify tubercle bacilli (M. tuberculosis). AFB have a cell wall that resists decolorization by acid treatment and retain the stain

applied to the specimen, which is a diagnostic indicator of the organism. The smear aids in early detection of the organism and timely initiation of antituberculosis therapy. AFB cultures are the most accurate means of identifying and confirming both positive and negative results of AFB smears. However, because the tubercle bacillus is a slow-growing organism, the culture results may take weeks to provide findings of the organism. A new test for TB is the nucleic acid amplification (NAA), a rapid diagnostic test. Test results are available in a few hours. Although it does not replace routine sputum smears and cultures, it offers a health care provider increased confidence in the diagnosis.

The following are prescribed:

- Isoniazid (Nydrazid) (INH) 300 mg PO daily
- Rifampin (Rifadin) (RMP) 600 mg PO daily
- Pyrazinamide (PZA) (Tebrazid) 30 mg/kg PO daily
- Streptomycin sulfate (Streptomycin) 15 mg/kg IM single dose
- Pyridoxine HcL (Aminoxin) 100 mg PO daily
- Megestrol acetate (Megace) 200 mg PO q6h

8. **What are the purposes for the prescribed medications?** The combination chemotherapy for the treatment of TB is the standard of care and includes three or more antitubercular agents including *isoniazid, rifampin, streptomycin,* and *pyrazinamide*. They destroy the organism as quickly as possible and minimize the emergence of drug-resistance organisms, because resistant strains emerge rapidly when drugs are administered as monotherapy. *Isoniazid* is a primary agent for the treatment and prophylaxis of tuberculosis. It is effective with TB because it is highly selective for mycobacteria by killing the tubercle bacilli at concentrations 10,000 times lower than those needed and affecting gram-positive and gram-negative bacteria that are actively dividing. It suppresses bacterial growth by inhibiting synthesis of RNA and mycolic acid, which is a component of the mycobacterial cell wall. Because resistance usually develops when given alone, it is usually combined with other antitubercular drugs. *Pyridoxine HcL* is a vitamin B complex that is used prophylactically to prevent the neuropathy associated with the use of isoniazid. *Rifampin* inhibits DNA-dependent RNA enzyme activity in susceptible bacterial cells, thereby suppressing RNA synthesis. *Pyrazinamide* aids in the eradication of the mycobacteria by interfering with lipid and nucleic acid biosynthesis. *Streptomycin sulfate* is an aminoglycoside, bactericidal and bacteriostatic agent also classified as an antitubercular. It is particularly active against acid-fast organisms such as the mycobacteria tubercle bacillus, the organism that causes pulmonary tuberculosis. *Megestrol acetate,* a female synthetic hormone, also functions to improve appetite, but the mechanism by which it improves appetite is unclear.

9. **What are the most common adverse reactions of the prescribed medications?** The most common adverse reactions of *isoniazid* are paresthesia, peripheral neuropathy, nausea and vomiting, epigastric distress, and elevated liver function tests (AST and ALT). The most common adverse effects of *pyridoxine HcL* include unstable gait; decreased sensation to touch, temperature, and heat; drowsiness; and perioral numbness. The most common adverse reactions of *rifampin* are hepatotoxicity, heartburn, epigastric distress, nausea, vomiting, anorexia, flatulence, cramps, diarrhea, and red discoloration of body fluids. The most common adverse reactions of *pyrazinamide* are active gout, hepatotoxicity, abnormal liver function tests, and rise in serum uric acid level. The most common adverse reactions of *streptomycin sulfate* are pain and irritation if administered intramuscularly, labyrinthine damage, nausea, vomiting, anorexia, and nephrotoxicity. The most common adverse reactions of *megestrol acetate* include nausea, vomiting, diarrhea, oral moniliasis, insomnia, pruritis, hypertension, and edema.

10. **Discuss the drug-to-drug and drug-to-food/herbal interactions for the prescribed medications.** With *isoniazid,* drug-to-drug interactions may occur with the simultaneous use of other hepatotoxic drugs such as acetaminophen, rifampin, and drugs containing alcohol, which may increase the risk of hepatotoxicity. Additive central nervous system central nervous system (CNS) toxicity with other antituberculars may occur. The simultaneous use of isoniazid and BCG vaccine may alter the effectiveness of the drug. The simultaneous use

of phenytoin may inhibit the metabolism of phenytoin, and aluminum-containing antacids may decrease the absorption of isoniazid. It increases the requirements of niacin and pyridoxine. Aminosalicylic acid, atropine, and ethanol increase the serum levels of isoniazid. When used concurrently with anticoagulants and ketoconazole, isoniazid decreases the effectiveness of these agents. Increased serum levels of benzodiazepines, carbamazepine, chlorzoxazone, and cycloserine are seen when used with isoniazid. Drug-to-food interactions occur with the simultaneous intake of food and isoniazid, by decreasing the rate and extent of isoniazid absorption, the concurrent use with foods containing high concentrations of tyramine may cause severe reactions. There are no clinically significant drug-to-herbal interactions clinically established. With *pyridoxine HcL* drug-to-drug interactions may occur with the concurrent use of chloramphenicol, oral contraceptives, cycloserine, ethionamide, hydralazine, immunosuppressants, isoniazid, and peniciliamine, causing an increase in pyridoxine requirements. Pyridoxine HcL decreases the serum levels of phenobarbital and phenytoin. Drug-to-drug interaction may occur with the simultaneous use of *rifampin* and acetaminophen, aminophylline, amiodarone, oral anticoagulants, barbiturates, benzodiazepine beta-blocking agents, buspirone, chloramphenicol, clofibrate, oral contraceptives, corticosteroid, cyclosporine, delaviridine, digoxin, disopyramide, doxycycline, enalapril, estrogens, haloperidol, hydantoins, lamotrigine, methadone, mexiletine, morphine, nevirapine, nifedipine, ondansetron, protease inhibitors, propafenone, quinidine, repaglinide, sertraline, sulfapyridine, sulfone, tacolimus, theophylline, tocainide, tricyclic antidepressants, trimethoprim/sulfamethoxazole, verapamil, zidovudine, and zolpidem, resulting in decreased serum levels of these agents. Concurrent use of alcohol, isoniazid, halothane, and pyrazinamide may increase the risk of hepatotoxicity. The simultaneous use of aminosalycylic acid, propranolol, quinidine, ritonavir, warfarin, macrolide antibiotics, ketoconazole, protease inhibitors, and verapamil may lead to potential therapeutic failure of rifampin. In addition, use with amprenavir, fluconazole, fluoroquinolones, losartan, clarithromycin, quinine, and thyroid hormones may increase the levels of these agents. There are no clinically significant drug-to-food/herbal interactions established. With *pyrazinamide,* drug-to-drug interactions may occur with rifampin, resulting in decreased effectiveness of anti-gout medications and fatal hepatotoxicity. There are no clinically significant drug-to-food/herbal interactions established. Drug-to-drug interactions may occur with the simultaneous use of *streptomycin* and warfarin, which may potentiate the anticoagulant effects of warfarin, and increased nephrotoxicity, ototoxicity, and neurotoxicity with other aminoglycosides, amphotericin B, polymycin, vancomycin, ethacrynic acid, furosemide, mannitol, methoxyflurane, cisplatin, cephalosporins, and bacitracin. Use with non-depolarizing muscle relaxants and succinylcholine may increase the effects of these agents. There are no clinically significant drug-to-food/herbal interactions established. With *megestrol acetate,* drug-to-drug interactions may occur with the simultaneous use of warfarin. There are no clinically significant drug-to-food/herbal interactions established.

11. **Discuss the potential complications for the client with TB.** *Miliary or hematogenous tuberculosis* is the invasion of large numbers of organisms into the bloodstream that then spread to all body systems. The organisms come from the necrotic Ghon's complex that has eroded through a blood vessel. The client is usually acutely ill with fever, dyspnea, and cyanosis or chronically ill with systemic manifestations of weight loss, fever, and/or gastrointestinal (GI) disturbance. Hepatomegaly, splenomegaly, and generalized lymphadenopathy may be present. *Pleural effusion* and *empyema* may also develop. *Pleural effusion* is caused by the release of caseous material into the pleural space. The bacteria-containing material triggers an inflammatory reaction and a pleural exudate of protein-rich fluid. *Empyema* is less common but may occur from large numbers of organisms spilling into the pleural space, usually from rupture of a cavity. *Tuberculosis pneumonia* is another complication and may be acute in nature. It results from large amounts of tubercle bacilli being discharged from the liquefied necrotic lesion into the lung or lymph nodes. The clinical manifestations are similar to those of bacterial pneumonia, including chills, fever, productive cough, pleuritic pain, and leukocytosis.

12. **Discuss client education for TB.** The client should be informed that TB is infectious but may be cured if medications are taken as prescribed. Instruct the client on how TB is transmitted, that it can be reactivated, but that it is not transmitted on articles such as clothing, books, or eating utensils. Emphasize that the client should cover the nose and mouth when coughing, laughing, or sneezing and should wash the hands very

carefully after any contact with body substances, masks, or soiled tissues. Remind the client that sputum is highly contaminated, therefore, coughing into paper tissues and proper disposal is mandatory. Inform the client that treatment may be necessary for a long time but that medications should be taken as prescribed, and of the importance of reporting adverse effects (these should be written) to the primary care provider. Stress that the medications should not be stopped for any reason without the primary health care provider's instructions. Emphasize that compliance is of utmost importance for health and wellness to be accomplished.

References

Broyles, B.E. (2005). *Medical-Surgical Nursing Clinical Companion.* Durham, NC: Carolina Academic Press.

Corbet, J.V. (2004). *Laboratory Tests and Diagnostic Procedures with Nursing Diagnoses* (6th ed.). Upper Saddle River, NJ: Prentice Hall.

Deglin, J.H. and Vallerand, A.H. (2005). *Davis's Drug Guide for Nurses* (9th ed.). Philadelphia: F.A. Davis.

Gahart, B.L. and Nazareno, A.R. (2005). *2005 Intravenous Medications.* St. Louis: Mosby.

Huether, S.E. and McCance, K.L. (2004). *Understanding Pathophysiology* (3rd ed.). St. Louis: Mosby.

Lehne, R.A. (2004). *Pharmacology for Nursing Care* (5th ed.). Philadelphia: W.B. Saunders.

Lewis, S.M., Heitkemper, M.M., and Dirksen, S.R. (2004). *Medical-Surgical Nursing: Assessment and Management of Clinical Problems* (6th ed.). St. Louis: Mosby.

Skidmore-Roth, L. (2006). *Mobsy's Handbook of Herbs & Natural Supplements* (3rd ed.). St. Louis: Mosby.

Spratto, G.R. and Woods, A.L. (2005). *2005 Edition: PDR Nurse's Drug Handbook.* Clifton Park, NY: Thomson Delmar Learning.

CASE STUDY 4

Pulmonary Empyema

GENDER
- M

AGE
- 55

SETTING
- Hospital

ETHNICITY CULTURE
- Black American

PREEXISTING CONDITIONS
- Pericarditis

COEXISTING CONDITIONS
- Renal failure

LIFESTYLE
- Retired

COMMUNICATION

DISABILITY

SOCIOECONOMIC STATUS
- Low

SPIRITUAL/RELIGIOUS
- Baptist

PHARMACOLOGIC
- Cefuroxime sodium (Zinacef)
- Gentamicin sulfate (Garamycin)
- Morphine sulfate (Duramorph)
- Rabeprazole sodium (Aciphex)

PSYCHOSOCIAL

LEGAL
- Are there federal or state supplemental resources to cover hospital expenses for self-employed retired persons?

ETHICAL
- Insufficient Social Security income should not be a deterrent for quality health care.

ALTERNATIVE THERAPY
- Prayer

PRIORITIZATION
- Antibiotic therapy

DELEGATION
- RN
- Client education

THE RESPIRATORY AND IMMUNE SYSTEMS

Level of difficulty: Easy

Overview: This case involves the use of collaborative management and history assessment to determine recent febrile illness, chest pain, dyspnea, or unusual cough. The nurse must be skilled in managing clients in need of thoracic procedures and competent in respiratory assessment and caring for clients with chest tubes to underwater seal drainage.

Client Profile

Mr. J, a 55-year-old male and retired self-employed carpenter, is readmitted to the hospital after being discharged two weeks ago. He is 5'10" and weighs 230 pounds. At readmission he complains of pleuritic chest pain and generalized weakness. His vital signs on admission are:

- Blood pressure: 150/90
- Pulse: 100
- Respirations: 30
- Temperature: 101.0° F

Case Study

On physical assessment, Mr. J's chest wall motion is reduced, palpation and percussion reveal flat sounds, and breath sounds are decreased. Medical history reveals history of hypertension, past history of lung abscess and bacterial pneumonia, past history of pulmonary tuberculosis, recurrent left pneumothorax, and frequent upper respiratory infections. Mr. J reports gastric ulcer, which he relates to alcohol intake for several years, and allergies to contrast dye, radiographic dye, and thorazine. His social history involves several years of cigarette smoking. A chest X-ray is ordered and confirms pleural effusion. The health care provider determines the need to remove pleural fluid and explains the purpose and plan to Mr. J. An informed consent for a thoracentesis is signed by the client. The thoracentesis is done, and pleural fluid is sent to the lab for color, red blood cell count, white blood cell count and differential, and glucose and protein levels. The results are:

- Appearance: cloudy
- Red blood cell (RBC) count: >1000/mm^3
- White blood cell (WBC) count: >1000/mm^3
- pH: <7.4
- Glucose: 68 mg/dL
- Protein: >3.0 g/dL

A gram stain and acid fast stain are ordered and yields gram-negative species. Blood is positive for Staphylococcus aureus, and WBC is 15,000/mm^3. A diagnosis of pulmonary empyema is confirmed and a treatment plan is discussed with Mr. J that includes the placement of chest tubes attached to water-seal drainage and wall suction.

Questions and Suggested Answers

1. **Discuss the pathophysiology of empyema.** Pulmonary empyema is pleural fluid with a high WBC count and purulent fluid. The most common cause of the empyema is pulmonary infection, lung abscess, or infected pleural effusion due to debris of infection (microorganisms, leukocytes, and cellular debris) dumped into the pleural space by blocked lymphatic vessels.

2. **Discuss the findings on auscultation if pleural effusion is present with empyema.** Decreased tactile fremitus on palpation is elicited because of the thickness of the fluid. Tactile fremitus is a vibration in the chest wall. Vibratory sensations are palpated in conditions that allow for the transmission of sound. Thick secretions do not allow for transmission; instead, they blunt the transmission of sound. Flat or dull percussion and decreased breath sounds are elicited because of the thickness of the empyema fluid. Percussion is the use of the fingertips to tap the body lightly but sharply to determine position, size, and consistency of an underlying structure and the presence of fluid or pus in a cavity. Breath sounds involve normal and abnormal sounds. Normal breath sounds include bronchial and bronchovesicular sounds. Abnormal sounds include crackles (rales), wheezes, and rhonchi.

3. **What are management strategies for clients with pulmonary empyema?** Removing the infected pleural fluid to improve chest expansion and improve ventilation is a major intervention. Because the primary factor for impaired ventilation (gas exchange) is the infected fluid in the pleural space, chest tube to underwater drainage is inserted to remove the abnormal fluid. Antibiotics are administered to irradicate the infectious process, and prevent the development of complications.

4. **Discuss pleural abnormalities as they relate to pulmonary empyema.** Pleural effusion is the presence of fluid in the pleural space. The source of fluid is usually blood vessels or lymphatic vessels lying beneath either of the pleura, but occasionally an abscess or other lesion is draining into the pleural space. Like pneumothorax, pleural effusion can cause compression atelectasis and displace mediastinal contents. However, pleural effusion does not cause the lung to collapse, because there is no communication between the pleural space and environmental air. Therefore, pressure in the pleural space remains negative and atelectasis is caused solely by pressure exerted by the effusion. Pleurisy (pleuritis) is inflammation of the pleura, which become reddened and covered with an exudate of lymph, fibrin, and cellular elements. Common signs of pleurisy are chills, fever, and pain on inspiration, and often a pleural friction rub can be heard over the affected area. Pleurisy is often preceded by upper respiratory infection.

5. **How would the health care provider determine that the client is experiencing compression of lung tissue due to the effusion?** Pleural fluid normally seeps continually into the pleural space from the capillaries lining the parietal pleura and is reabsorbed by the visceral pleural capillaries and lymphatic system. Any condition that interferes with either secretion or drainage of this fluid leads to pleural effusion. The health care provider would anticipate that the client is experiencing compression of lung tissue due to manifestations of dyspnea; a dry, nonproductive cough; and decreased tactile fremitus, because the extent of the exudate has caused restriction of chest expansion resulting in ineffective airway expansion.

The following are prescribed:

- Cefuroxime sodium (Zinacef) 1.5 g IV before the procedure/750 mg IV q8h × 24 hours
- Gentamicin sulfate (Garamycin) 2.5 mg/kg IV q8h
- Morphine sulfate (Duramorph) 2 mg IV q1–2h PRN
- Rabeprazole sodium (Aciphex) 60 mg PO once daily
- Chest tube to 20 cm wall suction via Pleur-evac

6. **What are the purposes for the prescribed medications?** *Cefuroxime sodium* is a cephalosporin used to treat organisms in the lower respiratory tract. It preferentially binds to one or more of the penicillin-binding proteins located on cell walls of susceptible organisms, inhibiting the third and final stage of bacterial cell wall synthesis, thus killing the bacterium. *Gentamicin sulfate* is an aminoglycoside antibiotic used to treat serious respiratory infections. It is bacteriocidal against specific gram-negative bacteria. *Morphine sulfate* is an opioid analgesic that effectively relieves pain associated with empyema and post-procedural pain by binding to opiate receptors in the central nervous system, altering the perception and response to painful stimuli. *Rabeprazole sodium* suppresses gastric acid secretion and relieves gastric upset. It is a gastric proton pump inhibitor that specifically suppresses gastric acid secretion by inhibiting H^+/K^+ ATPase, an enzyme on the surface of the gastric parietal cells of the stomach, which actively secretes hydrogen. When gastric pH is increased, gastric secretions are reduced. Having *chest tube to 20 cm wall suction via Pleur-evac* helps reinflate the lung by removing air and drainage from the intrapleural space. The Pleur-evac is a closed water-seal drainage system.

7. **What are the most common adverse reactions, drug-to-drug, drug-to-food/herbal interactions of the prescribed medications?** The most common adverse reactions of *cefuroxime sodium* are diarrhea, abdominal cramps, pruritus, phlebitis, and redness at the peripheral infusion site, especially if the agent is infused too rapidly for the site. Drug-to-drug interactions may occur with the simultaneous use of probenecid, which decreases renal elimination of cefuroxime sodium and potentiates toxicity. Risk of nephrotoxicity increases with the concurrent use of aminoglycosides and loop diuretics. Cefuroxime sodium may inhibit the bacteriostatic action of chloramphenicol, erythromycin, and tetracyclines. Large amount of any cephalosporin

and/or salicylates may cause hypoprothrombinemia and nonsteroidal anti-inflammatory agents (NSAIDs), naproxen, and sulfinpyrazone may increase the risk of hemorrhage because of the gastrointestinal (GI) ulcerative effects and antiplatelet activity. There are no clinically established drug-to-food interactions established. The most common adverse effects of *gentamicin sulfate* are hypersensitivity and eighth cranial nerve irritation. Drug-to-drug interactions may occur with the simultaneous use of beta-lactam antibiotics and vancomycin, having a synergistic effect with these agents. Penicillin inactivates gentamicin and should be avoided. Dangerous additive effects may occur with the concurrent use of anesthetics, neuromuscular blocking antibiotics, loop diuretics, and vancomycin. Gentamicin is potentiated by anticholinesterases and antineoplastic agents. It increases the effects of carbenicillin and ticarcillin when used to treat pseudomonas infections. As with cefuroxime, gentamicin antagonizes the effects of bacteriostatic antibiotics. No clinically significant drug-to-food/herbal interactions have been established. The most common adverse reactions of *morphine sulfate* are sedation, hypotension, constipation, and nausea. Drug-to-drug interactions may occur with the simultaneous use of central nervous system depressants, sedatives, antidepressants, hypnotics, histamine-2 antagonists, some phenothiazines, and barbiturates causing increased central nervous system (CNS) depression. Anticholinergics and antidiarrheals increase the risk of constipation and loop diuretics, antihypertensives, antidepressants, benzodiazepines, adrenergic blocking agents, calcium channel blocking agents, calcium, nitroprusside, and nitroglycerin increase the risk of hypotension when used concurrently with morphine. Rifampin may decrease the therapeutic effects of morphine and markedly reduce doses of monoamine oxidase (MAO) inhibitors are needed when used with opiates. Concurrent use with zidovudine may increase the toxicity of both agents and should be avoided. Respiratory depression is extended if morphine is used with neuromuscular blocking agents, such as succinylcholine, mivacurium, and tubocurarine. Morphine may potentiate the anticoagulant effects of warfarin (Gahart and Nazareno, 820). Drug-to-food interactions may occur with the simultaneous use of kava-kava, valerian, skullcap, chamomile or hops, which may increase CNS depression, and St. John's Wort, which may increase sedation. The most common adverse reactions of *rabeprazole sodium* include diarrhea, nausea, vomiting, dry mouth, and hypertension. Drug-to-drug interactions may occur with the simultaneous use of digoxin, which may increase digoxin levels and cause toxicity. It decreases the plasma levels of ketoconazole. Its simultaneous use with warfarin may increase the risk for bleeding. No significant drug-to-food/herbal interactions have been noted.

8. **A tube thoracotomy is done, with chest tube for drainage. What are specific nursing interventions for managing chest drainage systems?** Students could be assigned to draw a picture of a Pleur-evac or an atrium drainage system, in demonstrating their understanding of the chest tube drainage system, and their abilities to assist with reinforcing safety measures for the chest tube to the client. It is important to measure and document the amount of drainage coming from the pleural space, since planning for blood replacement is dependent on the amount of drainage that occurs in the first two hours of insertion (100–200 mL) and should lessen after this time. Blood pressure and pulse should be monitored because a drop in blood pressure and a rapid pulse rate are indicators of hemorrhage. If the drainage remains grossly bloody for longer than two hours, the health care provider should be notified promptly. The water-seal drainage port should be monitored for tidaling or fluctuation, since tidaling or fluctuation indicates patency of the tube and proper functioning of the apparatus. If tidaling does not occur soon after the procedure, there may be a kink or obstruction in the chest drainage tubes. The nurse should check to be sure the tubes are not kinked or compressed. Position the tubes in a dependent position to allow blood to flow by gravity, change the client's position, then have the client deep breathe and cough. If these measures do not restore tidaling, notify the surgeon. Observe for bubbling in the water-seal compartment, which is a result of air passing out of the pleural space into the fluid in the water-seal compartment. Bubbling should be intermittent, indicating that air is being removed from the pleural space. Intermittent bubbling occurs with normal expiration, because expiration increases intrapleural pressure and forces air out through the tube. Continuous bubbling during inspiration and expiration indicates that air is leaking into the drainage system or the pleural cavity. This must be corrected promptly, because air entering the system also enters the pleural space. The nurse must locate the source of the air leak, and repair if possible. The nurse begins to locate the source by inspecting

the chest wall where the catheters are inserted. If a chest tube is loose, the nurse gently squeezes the skin around the catheter or applies sterile petrolatum gauze around the insertion site. If this measure does not stop the continuous bubbling, the tubing should be checked inch by inch, and all connections should also be checked, and sealed with tape as needed. If the leak cannot be located, it may be necessary to replace the water-seal drainage apparatus. The nurse then notifies the surgeon, while having a new Pleur-evac initiated. Rapid bubbling in the absence of an air leak indicates considerable loss of air, such as from an incision or tear in the pulmonary pleura. The health care provider must be notified immediately so that appropriate intervention is taken to prevent collapse of the lung or mediastinal shift. If a thoracotomy was done, assisting the client with range-of-motion exercises to the affected arm and shoulder will prevent frozen shoulder. Frozen shoulder may develop because the client does not mobilize the extremity because of fear of pain. Keep the chest tube drainage apparatus below the client's chest. Pleur-evac should be taped to the floor to avoid tipping over and compromising the accuracy of the drainage. Rubber tips hemostats are required bedside equipment.

9. **What are common nursing diagnoses for post-chest tube insertion?**

    - Acute pain R/T incision, drainage tubes, and the surgical procedure
    - Impaired gas exchange R/T lung impairment and surgery
    - Ineffective breathing pattern R/T pain at site of surgical procedure
    - Deficient knowledge R/T condition, treatment, and home care

10. **Discuss client education for pulmonary empyema.** Assess the current knowledge of the client and significant others. Instruct the client about medications prescribed including dosage, schedule, adverse effects, and the importance of completing the entire prescription of antibiotics. Emphasize the importance of reporting change in respiratory status to the health care provider, such as increasing shortness of breath, fever, changes in mental or cognitive status, change in the amount or color of sputum, bleeding or unusual drainage from the chest tube exit site, or increased chest pain. Stress the importance of rest and decreased energy expenditure during recovery and of avoiding smoking or contact with secondhand smoke. The importance of regular hand washing and the appropriate technique should also be emphasized, as well as the importance of follow-up care with the health care provider.

References

Broyles, B.E. (2005). *Medical-Surgical Nursing Clinical Companion.* Durham, NC: Carolina Academic Press.
Cavanaugh, B.M. (2003). *Nurse's Manual of Laboratory and Diagnostic Tests.* Philadelphia: F.A. Davis.
Corbet, J.V. (2004). *Laboratory Tests and Diagnostic Procedures with Nursing Diagnoses* (6th ed.). Upper Saddle River, NJ: Prentice Hall.
Deglin, J.H. and Vallerand, A.H. (2005). *Davis's Drug Guide for Nurses* (9th ed.). Philadelphia: F.A. Davis.
Gahart, B.L. and Nazareno, A.R. (2005). *2005 Intravenous Medications.* St. Louis: Mosby.
Harkreader, H. and Hogan, M.A. (2004). *Fundamentals of Nursing: Caring and Clinical Judgment* (2nd ed.). Philadelphia: W.B. Saunders.
Ignatavicius, D.D. and Workman, M.L. (2006). *Medical-Surgical Nursing across the Health Care Continuum* (5th ed.). Philadelphia: W.B. Saunders.
Spratto, G.R. and Woods, A.L. (2005). *2005 Edition: PDR Nurse's Drug Handbook.* Clifton Park, NY: Thomson Delmar Learning.

CASE STUDY 5

Non-Small Cell Adenocarcinoma of the Right Lung

GENDER
- F

AGE
- 60

SETTING
- Hospital

ETHNICITY/CULTURE
- African/Nigerian

PREEXISTING CONDITIONS
- Recurrent pneumonias
- Pulmonary fibrosis

COEXISTING CONDITIONS
- Chronic obstructive pulmonary disease

LIFESTYLE
- Smoked three packs of cigarettes per day for 15 years

COMMUNICATION

DISABILITY

SOCIOECONOMIC STATUS
- Middle

SPIRITUAL/RELIGIOUS
- Attends Sunday Mass
- Spiritual counseling

PHARMACOLOGIC
- Ibuprofen (Motrin)
- Vinorelbine tartrate (Navelbine)
- Ondansetron HcL (Zofran)

PSYCHOSOCIAL
- Anxiety
- Fear
- Denial

LEGAL

ETHICAL
- Is it a nurse's responsibility to educate clients and others on the dangers of "secondhand smoke"?

ALTERNATIVE THERAPY
- Meditation
- Herbalism

PRIORITIZATION
- Reduce anxiety
- Prepare client for diagnostic tests

DELEGATION
- RN certified in oncology management
- Client education

THE RESPIRATORY AND IMMUNE SYSTEMS

Level of difficulty: Moderate

Overview: This case involves a thorough assessment of the client's condition, past medical history, social habits, and current medications including herbal and over-the-counter drugs. The nurse must use critical thinking and prioritization to meet the immediate needs of clients who are diagnosed with different types of cancer at different stages of progression. Nurses must be vigilant with assessment skills when caring for clients receiving chemotherapeutic agents that suppress bone marrow.

Client Profile

Ms. Y is a 60-year-old female who is admitted by her primary health care provider to the hospital after her annual physical examination. Ms. Y has never been married and has been unemployed for the past three years. She was employed as a "private" home health aide, but after the death of that client, she was unable to find employment.

Case Study

During the initial nurse interview, Ms. Y reports seeking her primary health care provider's advice because of a persistent cough for the past month. Ms. Y reports a history of smoking three packs of cigarettes per day for 15 years. Ms. Y admits to being anxious but does not believe she has cancer. She denies weight loss or unusual physical changes except the unusual cough. She reports occasional use of Advil (ibuprofen) for infrequent headaches and use of herbal medicines, especially at breakfast and before retiring to bed. Admission vital signs are:

- Blood pressure: 140/84
- Pulse: 80
- Respirations: 18
- Temperature: 98.2° F

Auscultation reveals unilateral wheeze in the right lower lobe of the lung. Respiratory assessment is occasionally interrupted because of her need to cough. After the physical assessment is complete, the following diagnostic studies and labs are prescribed: cytologic examination of sputum; chest X-ray; pulmonary function tests (PFTs); computed tomography (CT) scan of the lung; positron emission test (PET); serum sodium, potassium (K+), and calcium, platelet count, hematocrit, hemoglobin, white blood cell count, and creatinine. The results of the diagnostic tests reveal: sputum for cytology with malignant cells; chest X-ray shows lesion on the right lung; vital capacity (VC) is 75%, FEV_1 80%, FEF 68%; CT scan identifies the lesion and scans and measures it at 10 cm; PET is negative for metastasis. Results of the serum labs are:

- Sodium (Na): 133
- Potassium (K+): 4.2
- Calcium: 8.4
- Platelet count (PLT): 2,500,153
- Hematocrit (Hct): 32.8%
- Hemoglobin (Hgb): 11.5 g/dL
- White blood cell (WBC) count: 10,000/mm^3
- Creatinine: 0.9 mg/dL

After the diagnostic tests and lab results are reviewed and discussed with the medical, surgical, and oncology teams, a diagnosis of non-small squamous cell adenocarcinoma of the right lung is made. The findings are discussed and explained with Ms. Y, and a decision for plan of care is made. Serum sodium, calcium, complete blood count will be done twice weekly.

Questions and Suggested Answers

1. **Discuss the pathophysiology of lung cancer.** Lung cancer is the leading cause of cancer-related deaths in men and women in the United States. It most commonly occurs in individuals more than 50 years of age who have a long history of cigarette smoking. The disease is found most frequently in persons 40–75 years of age, with peak incidence between 55 and 65 years of age. More than 90% of cancers originate from the epithelium of

the bronchus (bronchogenic) and grow slowly, taking from eight to ten years for a tumor to reach 1 cm in size, which on an X-ray is the smallest detectable lesion. Lung cancers occur primarily in the segmental bronchi or beyond and have a preference for the upper lobes of the lungs. Pathologic changes in the bronchial system show nonspecific inflammatory changes with hypersecretion of mucus, desquamation of cells, reactive hyperplasia of the basal cells, and metaplasia of normal respiratory epithelium to stratified squamous cells. Lung cancers metastasize primarily by direct extension and via the blood circulation and the lymph system. Certain lung cancers cause the paraneoplastic syndromes, which are caused by hormones, enzymes, or antigens. However, a major cause of lung cancer is cigarette smoking, although passive smoking from "secondhand smoke" is also a significant contributing factor, because passive smoking has many of the carcinogens found in the inhaled or "mainstream" tobacco smoke. Studies have also shown that the inhalation of abestos fibers is associated with higher cancer risks for both smokers and nonsmokers.

2. **Compare tobacco smoke, secondhand smoke, and environmental and occupational exposure and their effects on the development of lung cancer.** Studies continue to document that various irritants are responsible for the development of lung cancer. However, tobacco smoke is responsible for more than one of every six deaths from pulmonary and cardiovascular diseases in the United States. More than 85% of lung cancers are attributed to the inhalation of carcinogenic chemicals, such as cigarette smoke. Lung cancer is ten times more common in cigarette smokers than nonsmokers. The risk is determined by the pack-year history (number of packs of cigarette used each day, multiplied by the number of years smoked). Another factor is the type of cigarettes smoked (tar content, filtered versus nonfiltered). Secondhand smoke (passive smoking) has been identified as a possible cause of lung cancer in nonsmokers. Therefore people who are involuntarily exposed to tobacco smoke in a closed environment (home, car, building) are at increased risk for developing lung cancer as compared to unexposed nonsmokers. Various carcinogens have been identified in the atmosphere, including motor vehicle emissions and pollutants from refineries and manufacturing plants. Evidence suggests that the incidence of lung cancer is greater in urban areas as a result of the buildup of pollutants and motor vehicle emissions. Radon, a colorless and odorless gas that is found in rocks and soil and has been associated with uranium mines, is now believed to seep into homes through ground rocks. Studies have shown that high levels of radon have been associated with the development of lung cancer, especially when combined with cigarette smoking.

3. **Discuss non-small cell lung cancer.** Non-small cell lung cancer is a squamous cell carcinoma that is almost always associated with cigarette smoking and is associated with exposure to environmental carcinogens (e.g., asbestos). It accounts for 30–50% of lung cancers and is more common in men. It arises from the bronchial epithelium and produces earlier symptoms because of bronchial obstructive characteristics. It does not have a strong tendency to metastasize, and metastasis is locally by direct extension, causing cavitating pulmonary lesions. Life expectancy is better than for small cell lung cancer.

4. **Discuss clinical manifestations of lung cancer.** Clinical manifestations of lung cancer are usually silent for most individuals, appearing late in the disease process. A *smoker's cough* and *persistent pneumonitis* may be the earliest manifestations of lung cancer. However, a persistent cough that may be productive of sputum is one of the most significant symptoms. If blood-tinged sputum is produced, this is because of bleeding caused by malignancy, but hemoptysis is not a common early symptom.

5. **Discuss the different stages of lung cancer as designated by the tumor-mode-metastasis (TNM) classification system.** *Stage IA* (T1N0M0): tumor is 3 cm or less in diameter with no metastases to regional lymph nodes and no distant metastasis. *Stage IB* (T2N0M0): tumor is greater than 3 cm in diameter or is any size that either invades the visceral pleura or has associated atelectasis or obstructive pneumonitis extending to the hilar region; however, there are no metastases to lymph nodes or distant metastasis. *Stage IIA* (T1N1M0): tumor is 3 cm or less in diameter with metastasis to lymph nodes in the peribronchial or ipsilateral hilar region, or both, without distant metastasis. *Stage IIB* (T2N1M0): tumor is greater than 3 cm in diameter or is any size that either invades the visceral pleura or has associated atelectasis or obstructive pneumonitis extending to the hilar region, with metastasis to lymph nodes in the peribronchial or ipsilateral hilar region,

or both, without distant metastasis. ***Stage IIIA*** (T2N2M0): tumor is greater than 3 cm in diameter or is any size that either invades the visceral pleura or has associated atelectasis or obstructive pneumonitis extending to the hilar region, with metastasis to ipsilateral mediastinal or subcarinal nodes without distant metastasis.

6. **Discuss diagnostic tests used to confirm lung cancer.** ***Chest X-rays*** are widely used for early identification of lung lesions. The findings may show the presence of the tumor or abnormalities related to obstructive features of the tumor such as atelectasis and penumonitis. X-rays can also show evidence of metastasis to the ribs or vertebrae and the presence of pleural effusion. ***CT scan*** is the single most effective non-invasive technique for evaluating lung cancer. With the use of the CT scan, the location and extent of masses in the chest can be identified. Usually the entire chest is scanned and suspicious areas are then scanned for highest resolution. ***Magnetic resonance imaging (MRI)*** may be used in combination with or instead of CT scans. ***PET*** is a useful diagnostic tool for early clinical staging. It allows measurement of differential metabolic activity in normal and diseased tissues. A definitive diagnosis of lung cancer is made with the use of a ***cytologic examination*** of early morning sputum, to identify tumor cells. However, since cancer cells may not be present in the sputum, sputum for cytology alone cannot confirm the diagnosis. ***Pulmonary angiography*** helps determine the overall respiratory status and ***fine needle aspiration*** is used to determine tumor histology. ***Staging*** of lung cancer provides information on tumor size, location, and degree of invasion. ***Staging*** assists in estimating prognosis and determining the appropriate therapy.

The following are prescribed:

- Vinorelbine tartrate (Navelbine) 30 mg/m^2 weekly at oncology clinic
- Ondansetron HcL (Zofran) 8 mg PO 30 minutes before chemotherapy

7. **What are the purposes for the prescribed orders?** ***Vinorelbine tartrate*** is to prevent cancer cells from reproducing. It arrests cancer cells at the metaphase of the cell cycle. In the metaphase cycle, mitosis, or division of cells, takes place and chromosomes are easily visualized during this phase. If cancer cells are not arrested at this phase, they will be arranged with normal chromosomes, which could result in chromosome aberrations and associated diseases. ***Ondansetron HcL*** prevents nausea and vomiting associated with the initial dose of chemotherapy. It is a serotonin blocker that increases tolerance to chemotherapy by blocking 5-HT3 receptor in the gastrointestinal (GI) tract, CTZ, and vomiting center.

8. **What are the most common adverse reactions, drug-to-drug, drug-to-food/herbal interactions of the prescribed medications?** The most common adverse reactions of ***vinorelbine tartrate*** are decreased deep tendon reflexes, paresthesia, fatigue, asthenia, peripheral neuropathy, constipation, nausea, anemia, neutropenia, irritation at the IV site, neurotoxicity, vomiting, and diarrhea. Drug-to-drug interactions may occur with the simultaneous use of cisplatin, mitomycin, and paclitaxel, and may increase neuropathy. There are no clinically significant drug-to-food/herbal interactions established. The most common adverse reactions of ***zofran*** are dizziness, headache, sedation, and diarrhea. Drug-to-drug interaction is seen when used simultaneously with rifampin. There are no clinically significant drug-to-food/herbal interactions established.

9. **What process does the nurse use when administering medications to this client?** The nursing process when administering medications to clients involves implementing the "seven rights":

    RIGHT DRUG: *Is this the drug that was prescribed, and is this the right drug for this client?* Vinorelbine tartrate is an antineoplastic, vinca alkaloid drug approved to treat non-small cell lung cancer. To avoid error, the nurse should check the drug label three times: (1) with first contact with the drug container, (2) after hanging the infusion bag, and (3) before starting the infusion.

    RIGHT DOSE: *Is this the dose that is prescribed, and is this a safe dose for the client?* The prescribed dose is in the standard range and is a safe dose for IV administration, and safe for the client. ***Vinorelbine tartrate*** adult dose is in the range of 25–30 mg/m^2 over six to ten minutes/q weekly. The dose is adjusted based on the WBC count. The nurse should know the recommended dosage range for the drug. Occasionally a drug is ordered by the health care provider using one measurement system, but it has a label from another. When in doubt, check with another nurse, the *Physician's Desk Reference,* the pharmacist, or the prescribing health care provider. *Zofran* is in the safe adult range and is to be administered 30 minutes before chemotherapeutic implementation. *Zofran* IV is 32 mg over 15 minutes pre-chemotherapeutic implementation.

RIGHT CLIENT: *Is this the right client for which this medication has been prescribed?* The nurse should check the health care provider's prescription on the client's medical record, compare the order on the medication administration record of the client, check the label on the infusion bag sent from the pharmacy for the correct client's name, drug, dosage, and correct solution. The last step in determining the "right client" is to ask the client to verbalize her full name then check her identification (ID) band for accuracy of names. Any ID bracelet that is smudged or cannot be easily read should be replaced immediately. This practice should be strictly followed even when nurses come to know the client.

RIGHT TIME: *Is this the correct time according to the prescription?* The nurse administers the drug at the specified times, documenting any delay or omission of the drug. This drug will be administered weekly. The nurse should know the nature and purpose of the medication so optimal timing will be ensured.

RIGHT ROUTE: *Is this the appropriate route to administer this medication?* This drug is administered by the intravenous route. The nurse validates the vascular access for patency or signs of infiltration or thrombophlebitis. Clients receiving chemotherapeutic agents usually have a peripheral inserted central catheter (PICC), which is a central venous catheter that is designed for long- or short-term use for drugs that are highly irritating in nature. The drug should be administered within a time frame that is based on the drug's absorption, biotransformation, half-life, and elimination in and from the body.

RIGHT DOCUMENTATION: *The administration documentation should consist of the drug name, dosage, route, and time of administration, as well as the client's response.* After administering the medication, the nurse should chart it immediately on the medication administration record (MAR) or computerized medical record. Medications should never be charted before administration.

RIGHT TO REFUSE: *The client has the right to refuse any medication.* If the client refuses the medication, follow the agency's protocol in documenting the refusal. If there are no areas on the MAR, write a follow-up note in the client's medical record indicating the reasons for the refusal and inform the prescribing health care provider of the refusal. Most refusals of medications are based on lack of or inaccurate information, so the nurse needs to always inform the client what type of drug is being implemented and the purpose for its administration.

10. **Discuss client education for lung cancer.** If the client smokes any form of tobacco, smoking should be discontinued completely. The client should have adequate rest and exercise. The client should stay away from factors that may cause lung irritation, increase protein intake with meals, drink plenty of fluids but minimize caffeinated beverages, take anti-emetic medication (Zofran) 30 minutes before chemotherapy, and schedule means of transportation 30 minutes early so as to keep scheduled appointments up-to-date.

References

Broyles, B.E. (2005). *Medical-Surgical Nursing Clinical Companion.* Durham, NC: Carolina Academic Press.
Corbet, J.V. (2004). *Laboratory Tests and Diagnostic Procedures with Nursing Diagnoses* (6th ed.). Upper Saddle River, NJ: Prentice Hall.
Gahart, B.L. and Nazareno, A.R. (2005). *2005 Intravenous Medications.* St. Louis: Mosby.
Huether, S.E. and McCance, K.L. (2004). *Understanding Pathophysiology* (3rd ed.). St. Louis: Mosby.
Ignatavicius, D.D. and Workman, M.L. (2006). *Medical-Surgical Nursing: Critical Thinking for Collaborative Care* (5th ed.). Philadelphia: W.B. Saunders.
Maghfoor, I. and Perry, M. (2005). *Lung Cancer: Oat Cell (Small Cell).* Available at www.emedicine.com/med/topic1336.htm.
Shuey, K.M. and Brant, J.M. (2004). "Hypercalcemia of Malignancy: Part II." *Clinical Journal of Oncology Nursing* 8(3): 321–323.
Spratto, G.R. and Woods, A.L. (2005). *2005 Edition: PDR Nurse's Drug Handbook.* Clifton Park, NY: Thomson Delmar Learning.

CASE STUDY 6

Pulmonary Emphysema

GENDER
- M

AGE
- 62

SETTING
- Hospital

ETHNICITY/CULTURE
- Italian American

PREEXISTING CONDITIONS
- History of cigarette smoking

COEXISTING CONDITIONS
- Hyperinflated lung

LIFESTYLE
- Supervisor, 20 years in garment industry

COMMUNICATION

DISABILITY
- Easy fatigability
- Dyspnea on slight exertion

SOCIOECONOMIC STATUS
- Middle

SPIRITUAL/RELIGIOUS
- Catholic

PHARMACOLOGIC
- Theophylline ethylenediamine
- Methylprednisolone sodium succinate (Solu-Medrol)
- Cromolyn sodium (Intal)
- Albuterol (Proventil)
- Ampicillin sodium/sulbactam sodium (Unasyn)
- Pneumococcal 0.5 mL and influenza vaccine
- Metered-dose inhaler – Albuterol (Proventil)

PSYCHOSOCIAL
- Depression
- Anxiety

LEGAL

ETHICAL

ALTERNATIVE THERAPY
- Fish oil
- Garlic

PRIORITIZATION
- Airway management
- Prevent respiratory failure

DELEGATION
- RN
- CNA

MODERATE

THE RESPIRATORY AND IMMUNE SYSTEMS

Level of difficulty: Moderate

Overview: This case involves a thorough assessment of the client's condition including recent exposure to risk factors, pattern of symptom development, past medical history, current medications, and available social and family support. It involves prioritization of care. The nurse must be skilled at assessing respiratory status and competent in managing respiratory emergencies. The certified nursing assistant (CNA) can take height and weight, vital signs, and assist with hygiene care as needed.

Client Profile

Mr. X is a 62-year-old thin, underweight male who is accompanied by his wife to the respiratory unit after brief triage in the emergency department (ED). His wife is in the waiting room of the unit while the receiving nurse makes Mr. X comfortable before initiating the history and physical.

Case Study

Report from the triage nurse indicates that on arrival to the ED, Mr. X demonstrates signs of mild anxiety but his chief complaint is "increased difficulty breathing after climbing three flights of stairs today." He reports that his breathing has become progressively worse to the point where it interferes with activities of daily living (ADL). He concludes by saying that the breathing is worse today, which is the reason he came to the ED. His vital signs are:

- Blood pressure: 140/78
- Pulse: 88
- Respirations: 24
- Temperature: 99.8° F

On assessment, he has a barrel chest and uses his accessory muscles of respiration to assist with breathing. He frequently does pursed-lip breathing during the interview and coughs and expectorates moderate amount of yellowish sputum. He has auscultatory rales at the base of the lung fields. His social history includes smoking three packs of cigarettes per day for 40 years.

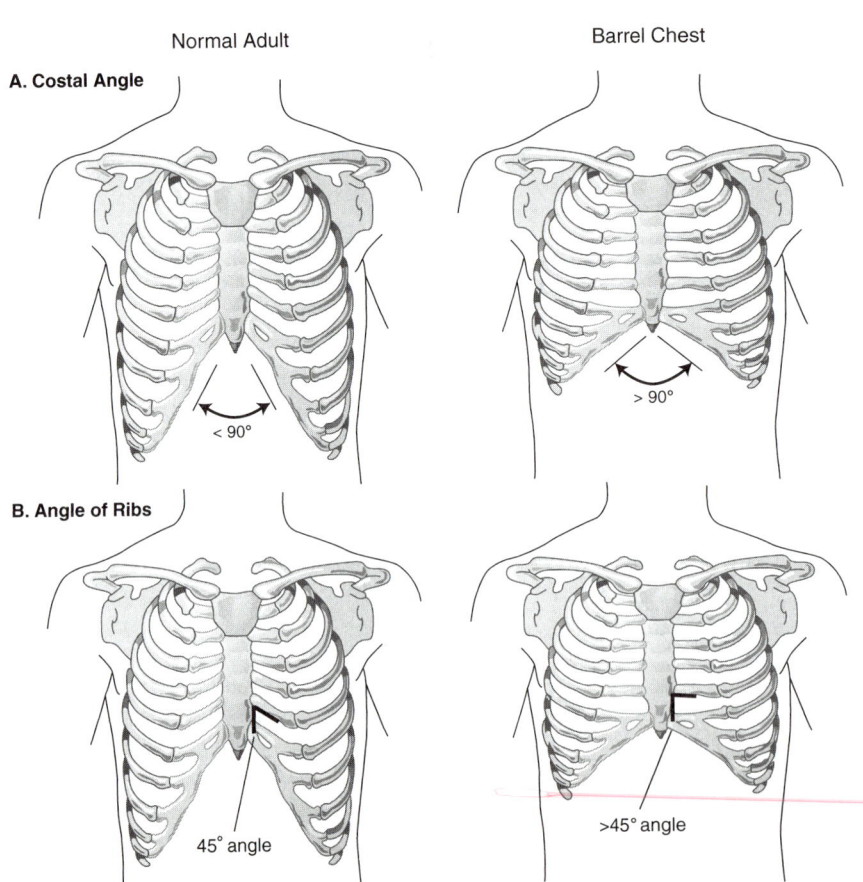

Mr. X reports not having gotten the pneumococcal and influenza vaccines for a long period of time but is not specific about the length of time. A health care provider completes the history and physical and orders a stat arterial blood gas (ABG) and complete blood count (CBC). The results of the ABG tests are:

pH: 7.36

$PaCO_2$: 48 mm Hg

PaO_2: 80%

HCO_3: 25

Complete blood count (CBC):

    White blood cell (WBC) count: 7.1

    Hematocrit (Hct): 38%

    Hemoglobin (Hgb): 15 mg/dL

Two liters of oxygen via nasal cannula are initiated. A chest X-ray shows a flattened diaphragm but no infiltrates. Pulmonary function studies reveal FEV-1/FVC 60% and increased residual volume (RV). Sputum analysis identifies Haemophilus influenza. A diagnosis of chronic obstructive pulmonary disease (pulmonary emphysema) is confirmed. Mr. X is admitted to the hospital for respiratory and oxygen therapy and pharmacological therapy.

Questions and Suggested Answers

1. **Discuss the types of emphysema and the most common risk factor for the development of pulmonary emphysema.** *Panlobular emphysema* affects both the bronchioles and alveolar and most commonly involves the lower lungs. This form occurs most often in smokers. *Centrilobular* (centriacinar) *emphysema* is the most common type and produces destruction in the bronchioles, usually in the upper lung regions. Inflammation develops in the bronchioles, but usually the alveolar sac remains intact. *Paraseptal (or panacinar) emphysema* destroys the alveoli in the lower lobes of the lungs, resulting in isolated blebs along the lung periphery. It is believed to be a likely cause of spontaneous pneumothorax. It occurs in the elderly and in clients with an inherited deficiency of alpha-1-a antitrypsin (AAT) enzyme. Normally, AAT inhibits the action of enzymes that break down proteins. Clients without AAT are at increased risk for pulmonary emphysema because the walls of the lung are at higher risk for destruction. Cigarette smoking is thought to alter the balance of these enzymes and increase destruction of lung tissue.

2. **Discuss the complications associated with emphysema.** Respiratory infections commonly develop in clients with pulmonary emphysema. The development is a result of alterations in the normal respiratory defense mechanisms and decreased immune resistance. Because respiratory status is already compromised, infection frequently leads to acute respiratory failure. Spontaneous pneumothorax may develop from rupture of an emphysematous bleb. This rupture results in a closed pneumothorax and requires insertion of a chest tube for reexpansion of the lung.

3. **Discuss the enzyme inhibitor that predisposes young clients who do not smoke to rapid development of lobular emphysema.** The alpha-1-a antitrypsin is the enzyme that predisposes young clients who are not smokers to the development of lobular emphysema. It is one of the most genetically linked lethal diseases among white people.

4. **Pulmonary function tests (PFTs) are used to confirm pulmonary emphysema. What are the specific findings of the PFTs?** The forced expiratory volume (FEV), or the volume of air that the client can forcibly exhale in one second (FEV_1), and the forced vital capacity (FVC), the maximum amount of air that can be forcefully exhaled after a full inspiration, is less than 70%. The normal value is 81–83%.

5. **Discuss the clinical manifestations of pulmonary emphysema.** Dyspnea is the presenting symptom in emphysema and has an insidious onset. If there is a long history of cigarette smoking, the client may present with chronic cough, wheezing, and increased shortness of breath. After the development of infections, the client

experiences a prolonged wheezing on expiration, anorexia, weight loss, and weakness. The client's typical posture tends to lean forward and the use of accessory muscles of respiration to breathe is evident, both of which force the shoulder girdle upward, causing the supraclavicular fossae to retract on inspiration. The general appearance is thin, pink skin color ("pink puffer"), flattened diaphragm, barrel chest, and pursed-lip breathing.

6. **What are common nursing diagnoses for clients with pulmonary emphysema?**

   - Ineffective airway clearance R/T expiratory airflow obstruction, ineffective cough, decreased airway humidity, and infection in the airways
   - Impaired gas exchange R/T alveolar hypoventilation as manifested by headache on awakening
   - Risk for infection R/T decreased pulmonary function, possible corticosteroid therapy, ineffective airway clearance
   - Imbalanced nutrition: less than body requirements R/T poor appetite, lowered energy level, shortness of breath, gastric distention, sputum production, and depression
   - Disturbed sleep pattern R/T anxiety, dyspnea, depression, hypoxemia, and/or hypercapnia
   - Deficient knowledge R/T condition, treatment, and health maintenance.

The following are prescribed:

- Albuterol (Proventil) aerosol metered-dose inhalant (MDI) two puffs stat and q4h PRN
- Oxygen/nasal cannula to maintain oxygen saturation greater than 89% but not to exceed two liters
- Dextrose 5% and 0.45% sodium chloride intravenous infusion at 100 mL/hr
- Theophylline ethylenediamine (with 20 mg theophylline, 25 mg aminophylline) 0.3 mg/kg/hr continuous intravenously administration
- Ampicillin sodium/sulbactam sodium (Unasyn) 1.5 gm IV q6h
- Cromolyn sodium (Intal) two metered sprays q6h
- Pneumococcal 0.5 mL single dose and influenza vaccine 0.5 mL single dose prior to discharge

7. **What are the purposes for the prescribed orders?** *Albuterol* is a selective beta$_2$-adrenergic bronchodilator that is very effective in opening the airways and improving breathing because of its rapid onset of action and efficacy. It relaxes the smooth muscles of bronchial tree, decreasing airway resistance, facilitating mucus drainage, and increasing vital capacity. Albuterol via MDI dilates the airways with a precise amount of medication that will be released with each activation of the canister. It does this by binding to specific beta$_1$-adrenergic receptors in airway smooth muscle, which when stimulated cause bronchodilation of the airways and enhance breathing. *Oxygen* increases the oxygenation to body tissues. Low-dose oxygen is needed to prevent the inhibition of the respiratory drive that relies on a decree of hypoxia to maintain this drive. *Intravenous fluids* are prescribed to provide hydration including helping to liquefy secretions, a source of carbohydrates, and the maintenance of an intravenous access. *Intravenous aminophylline* is a bronchodilator and respiratory stimulant that is used in conjunction with inhaled beta$_2$ selective agonist, such as albuterol, and systemic corticosteroids, such as methylprednisolone sodium succinate (Solu-Medrol) for the treatment of acute exacerbations of emphysema and other chronic obstructive pulmonary diseases. Aminophylline stimulates the beta$_1$ receptors of the bronchi to cause bronchodilation through smooth muscle relaxation. *Ampicillin/sulbactam sodium* is a penicillin and beta-lactamase inhibitor that destroys H. influenza, which is the organism identified in Mr. X's sputum. It is a broad-spectrum antibiotic that is effective against both gram-negative and gram-positive organisms. It is effective because it binds to the bacterial cell wall, resulting in cell death. The intravenous route of the medication will provide systemic and quick effect on the organism, which will help to alleviate the infectious process and shorten the exacerbation the client experiences that is associated with unusual sputum production at this time. *Cromolyn sodium metered doses* are used to "inhibit the degranulation of sensitized mast cells, which occur after exposure to certain antigens." (Spratto and Woods, 292). Cromolyn sodium is an antiasthmatic and antiallergenic agent employed as an adjunct to other respiratory agents in the treatment of emphysema exacerbations. *Pneumococcal vaccine* protects the client against the

major bacterium that causes pneumonia. It has 23 type-specific capsular polysaccharides that have a minimum protection of four years. The *influenza vaccine* helps to reduce the severity of pulmonary emphysema during flu season. It is prepared yearly to adjust for the specific immunologic characteristics that are present in the influenza viruses at the time.

8. **What are the most common adverse reactions of the prescribed medications?** The most common adverse reactions of *albuterol* are tachycardia and tremors. The most common adverse effect of *aminophylline* is tachycardia. Because it stimulates the beta$_1$ receptors of the bronchi to cause bronchodilation through smooth muscle relaxation, it also stimulates the beta$_1$ receptors in the heart. Other common adverse reactions of aminophylline include headache, insomnia, nausea, and vomiting, most commonly occurring when the peak serum levels are less than 20 mcg/mL. The most common adverse reactions of *ampicillin/sulbactam sodium* are rash, allergic reactions, diarrhea, nausea, and pain at infusion site. The most common adverse effects of *cromolyn sodium* include bronchospasms, cough, pharyngeal irritation, nasal congestion, and sneezing. The most common adverse reaction of *pneumococcal* and *influenza vaccines* is soreness at the injection site.

9. **Discuss the drug-to-drug and drug-to-food/herbal interactions of the prescribed medications.** Drug-to-drug interactions may occur with the simultaneous use of *albuterol* and epinephrine or other sympathomimetic bronchodilators. The simultaneous use of monoamine oxidase (MAO) inhibitors and tricyclic antidepressants potentiate their actions on the vascular system, which compound the toxic effects of *albuterol*. The simultaneous use of caffeine products with *albuterol* may increase the risk of tachycardia. Fir needle oil and pine needle oil increase the risk of bronchospasms if used concurrently with albuterol. Drug-to-drug interactions may occur with the simultaneous use of *aminophylline* and aminoglycosides, barbiturates, carbamazepine, isoproterenol, hydantoins, rifampin, and sulfinpyrazone because these agents increase theophylline clearance and decrease serum levels. The serum levels of *aminophylline* will increase with the simultaneous use of alcohol, allopurinol, beta-adrenergic blocking agents, cimetidine, clarithromycin, ciprofloxacin, disulfiram, erythromycin, estrogen-containing oral contraceptives, fluvoxamine, interferon alfa-A, methotrexate, mexiletine, pentoxifylline, propafenone, tacrine, thiabendazole, ticlopidine, troleandomycin, and verapamil. The simultaneous use of *aminophylline* with pancuronium will inhibit the action of pancuronium, requiring increased doses of pancuronium to accomplish neuromuscular blockade. Concurrent use of *aminophylline* with benzodiazepines, midazolam, and propofol may decrease their effects. The simultaneous use of *aminophylline* with halothane increases the risk of cardiac dysrrythmias and, when used concurrently with ketamine, may decrease *aminophylline* serum levels, and the use of caffeine may cause a false immunoassay diagnostic tests. Drug-to-drug interactions may occur with the simultaneous use of *ampicillin sodium/sulbactam sodium*, and drug-to-drug interactions may occur with the simultaneous use of allopurinol, which may increase the incidence of rash. If ampicillin sodium/sulbactam sodium is simultaneously used with aminoglycosides, the effectiveness of aminoglycosides may be impaired in patients with severe end-stage renal disease (ESRD). The simultaneous use of *ampicillin sodium/sulbactam sodium* with chloramphenicol, erythromycin, or tetracycline may reduce the bactericidal effects. If the bactericidal effects were reduced, this would have a significant negative effect on the organism, especially if the prescribed doses of ampicillin sodium/sulbactam sodium are low. The concurrent use with probenicid decreases renal excretion and increases blood levels of ampicillin. It may decrease the clearance and increase the risk of methotrexate toxicity and it decreases the effectiveness of oral contraceptives and can result in breakthrough bleeding in pregnant women. Concurrent use with beta-adrenergic blocking agents may decrease the effectiveness of therapy and increase the risk of anaphylaxis. There are no clinically significant drug-to-food/herbal interactions established. Drug-to-drug interactions may occur with the concurrent use of *cromolyn sodium* and corticosteroids, which results in synergistic actions. There are no clinically established drug-to-food/herbal interactions established for cromolyn sodium. With the *pneumococcal and influenza vaccines* no clinically significant drug-to-drug or drug-to-food/herbal interactions have been established. However, if the client is allergic to eggs, taking the influenza vaccine will cause allergic response and live vaccines should not be administered to clients who are immuno-suppressed. No specific drug-to-herbal interactions have been established for these vaccines.

10. **Discuss the surgical approaches that might be used for the client with emphysema.** Lung transplantation is performed for select clients with end-stage pulmonary emphysema. The more common surgical procedure for clients with pulmonary emphysema is lung reduction surgery. Lung reduction surgery can improve gas exchange in the client with pulmonary emphysema. The goal of this surgery is improvement of gas exchange through removal of hyperinflated lung tissue, because they are useless for gas exchange. After successful lung reduction, most clients have at least 75% improvement in FEV_1, decreased total lung capacity (TLC), and RV with noted increased activity tolerance. After lung reduction surgery, oxygen therapy may not be needed any more.

11. **Discuss client education for pulmonary emphysema.** The client should be taught the importance of compliance with prescribed medications, since these medications function to keep the airways open and facilitate breathing, or to eradicate infecting organisms in the event the client was exposed to an infectious agent that caused him or her to seek medical treatment. Discuss the proper use of MDIs and the effects of albuterol that should be reported to the primary health care provider in the event they occur. Some of these effects are tachydysrhythmias (fast or rapid heart rate), tremors, anxiety, and nausea. Teach the client the importance of gradual increase in exercise, slowly building up to a normal level of tolerance. Advise the client that the use of the MDI about ten minutes before exercise usually improves tolerance, and that the pulse rate should be checked after walking and should not exceed a normal rate of 100 beats per minute. Instruct the client to wait at least five minutes after completion of exercise before using the MDI, to allow a chance to recover. Remind the client that during this waiting period, pursed-lip breathing should be used. Emphasize that adequate sleep is extremely important. Instruct the client that if he is a restless sleeper, snores, stops breathing while asleep, or has a tendency to fall asleep during the day, these findings should be told to the primary health care provider, so the client can be evaluated for sleep apnea. The client may practice progressive relaxation technique such as listening either to a tape or to the client's own voice, while gradually beginning to tighten and relax muscle groups. The client should be advised to get an influenza vaccine yearly before the flu season to avoid exacerbation of emphysema. To minimize the amount of contaminants in the home, the client should keep windows open, if the weather permits, to help with ventilation; keep wood-burning stoves or fireplaces well ventilated, and avoid exposure to known allergens. Smoking cessation is mandatory, and the client should stay away from passive smoke as much as possible.

References

Broyles, B.E. (2005). *Medical-Surgical Nursing Clinical Companion.* Durham, NC: Carolina Academic Press.

Centers for Disease Control (2003). "Pneumococcal Vaccine." Available at www.cdc.gov.

Corbet, J.V. (2004). *Laboratory Tests and Diagnostic Procedures with Nursing Diagnoses* (6th ed.). Upper Saddle River, NJ: Prentice Hall.

Deglin, J.H. and Vallerand, A.H. (2005). *Davis's Drug Guide for Nurses* (9th ed.). Philadelphia: F.A. Davis.

Gahart, B.L. and Nazareno, A.R. (2005). *2005 Intravenous Medications.* St. Louis: Mosby.

Guyton, A.C. and Hall, J.E. (2006). *Medical Physiology* (11th ed.). Philadelphia: W.B. Saunders.

Lehne, R.A. (2004). *Pharmacology for Nursing Care* (5th ed.). Philadelphia: W.B. Saunders.

LeMone, P. and Burke, K.M. (2004). *Medical-Surgical Nursing: Critical Thinking in Client Care* (3rd ed.). Upper Saddle River, NJ: Prentice Hall.

Lewis, S.M., Heitkemper, M.M., and Dirksen, S.R. (2004) *Medical-Surgical Nursing: Assessment and Management of Clinical Problems* (6th ed.). St. Louis: Mosby.

Spratto, G.R. and Woods, A.L. (2005). *2005 Edition: PDR Nurse's Drug Handbook.* Clifton Park, NY: Thomson Delmar Learning.

CASE STUDY 7

Acute Respiratory Distress Syndrome

GENDER
- M

AGE
- 42

SETTING
- Hospital

ETHNICITY/CULTURE
- Black American

PREEXISTING CONDITIONS

COEXISTING CONDITIONS

LIFESTYLE
- Fireman

COMMUNICATION

DISABILITY

SOCIOECONOMIC STATUS
- Middle

SPIRITUAL/RELIGIOUS
- Catholic

PHARMACOLOGIC
- Lactated Ringers
- Enoxaparin (Lovenox)
- Midazolam HcL (Versed)
- Pancuronium bromide (Pavulon)
- Bumetanide (Bumex)

PSYCHOSOCIAL
- Anxiety

LEGAL
- Long-term financial support

ETHICAL

ALTERNATIVE THERAPY

PRIORITIZATION
- Maintain airway patency
- Maintain oxygenation

DELEGATION
- RN
- Client education

THE RESPIRATORY AND IMMUNE SYSTEMS

Level of difficulty: Difficult

Overview: This case involves a quick assessment of the client and presenting symptoms while maintaining airway patency. It involves prioritization of care to other clients when the burn client arrives on the unit. It involves a complete physical examination that includes the client's general appearance on arrival to the unit.

DIFFICULT

Client Profile

Mr. T is a 42-year-old firefighter assigned to an engine company located in a poor urban neighborhood. Mr. T has been acknowledged by the mayor of the city on three occasions for bravery, which includes going beyond the call of duty to save lives from actively burning buildings. One month ago, Mr. T was brought to the hospital emergency department (ED) for smoke inhalation after combating a fire for several hours. Mr. T was discharged and returned to work after clearance from his primary health care provider.

Case Study

Today, Mr. T is brought to the ED from his place of employment. On arrival at the ED, he is restless, complains of fatigue, headache, and difficulty breathing even when in an upright position. An arterial blood gas (ABG) test reveals:

pH: 7.30
PCO_2: 48
HCO_3^- done with a PaO_2 of 58

The test indicates respiratory acidosis. He is started on a non-rebreather mask and pulse oximeter to monitor oxygen saturation. Physical assessment by the nurse finds the use of accessory muscles with decreased breath sounds. Vital signs are:

Blood pressure: 100/72
Pulse: 114
Respirations: 22
Temperature: 99.4° F

Mr. T is 5'6" and weighs 205 pounds. Pulmonary function tests (PFTs) show decreased lung compliance with reduced vital capacity, minute volume and functional vital capacity. On auscultation of the lungs, the health care provider auscultates bilateral rales. Results of a chest X-ray done in the ED show diffuse haziness, "whited-out" (ground-glass) appearance of the lung. A repeat ABG reveals PaO_2 of 58 even after the implementation of four liters of oxygen. The client is intubated and placed on mechanical ventilation with positive-end expiratory pressure (PEEP) setting and placed in semi-Fowler's position. A pulmonary artery catheter is inserted. After review of physical findings, response to increase in oxygen, chest X-ray findings, and pulmonary capillary wedge pressure readings, the diagnosis of acute respiratory distress syndrome (ARDS) is made. Plans to initiate enteral feeding or parenteral nutrition (hyperalimentation) will be included in the treatment regimen.

Questions and Suggested Answers

1. **Discuss your understanding of the client's situation.** The initial defect of Mr. T's lungs occurred during the previous smoke inhalation, resulting in damage to the pulmonary capillary endothelium, which caused increased microvascular permeability. When the endothelium is damaged, fluid and proteins leak into the interstitium and then into the alveoli. Over a period of time, enzymes such as collagenase and elastase disrupt the elastic and collagen fibers in the interstitium and progress to the alveoli; the overall net effect is hypoxemia.

2. **Discuss the pathophysiology of ARDS and the leading cause of death in clients with ARDS.** ARDS is acute respiratory failure. It often occurs after an acute traumatic event in people with no previous pulmonary disease. However, there are many different causes for lung injury leading up to ARDS, but a systemic inflammatory response is the common finding in its development. The major site of injury in the lung is the

alveolar-capillary membrane, which is normally permeable to only small molecules. However, in ARDS, leakage via the capillary membrane develops, and lung fluid increases and contains high levels of proteins. Surfactant activity is also reduced in ARDS because the type II pneumocytes that produce pulmonary surfactant are damaged, resulting in the loss of lung compliance. As a result of the loss surfactant, the alveoli become unstable and tend to collapse unless they are filled with fluid. The alveoli can not participate in gas exchange, resulting in the formation of edema around terminal airways, which are compressed, closed, and can be destroyed. As fluid continues to leak in more lung areas, fluid, protein, and blood cells collect in the alveoli and the interstitial space between the alveoli. The lymph channels are compressed and ineffective, poorly ventilated alveoli receive blood but cannot oxygenate it, which increases the shunt, resulting in hypoxemia and ventilation-perfusion (V/Q) mismatch results. Because the leading cause of death in ARDS is sepsis, all signs of sepsis should be reported to the health care provider immediately so that prompt interventions are implemented.

3. **Discuss the usual cause of refractory hypoxemia in ARDS.** The client with ARDS responds poorly to high concentrations of oxygen (refractory hypoxemia) and often requires intubation and mechanical ventilation. The usual cause of refractory hypoxemia in ARDS is intrapulmonary shunting, which occurs because there is no contact between air and blood. Therefore, no matter how much oxygen the client is breathing, gas exchange does not occur.

4. **Discuss the purpose and benefits for the positive-end expiratory pressure (PEEP) setting on the ventilator.** The client with ARDS and refractory hypoxemia requires a mechanical ventilator with PEEP setting. PEEP maintains the intraluminal airway pressure above atmospheric pressure throughout exhalation, which increases the functional residual capacity. It also helps to stabilize partially collapsed alveoli, and may even open up completely collapsed alveoli. The overall effect is the reestablishing of contact between oxygen in the alveolus and blood in the pulmonary capillary, enabling gas exchange to take place. PEEP also increases oxygen transport by decreasing the shunt and increasing the amount of oxygen in the blood.

5. **Discuss the significance of pulmonary capillary wedge pressure (PCWP) in diagnosing ARDS.** Some of the clinical signs and symptoms of ARDS are similar to those of cardiogenic pulmonary edema. Therefore, to rule-out cardiogenic pulmonary edema from ARDS, a PCWP is analyzed. In cardiogenic pulmonary edema, a PCWP reading may be above 18 mm Hg; a normal PCWP reading should be less than 12 mm Hg. In ARDS, the PCWP is usually low or within the normal range, which is 8–13 mm Hg. PCWP is the most accurate, indirect indicator of left ventricular end-diastolic pressure or left ventricular preload. Elevations of PCWP greater than 18–20 mm Hg indicate increased left ventricular pressure as in left ventricular failure, which may coincide with the onset of pulmonary congestion. If the pressure is more than 30 mm Hg, this is an indication of pulmonary edema. Low PCWP suggests insufficient volume and pressure in the left ventricle, and may be an indication of pending or present hypovolemic shock.

6. **What are common nursing diagnoses for clients with ARDS?**
   - Anxiety R/T hypoxemia, life-threatening illness, and loss of control
   - Impaired gas exchange R/T disrupted pulmonary ventilation and perfusion
   - Fatigue R/T hypoxemia and systemic inflammation
   - Disturbed sleep pattern R/T the intensive care unit environment
   - Imbalanced nutrition: less than body requirements R/T presence of endotracheal tube, chemical paralysis, increased metabolic rate
   - Risk for injury R/T elevated F_IO_2 or barotrauma
   - Potential for ventilator-associated pneumonia

The following are prescribed:

- Lactated Ringers 1,000 mLs at 125 mLs per hour
- Enoxaparin (Lovenox) injection 40 mg/0.4 ML SC daily

- Midazolam HcL (Versed) 0.02 mg/kg/h by continuous infusion
- Pancuronium bromide (Pavulon) 0.1 mg/kg IV initial dose
- Bumetanide (Bumex) 1 mg IV q6h for 24 hours

7. **What are the purposes for the prescribed orders?** *Lactated Ringers* is a volume-expanding fluid use to expand vascular fluid volume and maintain adequate cardiac output and tissue perfusion. Lactate ions convert to bicarbonate to effectively treat acidosis and replace and maintain electrolyte balance. By increasing intravascular volume, blood pressure increases. *Enoxaparin* prevents thrombus formation, pulmonary embolus, and slows or halts the process of disseminated intravascular coagulation, which may develop if ARDS worsens. Enoxaparin is a low molecular weight heparin that works by binding to a substance called antithrombin III, which turns off activated II, IX, and X and, in doing so, turns off the coagulation pathway and prevents clots from forming. *Midazolam HcL* is a benzodiazepine that provides sedation, which will decrease the client's anxiety, and in doing so decrease oxygen consumption, allowing the ventilator to provide full ventilatory support. *Pancuronium bromide* is a neuromuscular blocking agent that temporarily paralyzes the client's muscles, so that breathing is totally dependent on the ventilator. This reduces oxygen consumption because the client does not perform any work on his own, enhancing the hypoxemic state. *Bumetanide* is a loop diuretic that eliminates pulmonary fluid/congestion by acting on the proximal and distal ends of the tubule and ascending limb of the loop of Henle to increase excretion of sodium and water.

8. **What are the most common adverse reactions of the prescribed medications?** The most common adverse reaction of *Lactated Ringers infusion* is infusion rate-related fluid overload. The most common adverse effects of *enoxaparin sodium* are bruising at the injection site (especially if it is not administered at a 90-degree angle), anemia, and thrombocytopenia. The most common adverse reaction of *midazolam* is drowsiness. Other common adverse effects include coughing, changes in vital signs, headache, hiccups, nausea and vomiting, and phlebitis at the injection site. The most common adverse reactions of *pancuronium* are increased pulse rate and blood pressure, decreased mean arterial pressure (MAP), and airway closure resulting from relaxation of the epiglottis, pharynx, and tongue muscles. The most common adverse reactions of *bumetanide* are hypovolemia, dehydration, hypochloremia, hypokalemia, hyponatremia, hypomagnesium, and metabolic alkalosis.

9. **Discuss the drug-to-drug and drug-to-food/herbal interactions of the prescribed medications.** Drug-to-drug interactions may occur with the simultaneous use of *enoxaparin* and warfarin, salicylates, other nonsteroidal anti-inflammatory agents (NSAIDs), dipyridamole, some penicillins, clopidogrel, ticlopidine, abciximab, eftifibatide, tirofiban, thrombolytics and dextran, may alter platelet function and increase the risk of hemorrhage. There are no clinically significant drug-to-food interactions established. Drug-to-herbal interactions may occur with the simultaneous use of garlic, anise, arnica, chamomile, clove, ginger, gingko, feverfew, horse chestnut and Panax ginseng, which may increase the risk of bleeding. Drug-to-drug interactions may occur with the simultaneous use of intravenous *midazolam HcL* and alcohol, central nervous system (CNS) depressants, inhalation anesthetics, opioid analgesics phenothiazines, thiopental, tricyclic antidepressants, and anticonvulsants, which may potentiate CNS depression. Azole antifungals, cimetidine, diltiaze, verapamil, macrolide antibiotics, omeprazole, and ranitidine decrease the clearance of IV midazolam, thus increasing its effects. Protease inhibitors may increase risk of prolonged sedation. Use with ritonavir is contraindicated because of the high risk of life-threatening sedation and respiratory depression. Drug-to-drug interactions may occur with the simultaneous use of *pancuronium bromide* and inhalation anesthetics, chronic use of tricyclic antidepressants, aminoglycosides (e.g., gentamicin), bacitracin, colistin, colistimethate, polymixin-B, tetracyclines, calcium salts, diuretics, diazepam, digoxin, magnesium sulfate, quinidine, morphine, lidocaine, meperidine, propranalol, and succinylcholine, which potentiate the action of pancuronium and increase neuromuscular blocking and duration of action. Recurrent paralysis may be seen if used with quinidine. Concurrent use with acetylcholine, anticholinesterases, aminophylline, azathioprine, carbamazepine, and potassium decrease pancuronium's effects (Gahart and Nazareno, 898). There are no clinically significant drug-to-food/herbal interactions established. Drug-to-drug interactions may occur with the simultaneous use

of antihypertensives, nitrates, which increases hypotension. The simultaneous use with aminoglycosides, cisplatin may increase risk of ototoxicity. The simultaneous use with probenecid may antagonize diuretic activity, and there is increased risk for hypokalemia when used simultaneously with diuretics, piperacillin, amphotericin B, stimulant laxatives, and corticosteroids. There are no clinically significant drug-to-food/herbal interactions established. Drug-to-drug interactions may occur with the simultaneous use of *bumetanide* and antihypertensives, nitrates, which increases hypotension. The simultaneous use with aminoglycosides, cisplatin, and ethacrynic acid, which may increase risk of ototoxicity. The simultaneous use with probenecid may antagonize diuretic activity, and there is increased risk for hypokalemia when used simultaneously with diuretics, piperacillin, amphotericin B, stimulant laxatives, and corticosteroids. Acyclovir, aminoglycosides, ciprofloxacin, cyclosporine, and vancomycin increase the risk of nephrotoxicity. Bumetanide may increase the effects of anticoagulants and thrombolytics and if used with lithium may result in lithium toxicity. Cardiac dysrythmias may occur with concurrent use with amiodarone or digoxin and the risk of cardiotoxicity increases with pimozide and sparfloxacin (Gahart and Nazareno, 191). Bumetanide may cause hyperglycemia if used with insulin or sulfonylureas and bumetanide's effects may be inhibited by ACE inhibitors, NSAIDs, probenecid, and salicylates (for clients with cirrhosis or ascites). There are no clinically significant drug-to-food/herbal interactions established.

10. **Discuss essential nursing responsibilities when caring for mechanically ventilated clients on neuromuscular blockers.** The health care team assumes full responsibility for maintaining the client's ventilation, because if the client accidentally extubates or if the ventilator fails, apnea will occur. Ventilator and cardiac alarms must be correctly set and checked frequently for proper functioning, and the client should be under direct observation of a qualified, professional nurse at all times. A complete Ambu bag must be set up and ready for immediate use in case a ventilator failure or accidental extubation occurs.

References

Black, J.M. and Hawks, J.H. (2005). *Medical-Surgical Nursing: Clinical Management for Positive Outcomes* (7th ed.). Philadelphia: W.B. Saunders.

Broyles, B.E. (2005). *Medical-Surgical Nursing Clinical Companion.* Durham, NC: Carolina Academic Press.

Deglin, J.H. and Vallerand, A.H. (2005). *Davis's Drug Guide for Nurses* (9th ed.). Philadelphia: F.A. Davis.

Gahart, B.L. and Nazareno, A.R. (2005). *2005 Intravenous Medications.* St. Louis: Mosby.

Heitz, U. and Horne, M.M. (2005). *Mosby's Pocket Guide Series: Fluid, Electrolyte and Acid-Base Balance* (5th ed.). St. Louis: Mosby.

Huether, S.E. and McCance, K.L. (2004). *Understanding Pathophysiology* (3rd ed.). St. Louis: Mosby.

Ignatavicius, D.D. and Workman, M.L. (2006). *Medical-Surgical Nursing across the Health Care Continuum* (5th ed.). Philadelphia: W.B. Saunders.

Rothenhaus, T. (2003). "Acute Respiratory Distress Syndrome." Available at http://www.emedicine.com/EMERG/topic15.htm.

Spratto, G.R. and Woods, A.L. (2005). *2005 Edition: PDR Nurse's Drug Handbook.* Clifton Park, NY: Thomson Delmar Learning.

CASE STUDY 8

Acquired Immunodeficiency Syndrome

GENDER
- M

AGE
- 40

SETTING
- Hospital

ETHNICITY/CULTURE
- Hispanic American

PREEXISTING CONDITIONS
- HIV

COEXISTING CONDITIONS
- Peripheral neuropathy
- Hepatitis C
- Recurrent bacterial pneumonia

LIFESTYLE
- Cab driver for eight years

COMMUNICATION
- Spanish and English as a second language

DISABILITY

SOCIOECONOMIC STATUS
- Low

SPIRITUAL/RELIGIOUS
- Nondenominational

PHARMACOLOGIC
- Interferon alfa-2b (Intron A)
- Amikacin sulfate (Amikin)
- Bleomycin sulfate (Blenoxane)
- Nystatin (Mycostatin)
- Trimethoprim/sulfamethoxazole (Bactrim)

PSYCHOSOCIAL
- Fear

LEGAL
- Financial support
- Advance directives
- Counseling

ETHICAL
- Discrimination and denial have decreased national response to the AIDS epidemic. Strong, positive leadership for care and prevention is needed.

ALTERNATIVE THERAPY
- Aloe vera
- Echinacea

PRIORITIZATION
- Body substance isolation
- Confidentiality

DELEGATION
- RN
- LPN
- CNA

THE RESPIRATORY AND IMMUNE SYSTEMS

Level of difficulty: Difficult

Overview: This case involves thorough knowledge of the complexities of acquired immunodeficiency syndrome (AIDS) and is void of values that cloud professional approach to delegation of assignments and optimum care (i.e., immediate and general). The nurse must be familiar with the mix of medications usually prescribed for Persons With AIDS (PWAs). The licensed practical nurse (LPN) can administer medications as prescribed after the registered nurse (RN) has completed the initial assessment. The certified nursing assistant (CNA) can provide routine hygiene care and take vital signs, reporting abnormal readings to the LPN.

Client Profile

Mr. C is a 40-year-old male who was diagnosed with human immunodeficiency virus (HIV) five years ago and has been under outpatient medical supervision at a community health center affiliated with a medical center in the community in which he resides. Mr. C lives with his aunt, who is 68 years old and is his primary caregiver. Mr. C was seen in the outpatient clinic two weeks ago with complaints of nausea, vomiting, and diarrhea. Review of laboratory data and diagnostic studies from previous clinic visits indicate progression of the disease as evidenced by axilary adenopathy, decrease in CD+W cells of 300 mm^3, and oral candidiasis.

Case Study

Today Mr. C is seen in the outpatient clinic with complaints of severe diarrhea for two days, fever, and dry, productive cough. He reports being able to walk for approximately four feet without assistance but becomes extremely fatigued afterward. The nurse practitioner completes a history and physical examination and, after reviewing Mr. C's previous clinic records, refers him to the hospital for further evaluation and possible admission. At the hospital, Mr. C's vital signs are:

Blood pressure: 110/86
Pulse: 106
Respirations: 28 and shallow
Temperature: 102.6° F

He is sent from the admission's department to the AIDS unit and is assigned to a private room. Mr. C is placed on three liters of oxygen as per the unit's protocol. An arterial blood gas (ABG) is done and reveals:

pH: 7.35
pCO_2: 45
HCO_3: 28
pO_2: 78

The health care provider is notified, and the nurse initiates a brief history and physical, taking into consideration the physical and emotional state of the client. The nurse briefly discusses the Patient's Bill of Rights and the American Health Insurance Portability and Accountability Act of 1996 (HIPPA) with Mr. C and informs him that the documents will be given to him before the completion of the nurse's work schedule. Mr. C is seen by a health care provider who continues with the history and physical assessment then reviews Mr. C's medical records sent from the clinic, which include a diagnosis of AIDS. Current laboratory data from the clinic indicate values of: CD+4/CD8+ ratio less than 2 and CD4+ count of 200/mm^3, positive ELISA and Western Blot tests. Current blood cultures reveal Escherichia coli, Pseudomonas aeruginosa, and Klebsiella pneumoniae. After the multidisciplinary team reviews current data and physical assessment findings, an admitted with diagnosis is made for AIDS complicated with pneumocystis carinii pneumonia (PCP), cytomegalovirus (CMV) retinitis, Kaposi's sarcoma (KS), and oral candidiasis.

Questions and Suggested Answers

1. **Define PCP.** PCP is a common opportunistic infection that is common in persons with HIV. Pneumocystitis carinii is a microorganism that causes pneumocytosis, a type of interstitial cell pneumonitis.

2. **Discuss clinical manifestations of PCP associated with AIDS.** The pneumonia begins with a nonproductive cough, progressing to a productive cough. Eventually the client has fever and dyspnea on exertion, then dyspnea at rest.

3. **Discuss the enteric pathogen that may occur in the stool of the client with AIDS.** *Salmonella species* invade the intestinal mucosa of the small bowel or colon, producing microscopic ulceration, bleeding, fluid exudate, and water and electrolyte loss. In the client with AIDS, salmonella species can result in AIDS wasting syndrome. Salmonellosis refers to food poisoning caused by ingesting raw or improperly cooked meat, poultry, eggs, and dairy products contaminated with Salmonella bacteria. The person may experience diarrhea that is violent with abdominal cramping, nausea, and vomiting. Treatment of symptoms includes trimethoprim-sulfamethoxazole, ampicillin, or ciprofloxacin for severe illness.

4. **Discuss the two cytokines that play important role in AIDS-related wasting syndrome.** *Tumor necrosis factor (TNF)* is one of the predominant factors that aid in the control of the macrophage response to inflammation. *Interleukin-1 (IL-1)* is a protein with numerous immune systems functions, including activation of resting T cells, endothelial cells, and macrophages; mediation of inflammation, and stimulation of the synthesis of lymphokines, collagen, and collagenase. The combination of TNF and IL-1 aids in providing a powerful feedback mechanism that control macrophage and neutrophil responses. The combination is involved in the initiation of tissue inflammation and proceeds to form large numbers of defensive white blood cells that help remove the cause of the inflammation.

5. **The Centers for Disease Control and Prevention (CDC) has included Kaposi's sarcoma (KS) in the classification of AIDS-related malignancies. Discuss how KS diagnosis is confirmed.** KS diagnosis is confirmed by biopsy of suspected lesions, and the prognosis depends on the extent of the tumor, presence of constitutional symptoms, and CD4 count. It is often the presenting symptom of disease. KS affects homosexual males with AIDS predominantly, occurring much less commonly in injection drug users and heterosexuals. At this time, the reason for the discrepancy is unknown. It presents as a vascular macules, papules, or violet lesions affecting the skin and viscera. The face is a common site for skin lesions, especially the tip of the nose and pinnae of the ears. Common sites of visceral disease include the gastrointestinal (GI) tract, lungs, and lymphatic system.

6. **Discuss priority nursing diagnoses associated with AIDS.**

   - Ineffective breathing pattern R/T congestion and weakness secondary to PCP, pulmonary KS, tuberculosis, mycobacterium avium complex – Nurses need to assess the client's respiratory status, maintaining a patent airway at all times, and administer prescribed oxygen to supplement oxygen needs. The head of the bed must be elevated and the client monitored frequently to lessen anxiety during times of dyspnea.
   - Activity intolerance R/T fatigue, weakness, anemia, arthralgia, myalgia, dyspnea, fever, malnutrition, or motor dysfunction secondary to neurologic disease – A change in activity tolerance becomes a common finding as AIDS progresses. Nurses must assess the client's need for sleep and rest and assist the client with activities of daily living (ADLs). The client should be encouraged to eat and maintain an adequate dietary intake during periods of activity intolerance. The client must be taught energy conservation measures, and nurses should anticipate the client's needs to help with energy conservation.
   - Pain R/T lymphadenopathy, peripheral neuropathy, lymphedema secondary to KS, lymphoma, severe myalgia, headache secondary to central nervous system infection and psychogenic pain related to fear and anxiety over death – The pain experienced by clients with AIDS needs to be carefully assessed. Although clients with AIDS are expected to waste away without significant painful experiences, nurses need to perform a thorough pain assessment in collaboration with the pain management team, so that appropriate pain relief will be implemented.
   - Knowledge deficit R/T transmission of the disease and the need for proper nutrition, adequate rest and exercise, and good health practices – Nursing care of asymptomatic AIDS clients includes education strategies aimed at reducing the risk of transmission. This includes safe sex, counseling, avoidance of sharing of needles or instructions on cleaning the "works" (paraphernalia used in the injecting of drugs) or both, care of household items, and proper disposal of items soiled with body fluids. Health maintenance is also important at this stage, and includes instruction on maintaining adequate nutrition, weight management, exercise, and stress reduction.
   - Spiritual distress R/T terminal illness. Nursing care in the late stages focuses on palliative care, symptom management, and emotional support for the client, family, and significant others.

The following are prescribed:

- Interferon alfa-2b (Intron A) 20,000,000 IU/M² SC for five consecutive days pr week for four weeks
- Amikacin sulfate (Amikin) 7.5 mg/kg IV q12h
- Trimethoprim/sulfamethoxazole (Bactrim) 5mg/kg IV q6h for seven days and then PO q6h for seven days
- Bleomycin sulfate (Blenoxane) 0.5 U/kg IV × two weekly
- Nystatin suspension (Mycostatin) 500,000 U PO three times per day, swish and swallow
- Ondansetron 32 mg IV 30 minutes before bleomycin therapy
- Dextrose 5% in 0.45% normal saline at 125 mL/hr

7. **What are the purposes for the prescribed medications?** *Alfa-2b interferon* is a naturally occurring small proteins and glycoproteins that bind to specific membrane receptors on the cell surface initiating induction of immunological enzymes, suppression of cell proliferation, increasing phagocytic activity of the macrophages, inhibition of viral replication, and increasing cytotoxicity of lymphocytes for target cells (Gahart and Nazareno, 673) and used either intramuscular or subcutaneously in the treatment of Kaposi's sarcoma. ***Amikacin sulfate*** is an aminoglycoside that has been shown effective against E. coli, P. aeruginosa, and K. pneumoniae, which is currently in the client's blood as revealed by the blood culture. Amikacin works by inhibiting protein synthesis in bacterial cell, causing the organisms to die. ***Trimethoprim/sulfamethoxazole*** is an antibacterial and antiprotozoal combination and the agent of choice in the treatment of pneumocystic carinii pneumonia. In the hospitalized client, it is given intravenously and then orally when client is discharged. It is effective against both gram-positive and gram-negative organisms by blocking sequential steps in the folic acid pathways, preventing synthesis of required nucleic acid and proteins. ***Bleomycin sulfate*** is an antibiotic antineoplastic agent that provides systemic action on cancer cells such as those of Kaposi's sarcoma. It is beneficial in treating Kaposi's sarcoma, because it blocks DNA, RNA, and protein synthesis, preventing replication of cancer cells, and causes minimal myelosuppression. ***Nystatin suspension*** is an antifungal agent that rids the oral mucosa of the fungal infection (candidiasis). It does this by binding to sterol in fungal cell membrane, thereby changing membrane potential and allowing leakage of intracellular components. ***Ondansetron*** is an antiemetic $5HT_3$ receptor antagonist that prevents nausea and vomiting associated with the emetogenic effects of bleomycin sulfate. The ***IV infusion*** is to replace fluid loss and maintain fluid balance and provide access for medication therapy.

8. **What are the most common adverse reactions of the prescribed medications?** The most common adverse effects of *interferon alfa-2b* are common yet rapidly reversible following cessation of therapy and include alopecia, nausea, vomiting, anorexia, bleeding, coughing, diarrhea, dizziness, dyspnea, granulocytopenia, leukopenia, and thrombocytopenia. The most common adverse reactions of ***amikacin sulfate*** are ototoxicity, fever, headache, nausea and vomiting, paresthesias, skin rash, tremor, hypersensitivity, and vestibular dizziness. The most common adverse effects associated with the use of ***trimethoprim/sulfamethoxazole*** include nausea, vomiting, and rash, although allergic reactions do occur. The most common adverse reactions of ***bleomycin sulfate*** are alopecia, anorexia, chills, dyspnea, fever, hypotension, nausea, tumor site pain, weight loss, hyperpigmentation, and patchy hyperkeratosis. ***Nystatin suspension*** has few adverse effects including epigastric distress, nausea and vomiting, and diarrhea. The common adverse reactions of ***Ondansetron*** are infrequent but may include abdominal pain, constipation, cramps, diarrhea, headache, flushing, dyspnea, and cardiac dysrhythmias.

9. **Discuss the drug-to-drug and drug-to-food/herbal interactions of the prescribed medications.** With ***alfa-2b interferon,*** drug-to-drug interactions occur with simultaneous use of aminophylline by increasing the risk of aminophylline toxicity. Used concurrently with cisplatin, zidovudine, and other agents that cause myelosuppression may result in severe complications including life-threatening infections, bleeding, and anemia. No specific drug-to-food/herbal interactions have been established. Drug-to-drug interactions may occur with the simultaneous use of ***amikacin sulfate*** and other ototoxic or nephrotoxic agents and may produce additive effects if used concurrently with anesthetics, neuromuscular blocking agents, diuretics, and succinylcholine. The following agents potentiate aminoglycosides and include anticholinesterases, antineoplastics, balactam

antibiotics, and vancomycin. Chloramphenicol, erythromycin, and tetracyclines may antagonize the effects of amikacin. There are no clinically significant drug-to-food/herbal interactions established. With *trimethoprim/sulfamethoxazole,* drug-to-drug interactions may occur with the concurrent use of hydantoins and methotrexate and should not be used. It may be potentiated by probenecid and may inhibit cyclosporine, increasing the risk of nephrotoxicity. It may potentiate the action of dapsone, oral hypoglycemics, phenytoin, and zidovudine. Decreased serum levels of tricyclic antidepressants are seen when used with trimethoprim/sulfamethoxazole as well as decreasing treatment with leucovorin. The risk of leukopenia and thrombocytopenia is increased when used with busulfan, cisplatin, amphotericin B, and ganciclovir. Trimethoprim/sulfamethoxazole may increase serum levels increasing the risk of toxicity of digoxin, doxapram, nethyldopate, procainamide, and quinidine. If used with alatrofloxacin, amiodarone, erythromycin, and fluconazole, the risk of nephrotoxicity is increased. Concurrent use with rifampin decreases the serum levels of trimethoprim. No clinically significant drug-to-food/herbals interactions have been established. With *bleomycin sulfate,* drug-to-drug interactions may occur with the simultaneous use of other antineoplastic agents, which may increase bone marrow toxicity. Simultaneous use of digoxin and phenytoin may decrease absorption of these agents and decrease serum levels. There are no clinically significant drug-to-food/herbal interactions established. There are no clinically significant drug-to-drug or drug-to-food/herbal interactions established for *nystatin suspension.*

With *ondansetron,* no specific drug-to-drug interactions requiring dose adjustments have been seen. However, in rare cases, decreased effects of ondansetron have been seen when used simultaneously with rifampin. There are no clinically significant drug-to-food/herbal interactions established.

10. **Discuss how the nurse can promote home- and community-based care.** The client, families, and significant others are instructed about the routes of transmission of HIV. The client is taught about precautions to prevent transmitting HIV (e.g., using condom during vaginal or anal intercourse; using dental dams or avoiding oral sex). The client is taught to avoid multiple sexual partners, individuals known to be HIV infected, people who use injection drugs, and sexual partners of people who inject drugs. Guidelines about infection and infection control, follow-up care, diet, rest, and activity should be emphasized. Personal hygiene should be discussed clearly, and those with pets should have another person clean areas soiled by the animals. The client with AIDS, or with partners who are HIV positive, should be reminded not to donate blood. The client and family should be encouraged to discuss end-of-life decisions, and to ensure that care is consistent with those decisions. Referrals to AIDS support resources should be made available for the client.

References

Black, J.M. and Hawks, J.H. (2005). *Medical-Surgical Nursing: Clinical Management for Positive Outcomes.* Philadelphia: W.B. Saunders.

Broyles, B.E. (2005). *Medical-Surgical Nursing Clinical Companion.* Durham, NC: Carolina Academic Press.

Corbet, J.V. (2004). *Laboratory Tests and Diagnostic Procedures with Nursing Diagnoses* (6th ed.). Upper Saddle River, NJ: Prentice Hall.

Deglin, J.H. and Vallerand, A.H. (2005). *Davis's Drug Guide for Nurses* (9th ed.). Philadelphia: F.A. Davis.

Gahart, B.L. and Nazareno, A.R. (2005). *2005 Intravenous Medications.* St. Louis: Mosby.

Huether, S.E. and McCance, K.L. (2004). *Understanding Pathophysiology* (3rd ed.). St. Louis: Mosby.

Ignatavicius, D.D. and Workman, M.L. (2006). *Medical-Surgical Nursing across the Health Care Continuum* (5th ed.). Philadelphia: W.B. Saunders.

Libster, M. (2002). *Delmar's Integrative Herb Guide for Nurses.* Albany: Thomson Delmar Learning.

Lilley, L.L., Harrington, S., and Synder, J.S. (2005). *Pharmacology and the Nursing Process* (4th ed.). St. Louis: Mosby.

Skidmore-Roth, L. (2006). *Mosby's Handbook of Herbs & Natural Supplements* (3rd ed.). St. Louis: Mosby.

Spratto, G.R. and Woods, A.L. (2005). *2005 Edition: PDR Nurse's Drug Handbook.* Clifton Park, NY: Thomson Delmar Learning.

PART THREE

The Cardiovascular and Lymphatic Systems

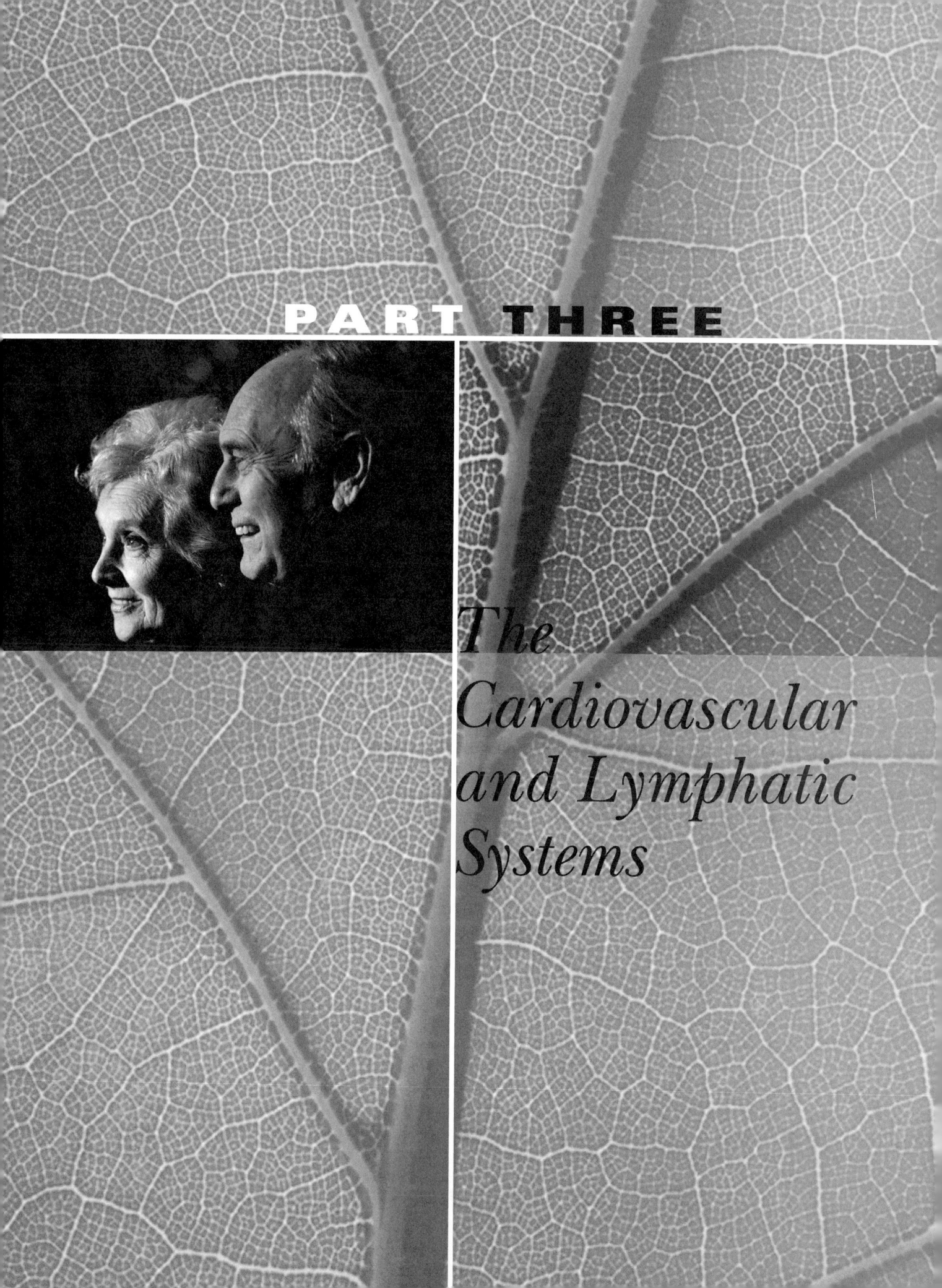

CASE STUDY 1

Primary (Essential) Hypertension

GENDER
- M

AGE
- 65

SETTING
- Hospital emergency department

ETHNICITY/CULTURE
- Black American

PREEXISTING CONDITIONS
- High blood pressure

COEXISTING CONDITIONS
- Family history: mother with history of hypertension died at age 70

LIFESTYLE
- Part-time school bus driver. Work hours are 11:00–3:00, three days per week.
- Diet includes moderate amount of sodium

COMMUNICATION

DISABILITY

SOCIOECONOMIC STATUS
- Low

SPIRITUAL/RELIGIOUS
- Baptist

PHARMACOLOGIC
- Furosemide (Lasix)
- Captopril (Capoten)
- Hydrochlorothiazide (HydroDIURIL)
- Spironolactone (Aldactone)
- Ezetimibe (Zetia)

PSYCHOSOCIAL
- Anxiety

LEGAL

ETHICAL

ALTERNATIVE THERAPY
- Listens to different kinds of music

PRIORITIZATION
- Interview
- Physical examination
- Evaluation of information
- Accurate monitoring of blood pressure

DELEGATION
- RN
- Client education

EASY

THE CARDIOVASCULAR AND LYMPHATIC SYSTEMS

Level of difficulty: Easy

Overview: This case involves understanding essential hypertension, monitoring blood pressure, administering prescribed medications, and clarifying the client's understanding of the disease. The case also involves client education and discharge planning with emphasis on follow-up care at the clinic or primary health care provider.

Client Profile

Mr. J is a 65-year-old male who has been visiting his primary health care provider yearly for annual examinations specifically related to history of mild congested heart failure (CHF). Over the past year, Mr. J notices that he gets infrequent headaches even though he is not stressed. Mr. J is 5'5" and weighs 240 pounds.

Case Study

Mr. J reports a family history of hypertension and was diagnosed with primary hypertension at the age of 64. He reveals he likes foods that are high in sodium content. His father is alive and well, but his mother died at age 70 from a cerebral vascular accident related to hypertension. His social history reveals alcohol consumption of beer during the day and a glass of wine at dinner. Mr. J is seen by a nurse practitioner (NP) at the community clinic for complaints of headache and dizziness, which he reports experiencing while shopping at a department store. Upon admission, his vital signs are:

- Blood pressure: 190/110
- Pulse: 104 and regular
- Respirations: 18
- Temperature: 98.4° F

He is transferred to the local hospital's emergency department (ED) for further evaluation. On arrival at the ED, he is seen by an NP who initiates a systems assessment and finds his blood pressure reading to be 180/110 × two readings with the use of appropriate blood pressure cuff size. Mr. J reports current medications of captopril and metoprolol tartrate. He is kept in the ED for three hours on continuous telemetry while awaiting a bed on a medical unit. He is later transferred to a medical unit for further evaluations. Lab values are prescribed and include: urine for urinalysis, complete blood count, serum potassium (K+), sodium (Na), glucose, blood urea nitrogen (BUN), creatinine, cholesterol and triglyceride levels, serum aldosterone, and 24-hour urine aldosterone. His body mass index (BMI) is done and is 35, indicating that Mr. J is moderately obese for his height. The following are Mr. J's laboratory results:

- Urinalysis: negative
- White blood cell (WBC) count: 8,500 cells/mm^3
- Hematocrit (Hct): 33%
- Hemoglobin (Hgb): 15 g/dL
- Platelet count: 150,000 cells/mm^3
- Glucose: 80 mg/dL
- Blood urea nitrogen (BUN): 14 mg/dL
- Creatinine: 1.2 mg/dL
- Potassium (K+): 3.7 mEq/L
- Sodium (Na): 158 mEq/L
- Albumin: 3.4 gm/dL
- Calcium: 9 mg/dL
- Cholesterol: 218 mg/dL
- Triglyceride: 180 mg/dL
- Urine aldosterone: 30 ug/24 hr
- Serum aldosterone: 28 ng/dL

A fundoscopic examination of the eyes is done and indicates the retinal structures of the eyes are within normal limits. A 12-lead electrocardiogram (EKG) shows sinus rhythm, and a chest X-ray reveals normal heart size and normal lung structures. The dietitian sees the client and performs a three-day dietary recall, and plans to suggest a two-gram sodium diet to the multidisciplinary team. After the health care provider, pharmacist, NP, RN, and dietitian review the diagnostic tests and the laboratory data, a diagnosis of primary hypertension is confirmed.

Questions and Suggested Answers

1. **What are specific cultural considerations in the United States for hypertension?** In the United States, as many as 50 million people experience hypertension. Hypertension affects one of every three black Americans and occurs most often in people over 35 years of age. Blood pressure management rates vary in minorities and are lowest in Mexican Americans and Native Americans/American Indians. One in four American adults has hypertension, and of those, 31.6% are not aware they have hypertension. Of those diagnosed, 14.6% are not receiving any treatment, 26.2% are receiving inadequate therapy, and 27.4% are using effective therapy. Socioeconomic and lifestyle factors may place significant barriers to controlling blood pressure in some minorities. There is a higher prevalence, incidence, and impact of hypertension among black individuals who also have a decreased treatment response with beta blockers, angiotensin-converting enzyme (ACE) inhibitors, or angiotensin receptor blockers when compared with diuretics or calcium-channel blockers.

2. **What are some common nursing diagnoses for clients with hypertension?**

    - Ineffective health maintenance R/T lack of knowledge of pathology, complications, and management of hypertension
    - Anxiety R/T complexity of management regimen, possible complications, and lifestyle changes associated with hypertension
    - Sexual dysfunction R/T effects of antihypertensive medication
    - Ineffective therapeutic regimen management R/T lack of knowledge, inconvenient schedule for taking medications, unpleasant side effects of medications.

3. **After the diagnosis of essential hypertension is confirmed with initial studies, what further evaluations are necessary?** After the confirmation of essential hypertension, further assessment is needed to determine additional risk factors for cardiovascular disease and the evaluating of factors to guide the selection of appropriate therapy and establishment of a baseline treatment. Further assessment of target organ damage such as the kidney should be evaluated, and renal function tests and cardiovascular screening tests should be included in the evaluating process to guide management effectively.

4. **What is the purpose of the registered dietitian in the multidisciplinary team conference with the client who is diagnosed with essential hypertension?** The dietitian usually reviews a three-day dietary recall with the client to identify whether sodium intake has been excessive and utilizes the information gathered to instruct the client on ways of lowering sodium intake in meals. The dietitian also uses the report of the BMI when discussing the reason for reducing and maintaining weight according to body frame. The Joint National Committee on Prevention, Detection, Evaluation, and Treatment of High Blood Pressure recommends a treatment plan based on cardiovascular disease risk factors, the presence or absence of target organ damage, and blood pressure levels. Emphasis is placed on adherence to the treatment plan to prevent long-term consequences of hypertension (e.g., stroke, heart failure, and renal failure). It is important for the dietitian to include during the conference the need for gradual lifestyle modification such as weight reduction, sodium restriction, dietary fat reduction, exercise, relaxation techniques, monitoring of blood pressure, and compliance with follow-up care.

The following are prescribed:

- Furosemide (Lasix) 40 mg IV stat
- Captopril (Capoten) 25 mg PO three times per day
- Hydrochlorothiazide (HydroDIURIL) 12.5 mg PO daily

- Spironolactone (Aldactone) 50 mg PO two times per day
- Ezetimibe (Zetia) 10 mg PO daily
- Two-gram sodium diet

5. **What are the purposes for the prescribed medications?** *Furosemide* is a loop diuretic that aids in the removal of excess sodium from the body, which is a major causative factor in hypertension. Furosemide inhibits reabsorption of sodium and chloride primarily in Henle's loop but also in the proximal and distal renal tubules. When sodium and chloride reabsorption is inhibited, intravascular volume is decreased and blood pressure is stabilized.

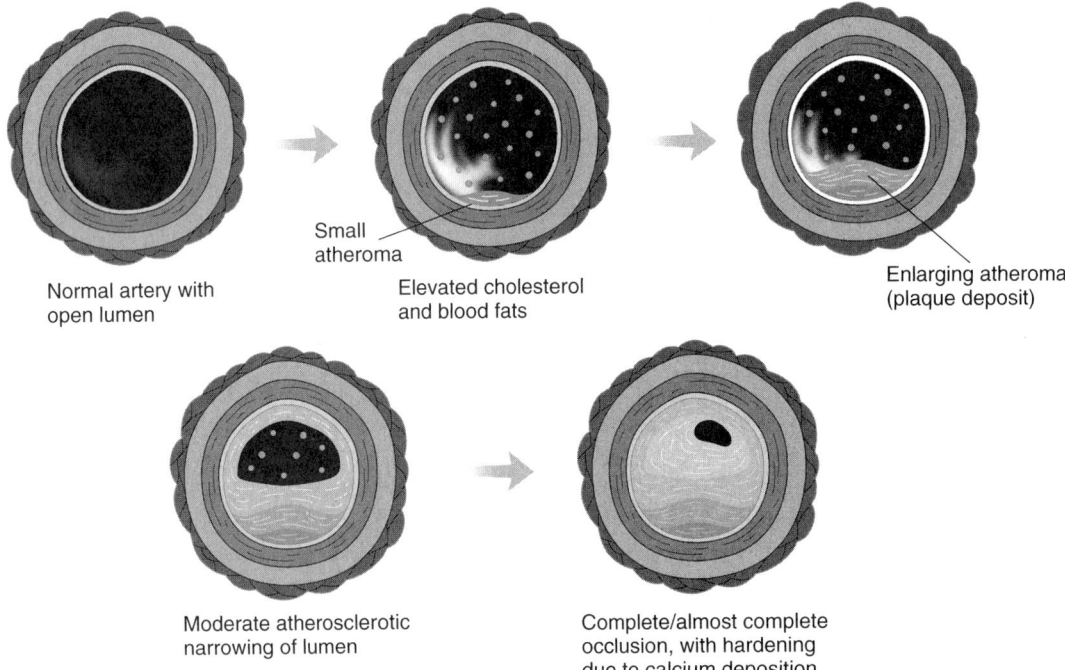

Normal artery with open lumen

Elevated cholesterol and blood fats — Small atheroma

Enlarging atheroma (plaque deposit)

Moderate atherosclerotic narrowing of lumen

Complete/almost complete occlusion, with hardening due to calcium deposition

Captopril is an antihypertensive agent that lowers blood pressure by specific inhibition of ACE, which is a major factor in hypertensive disease. Inhibition of the enzyme will help maintain blood pressure at a satisfactory level. *Hydrochlorothiazide* is a thiazide diuretic that aids in lowering blood pressure by interfering with the absorption of sodium ions across the distal renal tubular segment of the nephron. This action enhances excretion of sodium, chloride, and water, which helps to lower the pressure. *Spironolactone* is a potassium-sparing diuretic that retains potassium in the blood that helps to counteract the potassium-wasting effects of the furosemide and hydrochlorothiazide. Spironolactone helps to lower blood pressure by inhibiting aldosterone, since aldosterone is an active mineralocorticoid hormone that functions to increase sodium reabsorption by the kidneys and aids in regulating blood pressure. *Ezetimibe* lowers cholesterol by working at the lining of the small intestine inhibiting the absorption of cholesterol but does not inhibit cholesterol synthesis in the liver or increase bile acid excretion. Ezetimibe is an antilipidemic agent that decreases the amount of cholesterol available to the liver. Although cholesterol is a component of all cell membranes and intracellular organelles, high cholesterol levels cause substantial morbidity and mortality, requiring aggressive treatment to decrease morbidity and mortality. Consistent abnormally high cholesterol levels can result in hypertension and, eventually, vascular changes. When cholesterol levels remain elevated without treatment, plaques form in the arterial system and occlude vessels. A growing mass of plaque eventually narrows the lumen of the vessels and impedes blood flow to the vascular system. Over a period of time, destruction of the vascular system especially in the lower extremities develops, resulting in complications and need for surgical interventions. Consistently elevated cholesterol also results in hypertrophy of arterial smooth muscle, which over a period of time permanently narrows vessel lumens, resulting in failure of the vascular tone to return to normal. When peripheral resistance remains high, the vascular system is destroyed. A *two-gram sodium diet* helps maintain and stabilize blood pressure because the decreased sodium intake results in decreased water retention, and therefore, blood pressure decreases.

6. **What are the most common adverse reactions of the prescribed medications?** The most common adverse reactions of *furosemide* are hypokalemia, hypotension, dehydration, hyponatremia, hypomagnesemia, hypovolemia, and metabolic alkalosis. The most common adverse reactions of *captopril* are hypotension, cough, ataxia, drowsiness, and maculopapular rash with pruritis. The most common adverse reactions of *hydrochlorothiazide* are hypotension, hyperglycemia, hyperuricemia, and hypokalemia. The most common adverse reaction of *spironolactone* is hyperkalemia. The most common adverse reactions of *ezetimibe* include diarrhea, abdominal pain, headache, and dizziness.

7. **Discuss drug-to-drug and drug-to-food/herbal interactions for the prescribed medications.** Drug-to-drug interactions may occur with the simultaneous use of *furosemide* and other diuretics, which may enhance diuretic effects. The simultaneous use of digoxin, piperacillin, stimulant laxatives, and corticosteroids may increase the risk for hypokalemia and dysrhythmias. The simultaneous use of amphotericin B potentiates hypokalemia. The simultaneous use with insulin blunts the effects of hypoglycemia. The simultaneous use with aminoglycosides increases the risk of ototoxicity, and its use with warfarin or thrombolytic agents may increase the anticoagulant effect. Hydantoins, such as phenytoin, decrease the diuretic effects of furosemide, and clofibrate enhances its diuretic effect. Charcoal decreases the absorption of furosemide from the gastrointestinal (GI) tract. There are no clinically significant drug-to-herbal interactions established. Drug-to-drug interactions may occur with the simultaneous use of *captopril* and nitrates, diuretics, and antihypertensive, which enhances hypotensive effects. The simultaneous use of potassium-sparing diuretics (i.e., spironolactone and amiloride) increases potassium levels. The simultaneous use of probenecid decreases the elimination, and increases toxic effects. Drug levels of captopril may decrease used concurrently with corticosteroids, doxycycline, felbamate, quinidine, warfarin, estrogen-containing contraceptives, barbiturates, cyclosporine, benzodiazipines, theophylline, lamotrigine, valproic acid, bupropion, and haloperidol. Concurrent use with monoamine oxidase (MAO) inhibitors may result in hyperpyrexia, hypertension, seizures and death. Simultaneous use with verapamil, diltiazem, propoxyphene, erythromycin, clarithromycin, antidepressants, or cimetidine may increase captopril levels and risk of toxicity. Drug-to-food interactions occur with foods that decrease absorption of the drug such as with grapefruit juice. There are no clinically significant drug-to-herbal interactions established. Drug-to-drug interactions may occur with the simultaneous use of *hydrochlorothiazide* and amphotericin B, corticosteroids, piperacillin, or ticarcillin, which may increase hypokalemic effects and the simultaneous use with cholestyramine and colestipol may decrease thiazide absorption. Simultaneous use of kava, valerian, skullcap, chamomile, or hops can increase central nervous system (CNS) depression. Simultaneous use of licorice and stimulant laxative herbs (aloe, cascara sagrada, senna) may increase the risk of potassium depletion. Concomitant use with gingko may decrease antihypertensive effects. Drug-to-drug interactions may occur with the simultaneous use of *spironolactone* and other antihypertensives or nitrates that may increase hypotension. Simultaneous use with ACE inhibitors, angiotensin II receptor antagonists, indomethacin, potassium supplements, or cyclosporin may increase the risk of hyperkalemia. The simultaneous use with ammonium chloride, which may produce systemic acidosis, and concurrent use with didanosine may increase the risk of pancreatitis, while its use with digoxin increases the effects of digoxin and increase risk of toxicity. Aspirin may antagonize diuretic effects of spironolactone, and hyperkalemia may occur if potassium supplements are used simultaneously with spironolactone. The simultaneous use with zidovudine may cause antiretrovial antagonism. Drug-to-food interactions may occur with the simultaneous use of salt substitutes, which may increase the risk of hyperkalemia. There are no clinically significant drug-to-herbal interactions established. Drug-to-drug interactions may occur with the simultaneous use of *ezetimibe* and cholestyramine and/or antacids, which may decrease absorption. Ezetimibe should be taken two hours before or four hours after bile acid sequestrant drugs. The simultaneous use with cyclosporine or fenofibrate/gemfibrozil can significantly increase ezetimibe levels. There are no clinically significant drug-to-food/herbal interactions established.

8. **What is the ultimate goal of antihypertensive therapy?** The ultimate goal is to decrease cardiovascular mortality and morbidity by maintaining systolic blood pressure to less than 130 mm Hg and diastolic blood pressure to less than 90 mm Hg. Prevention and promotion of lifestyle changes such as weight loss, exercise, smoking cessation, reduction of stress, and the limiting of saturated fat in the diet will aid in the accomplishing of the ultimate goal. Because the ultimate goal cannot be achieved unless the client understands the disease process, its treatment, the need for participation in a self-care program, and the absence of complications, client education must focus on blood pressure monitoring, purpose and adverse effects of prescribed drugs, and the need for compliance. Emphasis should be placed on the need to seek medical attention immediately if there is edema of the hands and feet, and sudden weight gain.

9. **Discuss the effects of angiotensin-converting enzyme (ACE) on hypertension and nursing priority of care when caring for clients taking ACE inhibitor agents.** ACE reduces arterial pressure, primarily by decreasing total peripheral resistance without reflexively increasing cardiac output, contractility, or rate. ACE inhibitors are particularly helpful in conditions where hypertension is dependent upon renin-angiotensin II, such as with essential hypertension associated with high plasma renin activity and renal arterial disease. Clients using ACE inhibitors must be screened for renal arterial disease because in renal arterial disease, intrarenal compensatory mechanisms are absent or suppressed. Nurses should monitor serum creatinine and potassium levels before initiating ACE inhibitor therapy in clients with renal insufficiency.

10. **What are some complementary modalities clients with hypertension may use to decrease blood pressure?** Some complementary modalities to help decrease blood pressure in clients with hypertension include yoga, massage therapy, biofeedback, music therapy, and hypnosis. Because of the relationship between stress and hypertension, any activity that decreases stress will help decrease the blood pressure. The techniques of yoga seek to bring into balance the body, mind, and personality so that the client achieves energy, strength, and clarity of purpose by the whole being. Massage therapy includes benefits such as the increase of circulation to muscles and organs, and the flushing out of waste products such as lactic acid, and allowing oxygen in the blood to nourish the body cells. Massage therapy stimulates sensory receptors in the soft tissues and increases lymphatic flow. Massage may act directly on the source of pain to alleviate nociceptive stimulation, or act centrally to alter the processing of nociceptive input or to affect conduction of pain impulses in peripheral nerves.

11. **Discuss client education for a captopril (Capoten) prescription upon discharge to home.** Clients taking captopril should be provided with verbal and written instructions concerning the drug's use. This includes the dosage, frequency of administration, adverse effects, and potential drug or food interactions. The client should take captopril one hour before meals, on an empty stomach because food interferes with the drug's absorption. The client should report any of the following to the health care provider: onset of unexplained fever, unusual fatigue, sore mouth or throat, easy bleeding, or bruising. The client should consult health care access immediately if vomiting or diarrhea occurs. Impairment in taste may occur but usually reverses in two to three months, even with continued therapy. The client should be given a contact phone number and person they can call with questions. Stress the importance of compliance with therapy and of notifying the primary health care provider about plans to take over-the-counter medications with captopril.

References

American Heart Association. www.americanheart.org.

Corbet, J.V. (2004). *Laboratory Tests and Diagnostic Procedures with Nursing Diagnoses* (6th ed.). Upper Saddle River, NJ: Prentice Hall:

Broyles, B.E. (2005). *Medical-Surgical Nursing Clinical Companion.* Durham, NC: Carolina Academic Press.

Gahart, B.L. and Nazareno, A.R. (2005). *2005 Intravenous Medications.* St. Louis: Mosby.

Huether, S.E. and McCance, K.L. (2004). *Understanding Pathophysiology* (3rd ed.). St. Louis: Mosby.

Ignatavicius, D.D. and Workman, M.L. (2006). *Medical-Surgical Nursing across the Health Care Continuum* (5th ed.). Philadelphia: W.B. Saunders.

Spratto, G.R. and Woods, A.L. (2005). *2005 Edition: PDR Nurse's Drug Handbook.* Clifton Park, NY: Thomson Delmar Learning.

CASE STUDY 2

Coronary Artery Disease (Atherosclerosis)

GENDER
- F

AGE
- 68

SETTING
- Hospital's outpatient clinic

ETHNICITY/CULTURE
- White American

PREEXISTING CONDITIONS
- Obesity

COEXISTING CONDITIONS
- Peripheral vascular disease

LIFESTYLE
- Unemployed

COMMUNICATION

DISABILITY

SOCIOECONOMIC STATUS
- Low

SPIRITUAL/RELIGIOUS
- Anglican

PHARMACOLOGIC
- Lipid-lowering agents
- Diuretics
- Cardiotonic
- Vasodilator
- Calcium-channel blocker
- Anticoagulant

PSYCHOSOCIAL
- Anxiety

LEGAL
- Financial resources

ETHICAL

ALTERNATIVE THERAPY

PRIORITIZATION
- Accurate systems assessment
- Continuous telemetry

DELEGATION
- RN
- LPN
- Client education

EASY

THE CARDIOVASCULAR AND LYMPHATIC SYSTEMS

Level of difficulty: Easy

Overview: The nurse will elicit appropriate nursing history to more accurately identify appropriate nursing diagnoses. The nurse also will use critical-thinking skills in identifying the client's immediate needs during triage. Client education is important before discharge from the hospital.

Client Profile

Ms. Z is a 68-year-old female who is 5'5" and weighs 248 pounds. Her cardiologist refers her to the clinic of the community hospital after several complaints of fatigue and decrease in energy over the past month.

Case Study

Ms. Z is seen in the hospital outpatient clinic following the cardiologist's referral. She denies chest pain or palpitations on admission but reports frequent episodes of dizziness and inability to concentrate for "long periods of time." Her past medical history (PMH) includes hypercholesterolemia, chronic atrial fibrillation, episodes of syncope, occasional anginal type pain, and peripheral vascular disease (PVD). Past surgical history (PSH) includes a right femoral popliteal bypass. On initial assessment at the clinic, a complete physical examination is done and reveals bruits on auscultation of the left carotid artery. An electrocardiogram (EKG) shows atrial fibrillation. Her vital signs are:

- Blood pressure: 170/100
- Pulse: 78 and irregular
- Respirations: 20
- Temperature: 98.4° F

Lab reports from the clinic reveal:

- Prothrombin time (PT): 13.4 seconds, Control: 12.9 seconds
- Partial thromboplastin time (PTT): 30 seconds, Control: 29.9 seconds
- Glucose: 109 mg/dL
- Blood urea nitrogen (BUN): 9 mg/dL
- Creatinine: 0.8 mg/dL
- Sodium (Na): 136 mEq/L
- Potassium (K+): 3.9 mEq/L
- Calcium: 9 mg/dL
- Protein total: 7.8 g/dL
- Albumin: 3.2 g/dL
- Total bilirubin: 0.6
- White blood cell (WBC) count: 10,300/mm^3
- Red blood cell (RBC) count: 4.26 million/mm^3
- Hemoglobin (Hgb): 11.7 g/dL
- Hematocrit (Hct): 34.6%
- Platelet count: 258,000/mm^3
- Low-density lipoprotein (LDL): 127 mg/dL
- High-density lipoprotein (HDL): 46 mg/dL
- Total cholesterol: 257 mg/dL
- Triglyceride: 220 mg/dL

Medications taken at home are brought to the clinic and include: simvastatin, felodipine, lisinopril, hydrochlorothiazide, and aspirin 325 mg (EC). Carotid duplex ultrasonography is done and reveals marked narrowing of proximal left external carotid artery with area of plaque noted. Her ejection fraction is 30%. Magnetic resonance imaging (MRI) is done and compared with carotid duplex ultrasonography; the results are similar. After a complete history and physical and review of serum labs and diagnostic studies, the diagnosis of atherosclerosis is confirmed.

Ms. Z will be discharged to home and will return to the hospital as scheduled for possible carotid endarterectomy after reevaluation of current medication regimen and repeat carotid duplex ultrasonography. Ms. Z is referred to physical therapy for physical strengthening exercises.

Questions and Suggested Answers

1. **What are the most common cited coronary artery disease risk equivalents for atherosclerosis?**

   - Diabetes mellitus is a common risk equivalent of atherosclerosis because of the higher blood lipids and obesity that occurs, especially with type 2 diabetes mellitus. In addition, diabetes affects blood vessels, contributing to the process of atherosclerosis. In the presence of hyperglycemia, altered platelet function and elevated fibrinogen levels that eventually present themselves as the disease progresses enhance the risk for atherosclerosis.
   - Peripheral arterial disease is a common risk equivalent of atherosclerosis because it is a process that slowly occludes arterial flow of blood. The atherosclerotic process slowly starves the tissues of oxygenated blood, and gradually, complete occlusion of medium and large arteries develops, enhancing the risk of atherosclerosis.
   - Abdominal aortic aneurysm is another risk equivalent of atherosclerosis because of its risk factors such as cigarette smoking and hypertension, both of which initially cause narrowing of arteries, which alters blood in arteries, and eventually arteries are damaged. Good cholesterol (high-density lipoprotein, HDL) then cannot flow to the body as it should, and bad cholesterol (low-density lipoprotein, LDL) builds up, enhancing the problem of atherosclerosis.

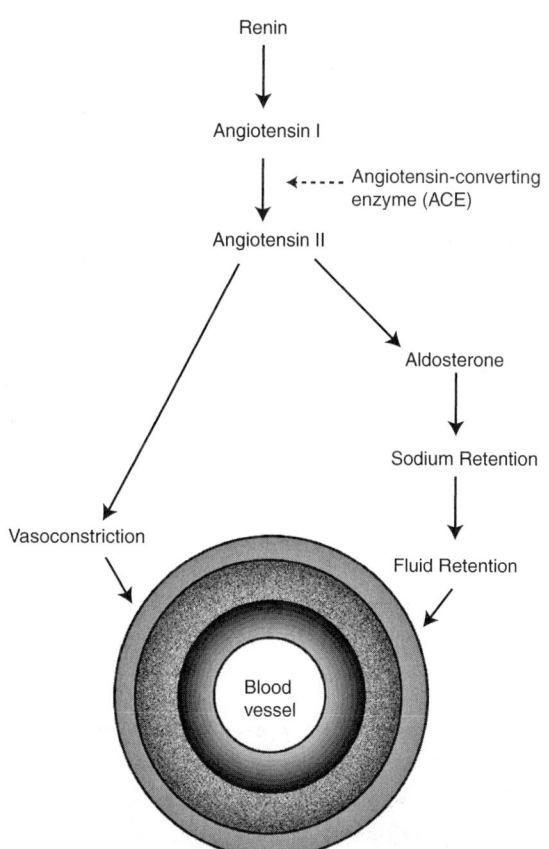

2. **What are prominent modifiable and nonmodifiable risk factors of atherosclerosis?** Prominent modifiable risk factors are environment, cigarette smoking, hypertension, elevated serum cholesterol, and diabetes. Prominent nonmodifiable risk factors include heredity, age, gender, and race.

3. **What are common nursing diagnoses for the client with atherosclerosis?**
   - Risk for altered tissue perfusion R/T fatty plaques
   - Altered nutrition: more than body requirements R/T intake of fats and calories
   - Deficient knowledge R/T condition, drug and diet therapy of hyperlipidemia, and home care.

The following are prescribed:

- Cholestyramine resin (Questran) 4 g PO four times per day, before meals
- Colestipol HcL (Colestid) 15 g two times per day, before meals and at bedtime
- Digoxin (Lanoxin) 0.125 mg PO daily
- Dipyridamole (Persantine) 75 mg PO four times per day
- Diltiazem HcL (Cardizem) 30 mg PO four times per day
- Warfarin sodium (Coumadin) 5 mg PO today

4. **What are the purposes for the prescribed medications?** *Choleystramine resin* is an antihyperlipidemic agent that prevents the reabsorption of the bile acids from the intestines. Because bile acids are necessary for the absorption of cholesterol, inhibiting the absorption of bile acids lowers the production of cholesterol levels and LDL cholesterol. *Colestipol HcL* also is an antihyperlipodemic agent that reduces the circulating cholesterol in the blood by binding with bile acids in the intestinal tract to form an insoluble complex that is excreted in the feces, lowering the cholesterol level. *Digoxin* is a positive inotropic cardiac glycoside that slows and strengthens cardiac contractility to promote better blood flow. This helps prevent stasis of blood that could cause clot formation. Digoxin helps control the ventricular rate, which improves ejection fraction. *Dipyridamole* is a platelet adhesion inhibitor (anti-platelet) that prevents platelet aggregation and slows the progression of atrial fibrillation. It prevents thromboxane A_2 formation, a substance that causes blood vessels to constrict and platelets to aggregate. When platelets do not aggregate, blood flow improves and tissue perfusion increases throughout the body. *Diltiazem HcL* is a calcium-channel blocking agent that lowers blood pressure by decreasing total peripheral vascular resistance and resulting in a reduction of arterial blood pressure. Further, it slows the progression of atrial fibrillation by dilating coronary artery and arterioles, resulting in better blood flow. *Warfarin sodium* is an anticoagulant that is used as prophylaxis for chronic atrial fibrillation. It inhibits clot formation and prevents clots from developing in the atria in the presence of incomplete emptying.

5. **What are the most common adverse reactions of the prescribed medications?** The most common adverse reaction of *choleystyramine* are abdominal discomfort, constipation, and nausea. The most common adverse reactions of *colestipol* are abdominal discomfort, heartburn, anorexia, flatulence, gastrointestinal (GI) bleeding, constipation, and nausea. The most common adverse reactions of *digoxin* are fatigue, bradycardia, anorexia, nausea and vomiting, diarrhea, pounding palpitations, visual disturbances, dizziness (due to decreased cardiac output), and digoxin toxicity. The most common adverse reactions of *dipyridamole* are headache, dizziness, hypotension, nausea, vomiting, diarrhea, abdominal pain, bruising, prolonged bleeding with breaks in skin or mucous membranes, and dyspesia. The most common adverse reactions of *diltiazem HcL* are headache, bradycardia, and peripheral edema. The most common adverse reaction of *warfarin sodium* is bleeding due to prolonged clotting.

6. **Discuss the drug-to-drug and drug-to-food/herbal interactions of the prescribed medications.** Drug-to-drug interactions may occur with the simultaneous use of *cholestyramine resin* and digoxin, oral anticoagulants, glipizide, imipramine, methyldopa, nicotinic acid, penicillin G, phenytoin, thiazide diuretics, thyroxine troglitazone, ursodiol, phosphate supplements, propranolol, tolbutamide, clofibrate, aspirin, furosemide, and tetracyclines by decreasing the absorption and effects of these drugs. Drug-to-food interactions may

occur with fat-soluble vitamins (A, D, E, K). Fat-soluble vitamins will be less efficiently absorbed, resulting in potential vitamin deficiencies. The simultaneous use of acetaminophen, amiodarone, gemfibrozil, corticosteroids, mycophenolate, methotrexate, nonsteroidal anti-inflammatory agents (NSAIDs), or warfarin may decrease the absorption of cholestyramine. There are no clinically significant drug-to-herbal interactions established. Drug-to-drug interactions may occur with the use of **colestipol HcL** and are basically the same as those with cholestyramine resin. There are no clinically significant drug-to-food/herbal interactions established. A wide variety of drug-to-drug interactions may occur with the simultaneous use of **digoxin** and loop and thiazide diuretics, which may increase digoxin-induced dysrhythmias. Angiotensin-converting enzymes (ACE) inhibitor medications may increase potassium levels and thereby decrease the therapeutic responses of digoxin. Sympathomimetics such as dobutamine increase the heart rate, which would further increase the contractile force of the myocardial muscle, since that is one of the properties of digoxin. Simultaneous use of digoxin and dobutamine would therefore enhance tachydysrhythmias. Quinidine, if used simultaneously with digoxin, can increase plasma levels of digoxin, which would displace digoxin from tissue binding sites, reducing renal excretion of digoxin, resulting in increase risk for digoxin toxicity. The simultaneous use of verapamil, a calcium-channel blocker, can significantly increase plasma levels of digoxin and counteracts the benefits of digoxin. Drug-to-herbal interactions may occur with the simultaneous use of hawthorn that contains natural cardiotonic ingredients. Hawthorn by itself increases the force of myocardial contraction and dilates blood vessels. The simultaneous use of hawthorn with digoxin increases the likelihood of toxic effects or the interference of the effectiveness of digoxin. If ginseng is taken with digoxin or oral antidiabetic agents, it may cause an increase in toxic effects of digoxin and hypoglycemia. If cascara sagrada is taken simultaneously with digoxin, it may increase potassium loss and toxic effects of digoxin. Drug-to-food interactions may occur if digoxin is taken simultaneously with high fiber meal. Drug-to-drug interactions will occur with the simultaneous use of **dipyridamole** and aspirin, anticoagulants, thrombolytic agents, NSAIDs, cefamandole, cefoperazone, cefotetan, plicamycin, valproic acid, and sulfinpyrazone, which will increase the risk of bleeding. The simultaneous use with theophylline may negate the effects of persantine during diagnostic thallium imaging. Evening primrose, feverfew, garlic, ginger, gingko biloba, ginseng, and grapeseed extract increase the antiplatelet effects of dipyridamole. Drug-to-drug interactions may occur with the simultaneous use of **diltiazem** and beta blockers, digoxin, disopyramide, or phenytoin, which may increase the metabolism of diltiazem and decrease its effectiveness. This also may have additive effects on the atrioventricular (AV) node conduction and cause prolongation of the AV node response. The simultaneous use of digoxin or quinidine may increase their levels, and the simultaneous use with cimetidine or ranitidine may increase diltiazem serum levels and increase toxicity. When used with amiodarone, a possible cardiotoxic effect may result. Diltiazem may increase serum levels of buspirone, cyclosporine, imipramine, methylprednisolone, moricizine, and theophyllines, resulting in increased risk of toxic effects of these agents. Drug-to-food interactions may occur with the simultaneous use of diltiazem and grapefruit juice. The list of drug-to-drug interactions with **warfarin sodium** is extensive. It includes interactions that may occur with the simultaneous use of heparin, thrombolytics, and NSAIDs, resulting in increased risk for hemorrhage. Use with antineoplastic agents, acetohexamide, acetaminophen, allopurinol, aminoglycosides, aminosalicylic acid, amiodarone, androgens, cephalosporines, chloral hydrate, chloramphenicol, cimetidine, clarithromycin, clofibrate, corticosteroids, celecoxib, cyclophosphamide, dextrothyroxine, diflunisal, moricizine, metronidazole, loop diuretics, ometrazole, hydantoins, hypoglycemic agents, indomethacin, penicillins, propafenone, propoxyphene, quinolones, thioamines, thyroid hormones, sulfonamides, tamoxifen, tetracyclines, and isoniazid also enhance bleeding tendencies by increasing warfarin's effects. A number of agents decrease the effects of warfarin, including cholestyramine, barbiturates, alcohol, dicloxacillin, etretinate, glutethimide, griseofulvin, nafcillin, rifampin, ritonavir, spironolactone, sucralfate, thiopurines, and trazodone. Drug-to-food interactions may occur with the simultaneous use of vitamins C and K. Drug-to-herbal interactions may occur with the simultaneous use of capsicum, celery, chamomile, clove, devil's claw, dong quai, echinacea, fenugreek, garlic, ginger, gingko, horse chestnut, licorice root, passionflower, herb, tumeric, and willow bark, which may increase the risk of bleeding. The simultaneous use of evening primrose, grapeseed extract, feverfew, ginseng, green tea, and St. John's Wort may decrease the effectiveness of warfarin.

7. **What are some physical findings in carotid stenosis?** Some physical findings detected in carotid stenosis include eliciting of bruits on auscultation of the carotid arteries due to obstruction of blood flow through the vessels as a result of narrowing. The client may complain of dizziness, which is due to lack of blood supply to the brain.

8. **What are some psychosocial stressors that can worsen hypertension and affect the client's ability to collaborate with treatment?** A stressor that affects any aspect of a person's being affects the whole self. Stress has a significant impact on various organ systems of the body. *Perception* is a psychosocial stressor that can affect the client's ability to collaborate with treatment. Once there is a person–environment relationship and the person appraises it as threatening, harmful, or challenging, an internal stress response occurs. When a person is stressed, the brain initiates the stress response by responding to the appraisal with the release of norepinephrine. Norepinephrine in turn stimulates the sympathetic nervous system centers located in the hypothalmus, and norepinephrine causes vasoconstriction of the blood vessels, which further increases the blood pressure. *Negative emotional response* can affect the disease process and participation in care, but it depends on the significance of the person–environment event to the person's well-being. A negative emotional response occurs when there is a threat to, delay in, or thwarting of a goal or a conflict between goals. Negative emotional response also triggers the autonomic nervous system, resulting in the release of vasoconstricting hormones, preventing the lowering of blood pressure. The effects of elevated blood pressure, such as a headache, can decrease the client's motivation toward participation in self-care. *Ineffective coping* can affect hypertension and also decreases the client's motivation toward participation in self-care. *Effective coping* is the process whereby a person manages the demands and emotions that are generated. If the client has not learned previous coping skills, in times of illness, which is a major stressor, effective coping will be difficult. A person who does not cope with stress successfully is at a higher risk for more serious physiologic changes.

9. **If Ms. Z is noncompliant with medical regimen after discharge and develops hypertensive crisis and is brought to the emergency department (ED), what are the indicators the nurse should focus on eliciting from the client on initial contact?** The nurse should assess the client for complaints of severe headaches, dizziness, feeling flushed, or having difficulty remembering. Blood pressure readings indicating severe hypertension and manifestations of disorientation may indicate a decrease in cardiac output secondary to increased vascular resistance.

10. **How should the nurse discuss discharge plans with Ms. Z in regards to her admission weight, at 5'5", of 248 pounds?** The nurse should find out what the client remembers and understands from what was initially discussed by the registered dietitian on initial interview then clarify misunderstandings as the client's needs are maintained as the priority. The nurse should discuss what entails an appropriate dietary intake per meal. Making recommendations for improved or modified eating behaviors as needed would be appropriate nursing interventions, as well as explaining the importance of balancing physical activity and food intake to decrease and maintain healthy weight for body frame and height. The primary health care provider should be consulted for the type of exercise the client should use given her medical problems. Reminding the client to read nutrition labels that appear on manufactured foods and teaching the client and significant others how to use the food guide pyramid (six or more servings per day of complex carbohydrate foods), fresh fruits and vegetables, and protein source more from plants than animals is very important. The nurse should remind the client that if chicken is to be used as a source of protein, the skin should be removed because the skin contains most of its fat. The client's salt intake should be limited, which will reduce water retention and decrease weight and blood pressure.

References

Broyles, B.E. (2005). *Medical-Surgical Nursing Clinical Companion*. Durham, NC: Carolina Academic Press.

Corbet, J.V. (2004). *Laboratory Tests and Diagnostic Procedures with Nursing Diagnoses* (6th ed.). Upper Saddle River, NJ: Prentice Hall.

Gahart, B.L. and Nazareno, A.R. (2005). *2005 Intravenous Medications*. St. Louis: Mosby.
Huether, S.E. and McCance, K.L. (2004). *Understanding Pathophysiology* (3rd ed.). St. Louis: Mosby.
Ignatavicius, D.D. and Workman, M.L. (2006). *Medical-Surgical Nursing across the Health Care Continuum* (5th ed.). Philadelphia: W.B. Saunders.
Lewis, S.M., Heitkemper, M.M., and Dirksen, S.R. (2004). *Medical-Surgical Nursing* (5th ed.). St. Louis: Mosby.
Spratto, G.R. and Woods, A.L. (2005). *2005 Edition: PDR Nurse's Drug Handbook*. Clifton Park, NY: Thomson Delmar Learning.

CASE STUDY 3

Chronic Vascular Ulcers of the Right Foot

GENDER
- M

AGE
- 78

SETTING
- Hospital

ETHNICITY/CULTURE
- Black American

PREEXISTING CONDITIONS
- Diabetes
- Hypertension

COEXISTING CONDITIONS
- Coronary artery bypass stroke

LIFESTYLE
- Retired

COMMUNICATION

DISABILITY
- Immobility

SOCIOECONOMIC STATUS
- Middle

SPIRITUAL/RELIGIOUS
- Baptist

PHARMACOLOGIC
- Rosiglitazone maleate (Avandia)
- Ticarcillin disodium/clavulanate potassium (Timentin)
- Gentamicin sulfate (Garamycin)
- Gabapentin (Neurontin)
- Enoxaparin (Lovenox)

PSYCHOSOCIAL
- Anxiety

LEGAL

ETHICAL

ALTERNATIVE THERAPY
- Prayer

PRIORITIZATION
- Microbiological control
- Metabolic control
- Vascular control
- Wound control

DELEGATION
- RN
- Wound care specialist
- CNA

MODERATE

THE CARDIOVASCULAR AND LYMPHATIC SYSTEMS

Level of difficulty: Moderate

Overview: This case involves accurate identification of weak or absent peripheral pulses; sensation of bilateral extremities; pain on toes, between toes, and on upper aspect of the foot. Critical-thinking skills are used to prioritize effective care.

Client Profile

Mr. M is a 78-year-old retired lieutenant of the U.S. Army. He is 5'10" and weighs 190 pounds. He is admitted from a nursing home with ulcers on the right great toe and plantar surface of the right foot.

Case Study

On admission to the hospital, Mr. M's vital signs are:

Blood pressure: 170/98
Pulse: 76
Respirations: 20
Temperature: 100.9° F

He is alert and oriented to time, place, and person. He has an indwelling Foley catheter in place to straight drainage, which is draining amber-colored urine. The following lab reports are sent from the nursing home:

White blood cell (WBC) count: 18,000/mm^3
Red blood cell (RBC) count: 3,000,000/uL
Hemoglobin (Hgb): 16.4 g/dL
Hematocrit (Hct): 34%
Platelet count (PLT): 298,000/mm^3
Glucose: 208 mg/dL
Blood urea nitrogen (BUN): 12 mg/dL

Past medical history (PMH) includes type 2 diabetes mellitus (non-independent diabetes mellitus [NIDDM]), peripheral vascular disease (PVD), hypertension, benign prostatic hyperplasia (BPH), depression, status-post (S/P) cerebrovascular accident (CVA) two years ago. Past surgical history (PSH) includes status-post (S/P) coronary artery bypass graft (CABG) and S/P femoral popliteal bypass and femoral endarterectomy one year ago. Medications sent with certified nursing assistant (CNA) who accompanied him to the hospital include: fluoxetine HcL, aspirin EC, ferrous sulfate, folic acid, gemfibrozil, finasteride, furosemide, metoprolol tartrate, omeprazole, and rosiglitazone maleate. Plans to review the medications brought to the hospital at a later time and renew them as appropriate are discussed by the health care provider and the primary nurse, the wound care specialist, and a pharmacist. Blood and wound culture is done and reveals Pseudomonas aeruginosa. The health care provider does a history and physical including a head-to-toe assessment. During the assessment of the lower extremities, the client reports pain in the lower right extremity during ambulation and at rest. Bilateral lower extremities are thoroughly assessed for color, temperature, pulses, odor, or drainage from the ulcer. An ankle brachial index (ABI) is done on both extremities and reveals an ABI 0.6 of the right lower extremity and a 0.9 of the left lower extremity. A surgical consult is requested and done, and the health care provider orders a duplex ultrasonography with color flow Doppler that shows chronic ischemic areas of the foot. After the multidisciplinary team reviews the labs and diagnostic reports, a medical diagnosis of vascular ulcers of the right foot is made. A discussion with Mr. M is done pertaining to management of the wound. Surgical débridement is discussed, and informed consent witnessed and signed by Mr. M. The débridement is scheduled for the next day. The débridement is successful. The client returns from the surgical procedure with an intact transparent wound barrier dressing to the foot and a vacuum-assisted pump applied with negative pressure to the ulcer area.

Questions and Suggested Answers

1. **Discuss risk factors and pathophysiology of vascular ulcers of the lower extremities.** Indirect effect results in malnutrition of the vessels and, subsequently, fibrosis of organs that the sclerotic arteries supply with

blood. Smoking may be the strongest risk factor. History of cigarette smoking, arteriosclerosis, atherosclerosis, hypertension, and diabetes mellitus result in initial narrowing of the arteries. After a prolonged period of time, the muscle fibers and the endothelial lining of the walls or small arteries and arterioles become thickened. Their indirect effect results in malnutrition of the vessels and, subsequently, fibrosis of organs that the sclerotic arteries supply with blood. Smoking may be the strongest risk factor because nicotine decreases blood flow to the extremities and increases heart rate and blood pressure by stimulating the sympathetic nervous system, causing vasoconstriction. In addition, it increases the chances of clot formation by increasing the aggregation of platelets, which eventually results in atrophy of the skin and underlying muscles. Because of the decreased arterial blood flow in the lower extremities, even minor trauma to the feet may result in wound infection, tissue necrosis, delayed wound healing, and the development of an ulcer.

2. **Discuss the clinical manifestations for vascular disease of the lower extremities.** The classic symptom of peripheral arterial disease of the lower extremity is *intermittent claudication*. Rest pain in the foot usually develops while the disease is still primarily in the stage of intermittent claudication and is described as numbness or a burning sensation, often feeling like a toothache. *Paresthesia*, a sensation of numbness or tingling occurring in the toes or feet, may occur due to nerve tissue ischemia. *Shiny skin* is another manifestation. The skin is taut with loss of hair, which is related to loss of blood supply that provides nutrients to the extremities. *Pallor* or *blanching* of the foot in response to elevation and *reactive hyperemia* (redness of the foot) are manifestations that occur when the extremity is hung in dependent position, resulting in dependent rubor.

3. **Discuss diagnostic studies used to confirm the diagnosis of vascular ulcers of the lower extremities.** *Doppler ultrasound* consists of a probe transducer containing a crystal that directs high-frequency sound waves toward the artery being examined. The sound waves bounce off the blood cells at a rate that corresponds with the velocity or speed of blood flow through the vessel. Recordings are made and reviewed to determine alteration in blood flow or occlusion of vessels. The continuous-wave (CW) Doppler ultrasound detects blood flow in peripheral vessels. Combined with computation of ankle or arm pressures, the CW Doppler ultrasound helps health care providers to characterize the nature of peripheral vascular disease and aids in the guiding of treatment. The *ABI* is the ratio of the ankle systolic blood pressure to the arm systolic blood pressure. It is an objective indicator of arterial disease that allows the health care provider to quantify the degree of stenosis. With increasing degrees of arterial narrowing, there is progressive decrease in systolic pressure distal to the involved sites.

4. **Discuss common nursing diagnoses for vascular ulcers of the lower extremities.** *Ineffective tissue perfusion (peripheral) related to decreased arterial blood flow.* Positioning of the client will improve tissue perfusion. However, before the client with peripheral vascular disease is positioned, the nurse must first learn whether the disorder is arterial or venous in nature. Because blood flows to dependent parts of the body (i.e., parts lower than the heart), clients with arterial disease must be positioned so that the blood flows toward their legs and feet. The nurse must teach the client the effects of vasoconstriction on disease vessels, and inform the client of factors that cause vasoconstriction (i.e., smoking, emotional upsets, stressors). *Impaired skin integrity related to decreased peripheral circulation, altered sensation, and increased susceptibility to infection.* Because of poor circulation, clients with chronic vascular ulcers are highly prone to ulcerations and infection of the extremities. Moreover, once a lesion develops, it tends to heal poorly, especially if the client has history of diabetes. Eventually, the client may require amputation of an extremity. General intervention involves keeping the area of ulceration clean and free from pressure and irritation. Foot care is an important part of the plan of care for clients with peripheral arterial disease. Excellent foot care should be an integral part of the daily routine of clients with peripheral vascular disorders. The client should be taught that there are no minor foot problems with peripheral vascular disease, especially since there is history of diabetes. Referral to a vascular specialist for care of corns, calluses, and nails are also integral part of the overall plan of care. *Acute pain related to tissue ischemia secondary to decreased peripheral circulation.* Any measure that increases circulation to the extremities will help alleviate ischemic pain. Pain can also be subdued by analgesics, and should be administered as scheduled, and evaluated for the need to increase dosage if

needed. The client may benefit from a bed cradle to keep pressure of bed sheets off the painful extremity. ***Activity intolerance related to imbalance between oxygen supply and demand.*** Assessment of the amount of exercise the client can tolerate before the onset of pain is necessary to provide baseline for evaluation. Collaborate with a physical therapist and the client in developing a structured program that will enhance mobility and improve oxygen utilization in the tissues. ***Ineffective therapeutic regimen management related to lack of knowledge of disease and self-care measures.*** The nurse must identify factors that influence learning, such as perception of the severity of the problem, cognitive ability, age appropriateness, and physical ability to provide self-care. Teach client and significant others about the disease, treatment, and activity restrictions. Emphasize the importance of smoking cessation and the need for a balanced diet with increased protein and foods high in vitamin C and zinc to enhance wound healing. Stress the importance of compliance with medication prescriptions and follow-up care.

The following are prescribed:

- Morphine sulfate (Duramorph) 8 mg IM q4h PRN pain × three days
- Ticarcillin disodium/clavulanate potassium (Timentin) 3.1 g q6h
- Rosiglitazone maleate (Avandia) 8 mg PO daily
- Metoprolol tartrate (Lopressor) 75 mg PO daily
- Furosemide (Lasix) 49 mg PO daily
- Gabapentin (Neurontin) 400 mg PO q8h
- Enoxaparin (Lovenox) 30 mg/0.3 ML SC q12h
- Oxycodone/acetaminophen (Endocet) 5/325 MG two tablets PO q4h PRN
- Fingerstick glucose every shift and PRN
- Serum labs: glucose, WBC

5. **What are the purposes for the prescribed orders?** ***Morphine sulfate*** relieves moderate-to-severe pain. It relieves pain by binding to the Mu receptor, which results in supraspinal analgesia and euphoria, resulting in pain relief. ***Ticarcillin disodium/clavulante potassium*** inhibits cell wall synthesis and thereby destroys the organism. It is also specified for Pseudomonas aeruginosa, the organism cultured from the client's blood. ***Rosiglitazone maleate*** lowers blood glucose by improving target cell response to insulin in Type II diabetes mellitus. It accomplishes this action by reducing cellular insulin resistance and decreasing hepatic glucose output. ***Metoprolol tartrate*** lowers and stabilizes blood pressure. It reduces secretion of renin, a potent vasoconstrictor, and in doing so, maintains blood pressure within normal limits. ***Furosemide*** removes excess sodium and water from body tissues. It is a potent loop diuretic that effectively aids in reducing and maintaining blood pressure by acting on Henle's loop and blocks chloride and sodium resorption, thus preventing retention of sodium and, therefore, retention of water, which would increase blood volume and pressure. ***Gabapentin*** relieves neuropathic pain related to diabetes mellitus. It is the analgesic effects of gabapentin that relieves neuropathic pain. It works by inhibiting specific neurons that normally elicit pain sensation. ***Enoxaparin*** prevents deep vein thrombosis (DVT) from forming in the lower extremities of persons on bedrest or whose mobility is altered. It is approved by the Food and Drug Administration (FDA) for the prevention of DVTs. Enoxaparin is effective in preventing DVT because, unlike the traditional heparin sodium, it does not specifically bind to proteins and tissues, and therefore is more available for anticoagulant actions once it is administered. ***Oxycodone/acetaminophen*** decreases pain and improves comfort by binding to receptors in various sites of the central nervous system (CNS) altering both perceptions of pain and emotional response to pain. The ***serum glucose*** provides information regarding hyperglycemia and the possible need for insulin coverage since the client has a history of type 2 diabetes mellitus and his glucose is elevated on admission. ***Fingerstick glucose*** provides random information of the need for insulin coverage. An elevated WBC count indicates infection and aids in guiding antibiotic regimen. The ***serum glucose*** monitoring provides information to determine the need for immediate insulin administration to prevent hyperglycemic complications.

6. **What are the most common adverse reactions, drug-to-drug, drug-to-food/herbal interactions of the prescribed medications?** The most common adverse reactions of ***morphine sulfate*** are constipation, sedation, and

hypotension. Drug-to-drug interactions may occur with the simultaneous use of monoamine oxidase (MAO) inhibitors, which will decrease the initial dose of morphine sulfate. The simultaneous use with alcohol, sedatives/hypnotics, clomipramine, barbiturates, tricyclic depressants, and antihistamines may increase CNS depression. Simultaneous use with partial-antagonist opioid analgesics may precipitate opioid withdrawal in physically dependent clients. Its use with buprenorphine, nalbuphine, butorphanol, or pentazocine may decrease analgesia, and simultaneous use of morphine and anticoagulants such as warfarin may increase anticoagulant effects. Simultaneous use of morphine with cimetidine decreases cimetidine metabolism and increases its effects. Drug-to-food interactions are not clinically established, but drug-to-herbal interactions are seen with the simultaneous use of kava, valerian, skullcap, chamomile, or hops, which may increase CNS depression. The most common adverse reactions of *ticarcillin disodium/clavulanate potassium* are diarrhea, nausea, sodium overload (e.g., congested heart failure), and bleeding. Drug-to-drug interactions may occur with the simultaneous use of anticoagulants, which may increase the risk of bleeding. Probenecid decreases elimination of ticarcillin and increases the risk of toxicity. There are no clinically significant drug-to-food/herbal interactions established. The most common adverse reactions of *rosiglitazone maleate* are fluid retention, edema, and weight gain. Drug-to-drug interactions may occur with the simultaneous use of insulins, which may increase the risk of edema or heart failure. If used simultaneously with oral hypoglycemic agents, it may enhance hypoglycemic effects. Drug-to-food/herbal interactions may occur with the simultaneous use of garlic and ginseng, both of which could potentiate hypoglycemic effects. The most common adverse reactions of *metoprolol tartrate* are dizziness, fatigue, insomnia, bradycardia, and heartburn. Drug-to-drug interactions may occur with the simultaneous use of verapamil, barbiturates, rifampin, cimetidine, and propylthiouracil, which may increase the adverse effects of metoprolol tartrate. There are no clinically significant drug-to-food/herbal interactions established. The most common adverse reactions of *furosemide* are hypokalemia, dehydration, and hypotension. Drug-to-drug interactions may occur with the simultaneous use of other diuretics, digoxin, and amphotericin B, which may increase digoxin toxicity. If furosemide is used simultaneously with insulins, it may blunt hypoglycemic effects. There are no clinically significant drug-to-food/herbal interactions established. The most common adverse reactions of *gabapentin* are drowsiness, dizziness, and fatigue. Drug-to-drug interactions may occur with the simultaneous use of phenytoin. Drug-to-food interactions may occur with the simultaneous use of gingko, kava, valerian, and skullcaps, which may increase CNS depression. The simultaneous use of antacids will reduce absorption of gabapentin. Drug-to-herbal interactions may occur with the simultaneous of gingko, which may decrease anticonvulsant effect. The most common adverse reactions of *enoxaparin* are rash and pruritus. Drug-to-drug interactions may occur with the simultaneous use of aspirin, ibuprofen, and warfarin, which may increase the risk of bleeding. Drug-to-food/herbal interactions may occur with the simultaneous use of ginger, gingko, feverfew, and horse chestnut, increasing the risk of bleeding. The most common adverse reactions of *oxycodone/acetaminophen* are dizziness, nausea, sedation, and constipation. Drug-to-drug interactions may occur with the simultaneous use of CNS depressant medications. Drug-to-food/herbal interactions may occur with the simultaneous use of St. John's Wort, which may increase sedating effects.

7. **Discuss surgical management for peripheral artery disease of the lower extremities.** Revascularization is usually reserved for clients with progressive, severe, or disabling manifestations including ischemia at rest. If revascularization is to be done, an angiography is commonly used before surgery to mark the level of inflow or areas of obstruction. A balloon angioplasty, femoral-popliteal bypass, or endarterectomy can be done with the goal being the removal of partial or total blockages. A *balloon angioplasty* is a procedure done to dilate or open obstructed blood vessel(s) by threading a small balloon-tipped catheter into the vessel. The balloon is inflated to compress arteriosclerotic lesions against the walls of the vessel, leaving a larger lumen through which blood can pass. *Femoral popliteal bypass* uses a graft and anastomoses or surgically connects the graft to any one of the three lower leg arteries such as the posterior tibial, anterior tibial, or peroneal artery. Postoperative care involves anticoagulant (heparin sodium), followed by warfarin sodium (coumadin), antibiotic therapy, dipyridamole (Persantine) to decrease platelet aggregation and increase blood flow to the graft site. The client is on bed rest with the leg flat in bed. The leg is wrapped with light

dressings or a vascular boot is applied. Leg swelling is common after revascularization related to reperfusion of ischemic muscles and surgical dissection around lymphatic drainage systems in the leg. Reclotting of the graft is possible, therefore peripheral tissue perfusion is assessed by neurovascular assessment of the limbs with the use of Doppler ultrasound flowmeter. The nurse should document all abnormal findings post-surgery and report appropriately to the surgeon. An endarterectomy may be done by opening the artery and removing the obstructed plaque. Antiplatelet agents are often used to prevent thrombosis after the procedure.

8. **Discuss client education for vascular ulcers of the lower extremities.** The client must be taught that tobacco/cigarette smoking must be discontinued, not only because of the effects of nicotine, but also because tobacco smoke impairs transport and cellular utilization of oxygen, which increases blood viscosity. Continued cigarette smoking also dramatically decreases the long-term patency rates of the bypass graft. Teach the client the importance of meticulous foot care to prevent injury. Any ulceration or inflammation should be reported to the primary health care provider. Thick or overgrown toenails should be cared for by a podiatrist. Shoes should not be laced tightly, and new shoes should be broken in gradually.

References

Broyles, B.E. (2005). *Medical-Surgical Nursing Clinical Companion.* Durham, NC: Carolina Academic Press.

Corbet, J.V. (2004). *Laboratory Tests and Diagnostic Procedures with Nursing Diagnoses* (6th ed.). Upper Saddle River, NJ: Prentice Hall.

Gahart, B.L. and Nazareno, A.R. (2005). *2005 Intravenous Medications.* St. Louis: Mosby.

Heitz, U. and Horne, M.M. (2005). *Mosby's Pocket Guide Series: Fluid, Electrolyte and Acid-Base Balance* (5th ed.). St. Louis: Mosby.

Huether, S.E. and McCance, K.L. (2004). *Understanding Pathophysiology* (3rd ed.). St. Louis: Mosby.

Ignatavicius, D.D. and Workman, M.L. (2006). *Medical-Surgical Nursing: Critical Thinking for Collaborative Care* (5th ed.). Philadelphia: W.B. Saunders.

Spratto, G.R. and Woods, A.L. (2005). *2005 Edition: PDR Nurse's Drug Handbook.* Clifton Park, NY: Thomson Delmar Learning.

CASE STUDY 4

Disseminated Intravascular Coagulation

GENDER
- F

AGE
- 56

SETTING
- Hospital

ETHNICITY/CULTURE
- Black American

PREEXISTING CONDITIONS
- History of intestinal obstruction

COEXISTING CONDITIONS

LIFESTYLE
- Health educator who lectures four days per week at a senior college

COMMUNICATION

DISABILITY

SOCIOECONOMIC STATUS
- Middle

SPIRITUAL/RELIGIOUS
- Evangelical

PHARMACOLOGIC
- Gentamicin sulfate (Garamycin)
- Clindamycin HcL (Cleocin Hydrochloride)
- Cryoprecipitate
- Aminocaproic acid
- Vancomycin HcL (Vancocin)
- Metronidazole (Flagyl)

PSYCHOSOCIAL
- Anxiety
- Pain

LEGAL

ETHICAL
- The right to make decisions related to care

ALTERNATE THERAPY
- Prayer

PRIORITIZATION
- Patent airway
- Improve circulatory volume
- Supportive therapy with blood components

DELEGATION
- RN
- Client education

MODERATE

THE CARDIOVASCULAR AND LYMPHATIC SYSTEMS

Level of difficulty: Moderate

Overview: The case involves critical-thinking skills to prioritize and delegate care efficiently and appropriately. It involves clinical expertise in caring for the client with potential for thrombi and bleeding, and acute renal failure (ARF). It requires a multidisciplinary team with a clear understanding of the physiological changes that occur in disseminated intravascular coagulation.

Client Profile

Mrs. L is a 56-year-old female who for the past month has experienced occasional nausea and dizziness. After returning home from her teaching assignment, Mrs. L experienced a moderately sharp pain across her umbilicus. She had a cup of tea then went to rest and fell asleep. Upon awakening, Mrs. L experienced a more severe, intolerable pain of the abdomen. She is accompanied by a neighbor to her family health care provider and, on arrival at the health care provider's office, is immediately transferred to the emergency department (ED) of a nearby hospital.

Case Study

In the ED, a quick systems assessment is done followed by an upper gastrointestinal radiographic series (UGIS), which is ineffective because she vomits contents of the barium sulfate, including fecal content seen in the vomitus. Mrs. L is transferred to a surgical unit, and a systematic approach is used in doing the nursing history. Serum, urine specimens, and blood cultures are collected and sent to the laboratory. A chest X-ray, abdominal X-ray, and electrocardiogram (EKG) are completed, and the informed consent is signed. The abdominal X-ray reveals large amounts of fecal contents resting in the small intestines. Mrs. L's husband is notified of the plans for surgery, and Mrs. L is prepared for emergency laparotomy. A nasogastric tube (NGT) is inserted and attached to low continuous suction, and a Foley catheter is inserted and placed to straight drainage. Mrs. L is transferred to the operating room (OR) with a tentative diagnosis of mechanical obstruction of the small intestines. The initial surgery is successful and Mrs. L is returned to the surgical unit. On arrival, there is gentamicin 80 mg IV, Ringers Lactate at 125 cc/hr, morphine sulfate via PCA at 1 mg continuous, 5 mg PCA dose every eight minutes, and Foley catheter draining amber-colored urine at 50cc/hr. Mrs. L is drowsy but responsive to name and painful stimuli. Vital signs are:

Blood pressure: 130/80
Pulse: 100
Respirations: 16
Temperature: 98.0° F

On post-op day one, a consultation is written for an infectious disease health care provider to approve intravenous clindamycin due to the large strains of gram-positive cocci, including E. coli and C. difficle, which were cultured from fecal contents of the intestines. Clindamycin 1500 mg is prescribed and is started on post-op day two. Within minutes after clindamycin is started, Mrs. L develops large wheals over her entire body, with pustules over the face and upper and lower extremities, and profuse watery diarrhea. Clindamycin is immediately discontinued and intravenous diphenhydramine HcL is administered. Ceftriaxone sodium IV is initiated. Mrs. L's condition worsens with evidence of high fever of 106.6° F, shaking chills, B/P 90/60, respirations 24, and pulse 120. She is immediately transferred to the surgical intensive care unit and is placed on four liters of oxygen via nasal cannula and 0.9% NaCL initiated at 150 mL/hr. Continuous monitoring of oxygen saturation with pulse oximeter, frequent arterial blood gases (ABGs), and accurate urinary output from indwelling catheter are maintained. On post-op day three, her condition deteriorates and a tentative diagnosis of sepsis-induced distributive shock is made. Laboratory data reveal:

Fibrinogen level: 200 mg/dL
D-dimer: 150 ng/mL
Bleeding time: 20 minutes
Platelet count (PLT): 100,000/mm^3
Prothrombin time (PT) with INR: 3.8
Activated partial thromboplastin time (aPTT): 80 seconds
Partial thromboplastin time (PTT): 90 seconds
White blood cell (WBC) count: 20,000/mm^3

After the labs are reviewed, a diagnosis of disseminated intravascular coagulation (DIC) secondary to sepsis-induced distributive shock is made.

Questions and Suggested Answers

1. **Discuss some specific factors that cause DIC.** Some factors that may cause DIC include the release of factor III into the circulation by fat emboli, such as may occur with fracture of a long bone, and tissue damage such as with extensive burns, resulting in the massive cell destruction that causes abnormalities in coagulation. All of these factors cause the release of thromboplastin substances that result in activation of thrombin, which in turn activates fibrinogen, and eventually, deposition of fibrin is spread throughout the microcirculation. The end result is the lysing of clots and depletion of clotting factors; the blood loses the ability to clot.

2. **Discuss common nursing diagnoses for clients with DIC.**
   - Ineffective tissue perfusion R/T bleeding and sluggish or diminished blood flow
   - Acute pain R/T bleeding into tissues and diagnostic procedures
   - Decreased cardiac output R/T fluid volume deficit and hypotension
   - Anxiety R/T fear of the unknown, disease process, and therapy

3. **What is the main purpose for the NGT to suction while the client was in the ED?** The purpose of the NGT was to decompress the bowel, draining fluid and air from the stomach and, as a result, preventing aspiration of stomach contents.

4. **What is the reason for withholding opioid analgesics from Mrs. L, even though she is complaining of severe abdominal pain on arrival to the ED?** Opioid analgesic medication is not administered on arrival to the ED because pain management is not the priority at this time. The key to managing potential intestinal obstruction is to make a quick but accurate history and physical assessment, perform emergency bowel series, insert NGT tube to decompress the bowel so as to avoid projectile vomiting that may cause aspiration. Opioid analgesic would change the character of the pain, which is needed to aid with the diagnosis and guide surgery.

The following are prescribed:

- Gentamicin sulfate (Garamycin) 2 mg/kg IV stat, followed by 3 mg/kg IV q8h
- Clindamycin HcL (Cleocin Hydrochloride) 1,500 mg q6h IV
- Metronidazole (Flagyl) 7.5 mg/kg q6h IV
- Diphenhydramine HcL (Benadryl) 50 mg IV stat
- Ceftriaxone sodium (Rocephin) 2 g q12h IV
- Fresh frozen plasma 1 unit IV
- Drotrecogin alfa (Activated) (Xigris) 24 mcg/kg/h continuous infusion × 96 h
- Daily serum labs: fibrinogen, D-dimer, bleeding time, PLT, PT, PTT

5. **What are the purposes for the prescribed medications post-surgery?** *Morphine sulfate* is an opioid analgesic that relieves moderate to severe pain by mimicking the actions of endogenous opioid peptides primarily at the delta receptors, where the opioid peptides and the morphine bind in the region of the brain and spinal cord that is associated with perception of pain. *Gentamicin* is a potent anti-infective and a broad-spectrum antibiotic that destroys bacteria by interfering with protein synthesis in bacterial cells by binding to ribosomal subunits, which eventually leads to rapid killing of organisms. It is effective against a wide variety of gram-negative and gram-positive organisms. *Clindamycin* is an antibiotic with both bactericidal and bacteriostatic properties. However, these properties are active depending on the concentration of the drug at the site of the infection and on the infecting bacteria. It destroys bacteria by inhibiting protein synthesis in bacteria by binding to the 50S ribosomal subunit. One of its indications is to treat intra-abdominal infections, and it is effective with most aerobic gram-positive bacteria. *Diphenhydramine HcL* is an antihistamine that stops the progression of an allergic reaction by directly competing with histamine for the H_1 receptors in

areas surrounding blood vessels and bronchioles. It blocks these receptors on the surfaces of basophils and mast cells, and thereby prevents the actions of histamine from these cells. **Metronidazole** is an antiprotozoal antibiotic that has especially good activity against anaerobic organisms and is widely used for intra-abdominal infections. It works by interfering with microbial DNA synthesis, inhibiting nucleic acid synthesis, resulting in death of organisms. It destroys both anaerobic and aerobic organisms. **Fresh frozen plasma** has the ability to increase colloid oncotic pressure and the plasma volume. It increases clotting factors V and VII, decreases deficiencies, and expands blood volume. **Ceftriazone sodium** is a cephalosporin antibiotic that preferentially binds to one or more of the penicillin-binding proteins located on the cell walls of susceptible organisms, which inhibits third and final stage of bacterial cell wall synthesis, killing the bacterium. **Drotrecogin alfa** is an immunomodulator, recombinant human-activated Protein C that inhibits clotting Factor V and VIII, limiting the thrombin-induced inflammatory responses and, in doing so, reduces the severity of sepsis and organ dysfunction.

6. **If the client has developed anaphylaxis due to adverse reaction to the clindamycin, what reversal agent would most likely be prescribed?** Epinephrine HcL intravenously would be prescribed, because it is the drug of choice to treat anaphylaxis. In drug-related anaphylaxis, immediate intervention is needed to prevent possible death. The symptoms of anaphylaxis include dyspnea, wheezing, stridor, tachycardia, and hypotension. During anaphylaxis, epinephrine constricts bronchial arterioles and inhibits histamine release, reducing the congestion and edema, and improves airflow.

7. **What are the most common adverse reactions of the prescribed medications?** The most common adverse reactions of *morphine sulfate* are pruritus, constipation, and nausea. The most common adverse reactions of *gentamicin sulfate* are decreasing creatinine clearance, ototoxicity, and nephrotoxicity. The most common adverse reactions of *clindamycin* are diarrhea, nausea, vomiting, and skin rashes. The most common adverse reactions of *metronidazole* are nausea and headache. The most common adverse reactions of *diphenhydramine HcL* are drowsiness, tachycardia, and dry mouth. The most common adverse reactions of *ceftriazone sodium* are diarrhea, nausea, and vomiting. The most common adverse reactions of *fresh frozen plasma* are transfer of hepatitis and human immunodeficiency virus (HIV). The most common adverse reaction of *drotrecogin alfa* is bleeding.

8. **Why are the specified serum labs ordered for Mrs. L?** *Serum fibrinogen* level provides information on specific clotting factors. If the level is lower than 200 mg/dL, this indicates alteration in Factors I, V, and VIII, warranting immediate intervention. *D-dimer* is specific for DIC because it is formed as a result of plasmin lysis, therefore an elevated value is highly specific for DIC. *Bleeding time* evaluates the vascular and platelet factors associated with hemostasis. However, because prolonged bleeding time does not prove with certainty that an abnormality exists, repeated evaluation should be done for accuracy. *Platelet count (PLT)* is important because platelets are decreased in DIC but are normal in fibrinolysis, which would guide accurate treatment of the client's bleeding condition. *Prothrombin time* measures the clotting ability of Factors I, II, V, VII, and X. If these factors are deficient, the PT is prolonged, indicating alteration in clotting factors. *Partial thrombolastin time* evaluates Factors I, II, V, VIII, IX, X, XI, and XII. If these factors are deficient, the PTT is prolonged, also indicating alteration in these factors, which are prominent in DIC and are the hallmark of DIC. Dosing of heparin sodium is based on PTT and INR.

9. **Discuss the drug-to-drug and drug-to-food/herbal interactions for the prescribed medications.** Drug-to-drug interactions may occur with the simultaneous use of *morphine sulfate* and alcohol, or *diphenhydramine HcL* may increase central nervous system (CNS) depressants, resulting in increased respiratory depression and hypotension. Its simultaneous use with monoamine oxidase (MAO) may produce a severe, fatal reaction. Drug-to-drug interactions may occur with the simultaneous use of *gentamicin sulfate* and other aminoglycosides, nephrotoxic, or ototoxic-producing medications, which may increase toxicity. Drug-to-drug interactions may occur with the simultaneous use of *clindamicin* and adsorbent antidiarrheals, which may delay absorption. Its use with chloramphenicol and erythromycin may antagonize the effects of *clindamicin* and

cause toxicity. Drug-to-drug interactions may occur with the simultaneous use of ***metronidazole HcL*** and alcohol, which may cause disulfiram-type reaction. Its use with oral anticoagulants may increase the anticoagulant effects and cause toxicity. The simultaneous use of ***diphenhydramine HcL*** with an anticholinergic agent may increase the anticholinergic effects of both drugs and increase toxic effects. Drug-to-drug interactions of ***ceftriazone sodium, fresh frozen plasma***, or ***drotrecogin alfa*** and other drugs have not been clinically established. There are no clinically significant drug-to-food/herbal interactions established for morphine sulfate, gentamicin sulfate, clindamicin, metronidazole HcL, diphenhydramine HcL, ceftriazone sodium, fresh frozen plasma, or drotrecogin. However, drotrecogin alfa should be used with caution when used concurrently with drugs that affect hemostasis.

10. **What is an important reminder for Mrs. L prior to discharge?** Mrs. L. should be reminded to always wear or carry a Medic-Alert card/bracelet indicating allergy to clindamycin. Immediate identification of the prior drug allergy will be known in the event Mrs. L has an emergency that requires administration of medications.

11. **You are a community-based nurse for a visiting nurse service. You are assigned to supervise home-care management in preparation for Mrs. L to return home upon discharge. A home health aide (HHA) is assigned to Mrs. L's care, with RN visits five days per week for the first week, three days per week for the second week, and one day per week for two additional weeks. Develop a community-based plan of care for the HHA to follow in the absence of the RN.** The HHA will assist Mrs. L with a daily bath using antimicrobial soap and will remind Mrs. L or assist her in taking her temperature at least once daily. The HHA will keep foods refrigerated and prepare foods appropriately. The HHA will report the following signs to the RN: temperature greater than 100° F, persistent cough with or without sputum, unusual amount of drainage from the abdominal site, urine that is cloudy or foul smelling. The HHA will remind Mrs. L, if needed, to take prescribed medications and will follow up on scheduled clinic or health care provider's appointments.

References

Broyles, B.E. (2005). *Medical Surgical Nursing Clinical Companion*. Durham, NC: Carolina Academic Press.
Corbet, J.V. (2004). *Laboratory Tests and Diagnostic Procedures with Nursing Diagnoses* (6th ed.). Upper Saddle River, NJ: Prentice Hall.
Dressler, D.K. (2004). Coping with a Coagulation Crisis. *Nursing 2004* 34(5): 58–63.
Gahart, B.L. and Nazareno, A.R. (2005). *2005 Intravenous Medications*. St. Louis: Mosby.
Huether, S.E. and McCance, K.L. (2004). *Understanding Pathophysiology* (3rd ed.). St. Louis: Mosby.
Ignatavicius, D.D. and Workman, M.L. (2006). *Medical-Surgical Nursing across the Health Care Continuum* (5th ed.). Philadelphia: W. B. Saunders.
Kozier, B., Erb, G., Berman, A., and Synder, S. (2004). *Fundamentals of Nursing: Concepts, Process, and Practice* (7th ed.). Upper Saddle River, NJ: Prentice Hall.
LeMone, P. and Burke, K.M. (2004). *Medical-Surgical Nursing: Critical Thinking in Client Care* (3rd ed.). Upper Saddle River, NJ: Prentice Hall.
Lewis, S.M., Heitkemper, M.M., and Dirksen, S.R. (2004). *Medical-Surgical Nursing Assessment and Management of Clinical Problems* (5th ed.). St. Louis: Mosby.
Spratto, G.R. and Woods, A.L. (2005). *2005 Edition: PDR Nurse's Drug Handbook*. Clifton Park, NY: Thomson Delmar Learning.

CASE STUDY 5

Unstable Angina Pectoris (Acute Myocardial Ischemia)

GENDER
- F

AGE
- 60

SETTING
- Hospital

ETHNICITY/CULTURE
- Hispanic American

PREEXISTING CONDITIONS
- Atherosclerosis
- Coronary spasms
- Anemia

COEXISTING CONDITION
- Hyperthyroidism
- Stimulant abuse

LIFESTYLE
- Accounting department supervisor

COMMUNICATION
- Spanish and English

DISABILITY

SOCIOECONOMIC STATUS
- Middle

SPIRITUAL/RELIGIOUS
- Nondenominational

PHARMACOLOGIC
- Nitrates
- Beta-adrenergic blockers
- Calcium-channel blockers
- Aspirin

PSYCHOSOCIAL
- Anxiety

LEGAL

ETHICAL

ALTERNATIVE THERAPY
- Acupuncture
- Ginseng

PRIORITIZATION
- Obtain description of client's chest discomfort
- Obtain 12-lead EKG
- Provide measures to enhance tissue perfusion

DELEGATION
- RN
- Client education

MODERATE

THE CARDIOVASCULAR AND LYMPHATIC SYSTEMS

Level of difficulty: Moderate

Overview: This case involves a thorough assessment and critical-thinking skills to identify the classic symptoms of unstable angina so that appropriate medical interventions can be implemented effectively and to prioritize clients, because clients with unstable angina can progress to myocardial infarction or even death.

Client Profile

Ms. T, a 60-year-old female, is brought to the hospital emergency department (ED) due to intolerable chest pain after climbing several flights of stairs at her place of employment. Ms. T is 5'5" and weighs 206 pounds. Ms. T is an accounting department supervisor. She is a good historian and is able to explain quality and intensity of the present symptoms that warranted her access to the hospital ED.

Case Study

Ms. T reports taking nitroglycerin (NTG) for chest pain but says she did not take her NTG tablets to work with her, therefore, the pain was worse than she had experienced with previous attacks. However, on arrival to the ED, she reports that the severity of the pain has subsided. Ms. T's vital signs on arrival to the ED are:

Blood pressure: 118/84
Pulse: 74 and irregular
Respirations: 22
Temperature: 98.2° F

A 12-lead electrocardiogram (EKG) is done and reveals ST depression, T-wave inversion, atrioventricular conduction delay, and atrial fibrillation. Ms. T presently denies any discomfort and is waiting to be seen by the nurse practitioner (NP). The NP in the ED is given the report of the 12-lead EKG and will collaborate with the health care provider. As the interview with the NP continues, Ms. T reports inability to walk more than two blocks without difficulty breathing. She further reports noticing these occurrences increasing over the past three weeks. Her past medical history (PMH) includes aortic stenosis and hyperlipidemia and a right- and left-heart catheterization seven years ago. She reports being monitored in a cardiology clinic by a team of cardiologists. Reports from her medical records indicate moderate stenosis of the left anterior descending (LAD) artery. She has mild pulmonary hypertension, mild coronary atherosclerosis, and a mildly increased left ventricular hypertrophy. Her right coronary artery (RCA) shows mild calcification, and the LAD and the circumflex artery have moderate lesions. She is admitted to the coronary care unit (CCU), and continuous telemetry is initiated. The health care provider prescribes an echocardiogram and exercise stress test. The findings are positive for myocardial ischemia with decreased ejection fraction noted. Current laboratory values reveal:

White blood cell (WBC) count: 10,000/mm^3
CK-MB: 132 U/L
Hematocrit (Hct): 32%
Hemoglobin (Hgb): 12 g/dL
Potassium (K+): 4 mEq/L
Sodium (Na): 145 mEq/L
Troponin: T$_1$ 0.1 ng/mL
LDH$_1$: 38%
LDH$_2$: 40%
Total serum cholesterol: 185 mg/dL
Triglyceride: 165 mg/dL

After review of diagnostic studies, laboratory data, physical assessment, and client's subjective data, a diagnosis of unstable angina pectoris is made. The health care team decides that Ms. T can return home, with follow-up care with her primary health care provider within two weeks from today's date. A repeat 12-lead EKG is done without any changes noted from the initial one. Ms. T is resting and her vital signs are:

Blood pressure: 118/78
Pulse: 74 irregular

Respirations: 18
Temperature: 98.2° F

The cardiologist and the NP discuss the discharge criteria with Ms. T, and she is to be discharged within 24 hours. The social worker and registered dietitian will visit with Ms. T in preparation for discharge.

Questions and Suggested Answers

1. **What is your understanding of the above situation?** The primary reason for seeking medical assistance is chest pain related to a diagnosis of unstable angina. However, Ms. T has multicardiac structure disorders that have resulted in the development of angina pectoris. For instance, she has history of hyperlipidemia, which may have developed as a result of high dietary fat intake, especially saturated fats. Untreated elevated lipids eventually affects the intima of the artery which over a prolonged period of time eventually narrows the artery sufficiently to compromise blood flow, resulting in diminished tissue perfusion to the coronary arteries causing angina pectoris. Ms. T's history of aortic stenosis over a prolonged period of time also contributes to the development of unstable angina because the stenosis results in resistance of blood flow from the left ventricle, resulting in decreased cardiac output. With decreased cardiac output, there is diminished blood flow to the coronaries, causing anginal attacks. Untreated aortic stenosis eventually results in left ventricular hypertrophy because the ventricle must work harder to compensate for the resistance of blood flow. Continued ventricular hypertrophy interferes with coronary artery perfusion because stroke volume is diminished, resulting in increase myocardial oxygen demand. The deprived coronary cannot manage the increase myocardial oxygen demand, resulting in more anginal attacks. The LAD artery delivers blood to portions of the left and right ventricles, and much of the interventricular septum, then travels down to the anterior surface of the interventricular septum toward the apex of the heart. The circumflex artery supplies blood to the left atrium and lateral wall of the left ventricle. When lesions are present in these arteries, blood flow is impaired and anginal attacks become more pronounced. One of the long-term results of these alterations in the normal cardiac function will be manifested in exercise intolerance, difficulty breathing, and chest pain with the potential for a myocardial infarction.

2. **What is the incidence according to the American Heart Association (AHA) in regard to being overweight and obesity?** According to the AHA, black Americans and Hispanics have the highest incidence of people who are overweight and obese. Asian/Pacific Islanders have the smallest incidence, and about two-thirds of all Americans are overweight or obesity.

3. **Discuss the relationship between gender and acute coronary syndrome (angina).** More women than men have angina. Many women experience atypical angina. Atypical angina can manifest itself as indigestion, pain between the shoulders, an aching jaw, or a choking sensation that occurs with exertion. Angina in women often has been diagnosed as panic disorder, stress, menopause-related problems, gastrointestinal disease, or hypochondriasis.

4. **Explain the two predominant types of angina.** The two predominant types of angina are *stable* and *unstable* angina. **Stable angina** is chest discomfort that occurs with moderate to prolonged exertion in a pattern that is familiar to the client. The frequency, duration, and intensity of symptoms remain stable over several months. Stable angina results in only slight limitation of activity and is usually associated with stable atherosclerotic plaque. It is usually relieved by NTG or rest and often is managed medically with agents such as calcium-channel blockers and beta-blocking medications. **Unstable angina**, or USA, is chest pain or discomfort that occurs at rest or with exertion and causes marked limitation of activity. The pain may last longer than 15 minutes or may be poorly relieved by rest or NTG.

5. **Discuss common nursing diagnoses for clients with angina pectoris.**

   - Acute pain R/T biologic injury agents (imbalance between myocardial oxygen supply and demand)
   - Ineffective cardiac tissue perfusion R/T interruption of arterial blood flow

- Activity intolerance R/T fatigue (caused by imbalance between oxygen supply and demand)
- Ineffective coping R/T effects of acute illness and major changes in lifestyle
- Deficient knowledge R/T condition, treatment, lifestyle changes

6. **If the following diagnostic tests were ordered for Ms. T, what would be the expected results?** The *chest radiography* would show calcification of aortic valve, left ventricular enlargement, and a prominent ascending aorta. The *echocardiogram* would show limited aortic valve movement and thickened left ventricular wall. It also could provide information about the heart's ejection fraction.

7. **When would surgical intervention be considered for Ms. T?** Surgical intervention would be considered when the pressure gradient in the coronary arteries is greater than 50 mm Hg or the valve orifice is less than 0.8 cm^2.

The following are prescribed at discharge:

- Nitroglycerin (NTG) tab 0.4 mg SL for chest pain PRN
- Propranolol HcL (Inderal) 40 mg PO two times per day
- Nifedipine (Procardia) 20 mg PO three times per day
- Clopidogrel bisulfate (Plavix) 75 mg PO daily

8. **What are the purposes for the prescribed medications?** *Sublingual nitroglycerin* is a coronary vasodilator that relieves pain by relaxing vascular smooth muscle resulting in dilation of both venous and arterial blood vessels. This leads to a decrease of myocardial oxygen demand and improved coronary tissue perfusion. *Propranolol HcL* is a beta-adrenergic blocking agent that decreases myocardial oxygen demand and the potential anginal attacks by working as an antagonist to block beta-receptor-mediated functions of the sympathetic nervous system. *Nifedipine* is a calcium-channel blocker that dilates coronary arteries and increases tissue perfusion to the myocardium. Nifedipine blocks calcium from entering into the cells and prevents spasms from occurring, allowing the dilation of the coronary arteries and increasing oxygen supply to the myocardium. *Clopidrogel* is an antiplatelet agent that prevents platelet aggregation, to delay clot formation. Clopidrogel bisulfate acts by selectively preventing the binding of adenosine diphosphate to its platelet receptor.

9. **What are the most common adverse reactions of the prescribed medications?** The most common adverse reactions of *nitroglycerine* are dizziness, headache, hypotension, and tachycardia. The most common adverse reactions of *propranolol* are bradycardia, confusion, fatigue, weakness, and paresthesia of the hands and impotence. The most common adverse reactions of *nifedipine* are dizziness, light-headedness, hypotension, facial flushing, heat sensation, peripheral edema, and diarrhea. The most common adverse reactions of *clopidrogel* are headache, dizziness, and fatigue, but it can cause intracranial hemorrhage, life-threatening bleeding, cardiac failure, and pulmonary hemorrhage.

10. **Discuss the drug-to-drug and drug-to-food/herbal interactions for the prescribed medications.** Drug-to-drug interactions may occur with the simultaneous use of *nitroglycerin* and drugs used the treat erectile dysfunction, such as sildenafil, which increases the risk of serious and potentially fatal hypotension. Additive hypotension occurs with the simultaneous use of antihypertensives, acute ingestion of alcohol, beta blockers, calcium-channel blockers, haloperidol, or phenothiazides. Simultaneous use with agents having anticholinergic properties such as tricyclic antidepressants, antihistamines and phenothiazines may decrease the absorption of NTG. There are no clinically significant drug-to-food/herbal interactions established. Drug-to-drug interactions may occur with the simultaneous use of *propranolol* and phenothiazides, haloperidol, hydralazine, propylthioracil, and other antihypertensives may cause hypotensive effects. Simultaneous use with IV phenytoin and verapamil may cause additive myocardial depression. Additive bradycardia may occur with the simultaneous use of digoxin. Phenobarbital may decrease propranolol's effects due to decreased liver breakdown. Smoking decreases serum levels of propranolol and increases its clearance from the body. The simultaneous use of antacids may decrease propranolol absorption. Concurrent use with thyroid administration may decrease the effectiveness of propranolol. Simultaneous use with insulin or oral hypoglycemic

agents may alter the effectiveness of these agents. There are no clinically significant drug-to-food/herbal interactions established. Clients receiving *nifedipine* may experience drug-to-drug interactions if client is concurrently receiving beta blockers, which may increase the risk of congested heart failure (CHF). Additive hypotension may occur when used simultaneously with fentanyl, other antihypertensives, nitrates, barbiturates, nafcillin, or quinidine which may decrease the effects of nifedipine. The simultaneous use with non-steroidal anti-inflammatory agents (NSAIDs) may decrease the antihypertensive effects. Nifedipine may increase risk for digoxin toxicity as well as increasing cyclosporine, diltiazem, itraconazole, magnesium sulfate, tacrolimus, theophylline, and vincristine serum levels. The use of propranolol and cimetidine simultaneously with nifedipine may decrease metabolism and increase the risk of toxicity. The use of grapefruit juice with nifedipine may increase nifedipine serum levels and effect. Drug-to-herbal interactions may occur with the simultaneous use of melatonin which may increase blood pressure and heart rate. Drug-to-drug interactions may occur with the simultaneous use of *clopidogrel bisulfate* and abciximab, eptifibatide, tirofiban, aspirin, NSAIDs, heparin, heparanoids, thrombolytic agents, ticlopidine, or warfarin, which may increase the risk of bleeding. The simultaneous use with phenytoin, tolbutamide, tamoxifen, torsemide, or fluvastatin may decrease metabolism and increase effects of these drugs. Drug-to-herbal interactions occur with the simultaneous use of anise, arnica, chamomile, clove, fenugreek, feverfew, garlic, ginger, gingko, grapeseed extract, evening primrose, and Panax ginseng, which may increase the risk of bleeding.

11. **Discuss client education for unstable angina and aortic stenosis?** Before discharge, the nurse should prepare detailed teaching material for the client concerning the therapeutic regimen, the disease process, factors contributing to symptoms, and the rationale for the intervention. The client needs information concerning prescribed medications, including a clear explanation of why the drugs are prescribed, dosages, side effects, and special considerations for their use. The nurse should stress that if chest pain develops and is not relieved with three nitroglycerin tablets, the emergency service (911) must be called immediately. By reviewing the prescribed exercise plan with the client and reminding the client that activity restrictions are needed for persons with aortic stenosis, the nurse provides vital discharge information. The client should be given a list of health care personnel to call if needed and their contact numbers. Finally, the nurse must stress the importance of complying with the schedule for follow-up appointments.

References

American Heart Association. www.americanheart.org.

Broyles, B.E. (2005). *Medical-Surgical Nursing Clinical Companion.* Durham, NC: Carolina Academic Press.

Corbet, J.V. (2004). *Laboratory Tests and Diagnostic Procedures with Nursing Diagnoses* (6th ed.). Upper Saddle River, NJ: Prentice Hall.

Gahart, B.L. and Nazareno, A.R. (2005). *2005 Intravenous Medications.* St. Louis: Mosby.

Ignatavicius, D.D. and Workman, M.L. (2006). *Medical-Surgical Nursing: Critical Thinking for Collaborative Care* (5th ed.). Philadelphia: W.B. Saunders.

Lewis, S.M., Heitkemper, M.M., and Dirksen, S.R. (2004). *Medical-Surgical Nursing: Assessment and Management of Clinical Problems* (5th ed.). St. Louis: Mosby.

Smeltzer, S.C. and Bare, B.G. (2004). *Textbook of Medical-Surgical Nursing* (10th ed.). Philadelphia: Lippincott Williams & Wilkins.

Spratto, G.R. and Woods, A.L. (2005). *2005 Edition: PDR Nurse's Drug Handbook.* Clifton Park, NY: Thomson Delmar Learning.

CASE STUDY 6

Sternal Wound Infection

GENDER
- M

AGE
- 66

SETTING
- Hospital

ETHNICITY/CULTURE
- White American

PREEXISTING CONDITIONS

COEXISTING CONDITIONS
- Coronary artery bypass graft

LIFESTYLE
- Self-employed construction worker

COMMUNICATION

DISABILITY

SOCIOECONOMIC STATUS
- Middle

SPIRITUAL/RELIGIOUS
- Catholic

PHARMACOLOGIC
- Morphine sulfate (Duramorph)
- Piperacillin sodium/Tazobactam sodium (Zosyn)
- Ciprofloxacin HcL (Cipro)

PSYCHOSOCIAL
- Anxiety

LEGAL

ETHICAL
- Quality care
- Decrease in income
- Health care benefits

ALTERNATIVE THERAPY
- St. John's Wort

PRIORITIZATION
- Room assignment
- Antimicrobial management

DELEGATION
- RN
- Wound care specialist
- CNA

MODERATE

THE CARDIOVASCULAR AND LYMPHATIC SYSTEMS

Level of difficulty: Moderate

Overview: This case focuses on the use of critical thinking to provide effective prioritization in a triage situation in a busy urban medical center emergency department. It also involves management of sternal wound infection secondary to post-coronary artery bypass graft. A wound care specialist is important to management of an infected wound. The certified nursing assistant (CNA) can help with assembling necessary equipment in preparation for wound care and can position the client for the performance of the wound care.

Client Profile

Mr. Y is a 66-year-old male who was discharged from the hospital six weeks ago after an emergency quadruple coronary artery bypass graft (CABG) surgery. His post-op recovery was uneventful, and he was discharged ten days after the surgery. He returns to the chief surgeon's private office on the tenth day post-discharge prior to readmission because the sternal incisional site is red and inflamed with an unusual odor from the site of the wound. He reports pain at the site during hygiene care and a temperature of 101.2° F during the five days prior to seeing the health care provider. Mr. Y believes the redness at the incisional site is normal after surgery. However, because of the unusual odor, he goes to the health care provider's office to have the wound evaluated. Mr. Y is 5′8″ and weighs 206 pounds.

Case Study

Mr. Y is referred to the hospital for further evaluation. On initial interview his vital signs are:

    Blood pressure: 130/84
    Pulse: 78 and regular
    Respirations: 20
    Temperature: 102.4° F

The sternal incision is red, raised, and moderately warm to touch. There are no signs of dehiscence although the wound edges are not completely approximated. Mr. Y reports a 30-year history of cigarette smoking, three packs per week. His past medical history (PMH) includes hyperlipidemia, stable angina, and past surgical history of left cardiac catheterization and percutaneous transluminal coronary angioplasty (PTCA) with stent two years ago. Lab test results sent from the health care provider's office reveal:

    White blood cell (WBC) count: 12,000/mm^3
    Red blood cell (RBC) count: 4.6/mm^3
    Calcium: 9 mg/dL
    Sodium (Na): 142 mEq/L
    Potassium (K+): 4.9 mEq/L
    Chloride: 100 mEq/L
    Blood urea nitrogen (BUN): 15 mg/dL
    Creatinine: 1.4 mg/dL
    Glucose: 130 mg/dL
    Platelet count (PLT): 300, 000/cm
    Prothrombin time (PT): 14 seconds, Control: 15.1 seconds
    Hematocrit (Hct): 42%
    Hemoglobin (Hgb): 16 g/dL
    Low-density lipoprotein (LDL): 130 mg/dL
    Total cholesterol: 200 mg/dL

Medications brought to the hospital include: lovastatin (Mevacor), nitroglycerin (NTG) sublingual, isosorbide dinitrate (Isordil), warfarin sodium (Coumadin) 7.5 mg, and rabeprazole sodium (Aciphex). Mr. Y is transferred to a cardio-thoracic unit. A computed tomography (CT) scan of the chest is done in the ED and there is no evidence of infection in the deeper structures of the thoracic cavity. On continued interview, Mr. Y reports self-medication with St. John's Wort whenever he feels anxious. His sternal wound is inspected by the receiving nurse who documents and reports the finding. Wound specimen for culture and sensitivity, and blood for gram stain are done and sent to the lab. An electrocardiogram (EKG) and a chest X-ray are done upon arrival to the unit, nursing assessment is completed, Mr. Y is placed on telemetry, and the nurse documents assessment findings. A nurse practitioner (NP) reviews the medications with the client and will discuss with the cardiologist before including them in current orders. The lab sends the report of the cultures, and the results are positive for Staphylococcus aureus and Enterococcus species. Mr. Y is informed that he will be admitted for further evaluation and antibiotic therapy. A diagnosis of sternal wound infection is made.

Questions and Suggested Answers

1. **What is a local factor that has affected Mr. Y's wound healing?** The local factor that has affected Mr. Y's healing is infection as evidenced by the assessment of his sternal wound that is red, raised, and warm to touch. In addition, he has an elevated temperature of 102°F on admission and an elevated WBC count of 12,000/mm^3. Further his wound culture reveals evidence of S. aureus and Enterococcus.

2. **How do age, chronic disease, and vascular problems delay Mr. Y's wound healing?** *Age* delays wound healing because there is decreased vascularity, the water content decreases, and the skin becomes drier. These changes increase the older adult's susceptibility to trauma and delay wound healing. *Chronic diseases* delay wound healing by slowing cell renewal, resulting in skin that has decreased elasticity. Chronic diseases such as bowel or bladder incontinence can contaminate wounds and delay healing. *Vascular problems* delay wound healing because when tissue cells are damaged, local blood vessels temporarily constrict and nutrient blood supply is altered.

3. **Discuss common nursing diagnoses related to wound management.**
   - Altered protection R/T infectious process
   - Impaired tissue integrity R/T sternal wound
   - Deficient knowledge R/T condition, treatment, and home care

The following are prescribed:

- Piperacillin sodium/tazobactam sodium (Zosyn) 3 g IV q8h
- Morphine sulfate (Duramorph) PRN 2 mg IV prior to each dressing change
- Oxycodone (Roxicodone) 5–10 mg q4h PRN for mild to moderate pain
- Lovastatin (Mevacor) 40 mg PO two times per day
- Isosorbide dinitrate (Isordil) 10 mg four times per day PO, before meals and at bedtime
- Rabeprazole sodium (Aciphex) 20 mg PO daily
- Warfarin sodium (Coumadin) 7.5 mg PO daily after checking PT level
- Wound irrigation with 0.9% normal saline solution two times per day, followed by a wet-to-moist packing with 0.9% normal saline solution

4. **What are the purposes for the prescribed medications?** *Piperacillin sodium/tazobactam sodium* is an extended-spectrum penicillin and beta-lactamase inhibitor that is used to treat infections caused by the organisms identified in the cultures. It is active against most gram-negative and many gram-positive anaerobic and aerobic organisms including *Clostridium, Klebsiella, Pseudomonas,* and *Proteus*. It destroys the organisms by interfering with bacterial cell wall synthesis and promoting the loss of their membrane integrity, resulting in death of the cells. *Morphine sulfate* is an opioid analgesic that relieves moderate to severe pain by mimicking the actions of endogenous opioid peptides, primarily at the delta receptors where the opioid peptoids and the morphine bind in the region of the brain and spinal cord that is associated with perception of pain. *Oxycodone* is a semi-synthetic opioid analgesic used to treat moderate pain. It acts by altering pain perception in the central nervous system (CNS). *Lovastatin* is an antihyperlipidemic, HMG-CoA reductase inhibitor that reduces cholesterol levels by interfering with the body's ability to produce its own cholesterol. Lovastatin reduces lipid levels by triggering induction of LDL receptors, which promotes removal of LDL and very low density lipoprotein (VLDL) remnants from plasma. When LDL and VLDL remnants are removed, high density lipoprotein

(HDL) plasma concentrations increase, and it collects excess cholesterol from body cells and transports it to the liver for secretion. *Isosorbide dinitrate* is a coronary vasodilator that relaxes vascular smooth muscle resulting in vasodilation. This increases blood flow to the coronary arteries and prevents anginal attacks that may occur even after CABG. *Rabeprazole sodium* is a proton pump inhibitor that suppresses acid secretion and is used prophylactically for Mr. Y. Many factors increase gastric acid secretion which, if left untreated, can result in gastric ulcer and predisposes the individual to gastric cancer. Rabeprazole sodium also is effective for dyspepsia and heartburn, which are adverse effects of lovastatin. Rabeprazole sodium suppresses gastric acid secretion by inhibiting H^+/K^+ ATPase, the enzyme that makes gastrin acid. *Warfarin sodium* is an oral anticoagulant that prevents the formation of new thrombus. Clients who are post-coronary artery bypass are usually placed on warfarin sodium or clopidogrel bisulfate to prevent formation of thrombus secondary to the use of the cardiopulmonary bypass machine during surgery which can damage the red blood cells causing them to aggregate more easily. Thrombus also may occur depending on the client's mobility. Warfarin functions to prevent the forming of new clots by indirectly interfering with blood clotting by depressing the hepatic synthesis of vitamin K-dependent coagulation Factors II, VII, IX, and X.

5. **What are the most common adverse reactions of the prescribed medications?** The most common adverse reactions of *piperacillin sodium/tazobactam sodium* are hypersensitivity, rashes, hypokalemia, prolonged prothrombin and partial thromboplastin times, and phlebitis (if infused too rapidly). The most common adverse reactions of *morphine sulfate* are pruritus, constipation, and nausea. Respiratory depression is very rare even in children. The most common adverse effects associated with *oxycodone* are dizziness, lightheadedness, nausea and vomiting, and sedation. The most common adverse reactions of *lovastatin* are flatulence, abdominal cramps, diarrhea, constipation, headache, and insomnia. The most severe adverse effects are hepatotoxicity and myopathy. Because of the risk of toxicity to the liver, clients should have liver function tests done prior to beginning therapy with lovastatin. The most common adverse reactions of *isosorbide dinitrate* are dizziness, headache, hypotension, tachycardia, confusion, disorientation, nausea, and vomiting. The most common adverse reactions of *rabeprazole sodium* are hot flashes, diarrhea, abdominal pain, flatulence, constipation, and dyspepsia. The most significant adverse reaction of *warfarin sodium* is hemorrhage that could occur from any body tissue or organ. Hepatotoxicity also is a risk when using warfarin.

6. **Discuss the drug-to-drug, drug-to-food/herbal interactions for the prescribed medications.** Drug-to-drug interactions may occur with the simultaneous use of *piperacillin sodium/tazobactam sodium* and antiprobenecid, which may decrease renal excretion of piperacillin/tazobactam and increase blood levels. The simultaneous use with lithium may alter excretion of lithium. Concomitant use with anticoagulants, thrombolytics, nonsteroidal anti-inflammatory agents (NSAIDs), dipyridamole, and dextran may increase the risk of bleeding, and its use with potassium-losing diuretics, corticosteroids, or amphotericin B may increase risk of hypokalemia. If used simultaneously with aminoglycosides in clients with renal impairment, it may decrease the half-life of aminoglycosides. This antibiotic may inhibit the effectiveness of oral contraceptives and may cause false positive glucose readings in the urine. There are no clinically significant drug-to-food/herbal interactions established. Drug-to-drug interactions may occur with the simultaneous use of *morphine sulfate* and other CNS depressants and monoamine oxidase (MAO) inhibitors, which may increase sedating effects. Simultaneous use with partial-antagonist opioid analgesics may precipitate opioid withdrawal in physically dependent clients. The simultaneous use of buprenorphine, nalbuphine, butorphanol, or pentazocine may decrease analgesia. The simultaneous use with warfarin sodium may increase anticoagulant effect and use with cimetidine may decrease metabolism and increase the effects of morphine sulfate. There are no clinically significant drug-to-food interactions established. Drug-to-herbal interactions may occur with the simultaneous use of kava-kava, valerian, skullcap, chamomile, hops, and St. John's Wort, which may increase CNS depression. Drug-to-drug interactions may occur with the simultaneous use of *oxycodone* and anticholinergic agents causing the client to experience a paralytic ileus. Tricyclic antidepressants and MAO inhibitors when used with oxycodone can result in an increased effect of either or both agents. Use of oxycodone with other CNS depressants (narcotic analgesics, phenothiazines, anxiolytics, sedative-hypnotics, anesthetics, and alcohol) will increase the CNS depression. As with most opiod analgesics,

drug-to-herbal interactions may occur with the simultaneous use of kava-kava, valerian, skullcap, chamomile, hops, and St. John's Wort, which may increase CNS depression. Drug-to-drug interactions may occur with the simultaneous use of ***lovastatin*** and clarithromycin, clofibrate, cyclosporine, flucanozole, erythromycin, gemfibrozil, ketoconazole, and niacin, which increase the risk of myopathy and rhabdomyolysis. The simultaneous use with warfarin may potentiate hypoprothrombinemia. Drug-to-food interaction may occur with the simultaneous use of grapefruit juice above one quart, which may result in increase risk for myopathy and rhabdomyolysis. There are no drug-to-herbal interactions established. Drug-to-drug interactions may occur with the simultaneous use of ***isosorbide dinitrate*** and agents used to treat erectile dysfunction, such as sildenafil, which may result in significant and potentially fatal hypotension. The simultaneous use of antihypertensives, beta blockers, calcium-channel blockers, and phenothiazines may cause additive hypotension. Aspirin may increase blood levels and effects of isosorbide dinitrate. There are no clinically significant drug-to-drug or drug-to-food/herbal interactions established. Drug-to-drug interactions may occur with the simultaneous use of ***rabeprazole sodium*** and ketoconazole may decrease plasma levels. Use with digoxin may increase the serum levels and increase the risk of digoxin toxicity. Its use with warfarin may increase the risk of bleeding. There are no clinically significant drug-to-food/herbal interactions established. Drug-to-drug interactions may occur with the simultaneous use of ***warfarin sodium*** and heparin, abciximab, androgens, capecitabine, cefoperazone, cefotetan, chloral hydrate, chloramphenicol, clopidrogel, disulfiram, fluconazole, fluoroquinolones, itraconazole, metronidazole, plicamycin, thrombolytic agents, epitifibatide, tirofiban, ticlopidine, sulfonamides, quinidine, quinine, NSAIDs, valproates, aspirin, acetaminophen, allopurinol, aminosalicylic acid, and amiodarone. All of these may increase the risk of bleeding. Drug-to-food/herbal interactions may occur with the simultaneous use of capsicum, celery, clove, chamomile, fenugreek, garlic, ginger, licorice root, green tea, Panax ginseng, St. John's Wort, and foods high in vitamin K.

7. **How do drugs such as corticosteroids, anti-inflammatory agents, and chemotherapy delay wound healing?** Corticosteroids, anti-inflammatory agents, and chemotherapy delay wound healing because of their ability to alter protein synthesis and cellular growth. Corticosteroids and anti-inflammatory agents slow wound healing because the anti-inflammatory effects of steroids prolong the inflammatory phase. When the inflammatory phase is prolonged, this results in delay of the phagocytic immune response (the first line of defense), the antibody immune response (the response that disables invaders), and the cellular immune response (which attacks pathogens). Chemotherapy delays wound healing by suppressing the function of the bone marrow, thereby altering oxygen-rich nutrients that are needed for wound healing.

8. **How do years of cigarette smoking delay wound healing?** Years of cigarette smoking can cause delayed wounding healing because smoking constricts blood vessels and reduces the blood's oxygen-carrying capacity, resulting in decreased tissue oxygenation. Smoking also increases platelet aggregation, which in turn may cause hypercoagulability with decreased perfusion to the skin or wound, which would delay wound healing.

9. **What are the benefits of wound irrigation?** Wound irrigation promotes wound healing by removing exudate, drainage, pus, and slough. Irrigation washes the wound without wiping delicate tissues with a fabric that might cause damage to newly forming granulation tissue. Irritation also penetrates tunnels or fissures in the wound. Irrigating with 0.9% normal saline speeds the healing process, because the normal saline solution is iso-osmolar, therefore it keeps the wound moist.

10. **Discuss the phases of wound healing.** The phases of wound healing are the inflammatory phase, the reconstruction phase, and the maturation phase. The ***inflammatory phase*** begins at the time of tissue injury and lasts for three to four days. During the inflammatory phase, phagocytosis (by neutrophils) moves into the wound and the neutrophils begin to ingest bacteria and wound debris. Monocytes change into macrophages and continue cleaning the wound and stimulate the formation of fibroblasts (connective tissue cells). This fibrin network provides a structure to aid in the formation of fibrous bridges as well as epithelial cells that move inward from the wound edges to create an epithelial layer. The ***reconstruction phase*** (or proliferative phase) of healing is the second phase, which lasts for several days (4–21 days). During this phase, collagen fills the wound bed, new blood vessels develop (angiogenesis), and granulation tissue is formed from fibroblasts,

giving the wound a bright red granular appearance. Progressive collagen accumulation during the second week of healing results in the basic structure of the scar, which does not achieve its full tensible strength for a long time. The third and final stage of wound healing is the ***maturation phase*** (or remodeling phase). Reorganization of collagen fibers, wound remodeling, and maturation of the tissues to approximate the skin's original strength characterizes the maturation or remodeling phase.

11. **Discuss client education at time of discharge for an unhealed wound.** Planning for discharge should begin several days before dismissal from the hospital so that the home situation can be appraised and necessary supplies and equipment can be obtained. The social worker should be included in the discharge plans to help with retrieving needed supplies and implementing community resources (e.g., visiting nurse service, home health) in the initial wound care on discharge. The client should be instructed about signs of infection and given directions about when and how to contact the primary health care provider in the event infection recurs. The client should be instructed to eat a balanced diet with frequent high-protein snacks, including vitamin and mineral supplements as prescribed by the health care provider. Proper use of dressing materials and supplies, as well as frequent hand washing, should be stressed. The importance of follow-up care as ordered by the primary health care provider should be stressed. All of these instructions should be both verbal and written.

References

Broyles, B.E. (2005). *Medical-Surgical Nursing Clinical Companion.* Durham, NC: Carolina Academic Press.

Corbet, J.V. (2004). *Laboratory Tests and Diagnostic Procedures with Nursing Diagnoses* (6th ed.). Upper Saddle River, NJ: Prentice Hall.

"Factors That Interfere with Wound Healing" (November 2005). Available at www.merckvetmanual.com/mvm/index.jsp?cfile=htm/bc/160706.htm.

Gahart, B.L. and Nazareno, A.R. (2005). *2005 Intravenous Medications.* St. Louis: Mosby.

Huether, S.E. and McCance, K.L. (2004). *Understanding Pathophysiology* (3rd ed.). St. Louis: Mosby.

Ignatavicius, D.D. and Workman, M.L. (2006). *Medical-Surgical Nursing: Critical Thinking for Collaborative Care* (5th ed.). Philadelphia: W.B. Saunders.

Lehne, R.A. (2004). *Pharmacology for Nursing Care* (5th ed.). Philadelphia: W.B. Saunders.

LeMone, P. and Burke, K.M. (2004). *Medical-Surgical Nursing: Critical Thinking in Client Care* (3rd ed.). Upper Saddle River, NJ: Prentice Hall.

Romo, T. and McLaughlin, L.A. (November 2005). "Wound Healing Skin." Available at www.emedicine.com/ent/topic13.htm.

Sholar, A. and Stadelmann, W. (May 2003). "Wound Healing, Chronic Wounds." Available at www.emedicine.com/plastic/topic477.htm.

Smeltzer, S.C. and Bare, B.G. (2004). *Textbook of Medical-Surgical Nursing* (10th ed.). Philadelphia: Lippincott Williams & Wilkins.

Spratto, G.R. and Woods, A.L. (2005). *2005 Edition: PDR Nurse's Drug Handbook.* Clifton Park, NY: Thomson Delmar Learning.

CASE STUDY 7

Valvular Heart Disease – Aortic Stenosis

GENDER
- M

AGE
- 56

SETTING
- Hospital

ETHNICITY/CULTURE
- Hispanic/American

PREEXISTING CONDITIONS
- Angina

COEXISTING CONDITIONS

LIFESTYLE
- Supervisor for a community department store

COMMUNICATION
- Spanish and English

DISABILITY

SOCIOECONOMIC STATUS
- Middle

SPIRITUAL/RELIGIOUS
- Catholic

PHARMACOLOGIC
- Calcium-channel blocker
- ACE inhibitor
- Cardiotonic
- Oxygen

PSYCHOSOCIAL
- Anxiety

LEGAL

ETHICAL

ALTERNATIVE THERAPY
- Holy Communion

PRIORITIZATION
- Maintain cardiac output
- Monitor vital signs
- Administer oxygen

DELEGATION
- RN
- Client education

MODERATE

THE CARDIOVASCULAR AND LYMPHATIC SYSTEMS

Level of difficulty: Moderate

Overview: This case involves the use of the nursing process and critical thinking to appropriately assess the client and delegate effectively so that care can be implemented. The case requires health care personnel who are competent in cardiac assessment, identifying heart sounds and dysrhythmias, and intervening effectively.

Client Profile

Mr. W is a 56-year-old male who is 5'6" and weighs 190 pounds. His past medical history includes childhood rheumatic heart disease with one occurrence of strep throat at the age of 30. Mr. W is married, and there is one young adult living at home with him and his wife. They live in a private home with four flights of steps going up to the bedrooms.

Case Study

Mr. W is referred to the hospital by his primary health care provider after frequent complaints of difficulty breathing when climbing stairs and a report of feeling tired after walking only two blocks. Mr. W also reports anginal-type chest pain and infrequent syncope. He reports loss of appetite and loss of 12 pounds over one month. On admission to the hospital, his vitals signs are:

Blood pressure: 150/68
Pulse: 64 and irregular
Respirations: 16
Temperature: 98.6° F

On auscultation, there is a harsh systolic murmur in the second intercostal space at the right sternal border. An arterial blood gas (ABG) is done and reveals hypoxemia. Oxygen, three liters via nasal cannula, is initiated. Mr. W denies surgical history but reports having a cardiac catheterization that was done two months ago at another hospital and chronic atrial fibrillation. The result of the catheterization is sent from Mr. W's primary health care provider's office. The report of the catheterization is:

Routine blood pressure in brachial artery: 120/50 mm Hg (normal = 90–140/60–90 mm Hg)
End-diastolic volume (EDV): 80 ml/m^2 (normal = 50–90 ml/m^2)
Ejection fraction: 0.58 (normal = 0.67 $\pm$ 0.07)
Cardiac output: (CO) 4 liters/min (normal = 3–6 liters/min)

A thorough history and physical is completed by a health care provider and a registered nurse (RN). A multidisciplinary team reviews the current data gathered from the history, physical, and reports of the previous diagnostic tests. A chest X-ray reveals mid-left ventricular enlargement, and echocardiography provides data of the cardiac structure, movement of the valve leaflets, and the size and function of the cardiac chambers, which aids in diagnosis. An EKG confirms chronic atrial fibrillation. Admission lab tests reveal:

White blood cell (WBC) count: 9,000/mm^3
Red blood cell (RBC): 3.4 million/mm^3
Hemoglobin (Hgb): 10 g/dL
Hematocrit (Hct): 28%
Platelet: 150,000/mm^3
Glucose: 116 mg/dL
Blood urea nitrogen (BUN): 15 mg/dL
Creatinine: 0.9 mg/dL
Sodium (Na): 135 mEq/L
Potassium (K+): 4.6 mEq/L
Albumin 3.3 mg/dL
Calcium 8.6 mg/dL
Digoxin level: 1.3 ng/dL

After review of collected data and collaborative discussion with the multidisciplinary team, a diagnosis of aortic stenosis is confirmed. The findings are discussed with Mr. W and his wife, and a surgical consultation is done. Elective surgery for aortic valve repair is planned and will be scheduled within three days. A prosthetic valve will be used. In preparation for the aortic valve repair, Mr. W is to be transfused as prescribed with two units of packed red blood cells (PRBCs) because of the low Hgb and Hct.

Questions and Suggested Answers

1. **Discuss common nursing diagnoses for clients with valvular heart disease.**

   - Decreased cardiac output R/T altered stroke volume
   - Impaired gas exchange R/T ventilation perfusion imbalance
   - Ineffective cardiopulmonary tissue perfusion R/T cardiac pathology
   - Activity intolerance R/T inability of the heart to meet metabolic demands during activity
   - Acute pain R/T physiologic injury agent (hypoxia)
   - Deficient knowledge R/T condition, treatment, and home care

2. **Why is cardiac catheterization usually done when clients are diagnosed with aortic stenosis?** Cardiac catheterization provides specific information about the anatomy and physiology of the heart. In the presence of abnormalities, it provides visualization of the severity of the stenosis. It traces cardiac circulation and visualization of the cardiac vasculature. Because of its invasive nature, the cardiac catheterization usually is preceded by an echocardiogram.

3. **Why is atrial fibrillation a common finding in aortic stenosis?** Atrial fibrillation develops in aortic stenosis because of left atrial dilation that prevents the atria from emptying adequately into the ventricles. Dilated atrial walls provide ideal conditions for a long conductive pathway as well as slowed conduction causing the sinoatrial (SA) node to not regulate the rate and the atrial contraction waves (P waves) to arise from different foci in the atria. This occurs so fast (350–600 atrial beats per minute) that they do not result in conduction to the ventricles.

4. **What is a long-term complication of aortic stenosis?** Left-sided heart failure is a long-term complication of aortic stenosis. As the stenosis progresses, cardiac output becomes fixed and unable to increase to meet the demands of the body during exertion. Eventually, the left ventricle fails, volume backs up in the left atrium, and the pulmonary system becomes congested, resulting in right-sided heart failure. Conduction defects also are complications, and if aortic stenosis is severe, sudden death could occur.

The following new medications are prescribed:

- Digoxin (Lanoxin) 0.125 mg PO
- Diltiazem (Cardizem) 40 mg PO two times per day
- Amiodarone HcL (Cardarone) 200 mg PO daily
- Warfarin sodium (Coumadin) 5 mg PO today

5. **What are the purposes for the prescribed orders?**
   Digoxin is a positive inotropic cardiac glycoside administered to increase the force of contraction and in doing so increase the ejection fraction to within the normal range. This improves tissue perfusion. Mr. W has aortic stenosis; therefore, there is alteration in aortic outflow, and a decrease in stroke volume resulting in a decrease in cardiac output. When cardiac output is decreased, there is the need for inotropic agents to help increase stroke volume and in doing so increase cardiac output, and digoxin has the abilities to improve these negative factors. *Diltiazem* is a calcium channel-blocking agent used to reduce the regurgitant flow for clients with aortic stenosis. It is highly effective because the drug is very effective on peripheral vascular smooth muscle, causing potent peripheral vasodilation and perfusion to the heart muscle in the presence

of the stenosis. It has antidysrhythmic properties that help convert atrial fibrillation to sinus rhythm. However, if there is resistance to conversion, diltiazem will slow the progression of atrial fibrillation. *Amiodarone HcL* is a class III antiarrhythmic agent used to decrease peripheral resistance and increase coronary blood flow in the presence of the stenosis. As an antiarrhythmic, it is used as prophylaxis for atrial fibrillation and other dysrhythmias that may occur due to the stenosis. Amiodarone HcL is also beneficial with aortic stenosis because it blocks the effect of sympathetic stimulation and works directly on smooth muscles, resulting in decreased peripheral resistance and increase in coronary blood flow even though there is stenosis of a valve. *Warfarin sodium* is an oral anticoagulant that prevents thrombus formation by depressing hepatic synthesis of vitamin K-dependent coagulation Factors II, VII, IX, and X. It is used as prophylaxis for atrial fibrillation with potential for embolization.

6. **What are the most common adverse reactions of the prescribed medications?** The most common adverse reactions of *digoxin* are bradycardia, nausea, anorexia, other dysrhythmias, and toxicity. The most common adverse reactions of *amiodarone HcL* are bradycardia and other conduction abnormalities, muscle weakness, fatigue, dizziness, hypotension, corneal microdeposits, anorexia, nausea, vomiting, constipation, photosensitivity, hypothyroidism, ataxia, involuntary movement, paresthesia, peripheral neuropathy, poor coordination, and tremor. The most common adverse effects associated with *diltiazen* include AV block, bradycardia, hypotension, syncope, palpitations, tachycardia, and peripheral edema. The most common adverse effects of *warfarin sodium* are bruising and prolonged bleeding.

7. **Discuss the drug-to-drug and drug-to-food/herbal interactions of the prescribed medications.** Drug-to-drug interactions may occur with the simultaneous use of *digoxin* and cholestyramine; colestipol, which may increase digoxin absorption; diuretics, corticosteroids, amphotericin B, laxatives, and sodium polystyrene sulfonate that may cause hypokalemia and increase the risk of digoxin toxicity. Calcium IV may increase the risk of dysrhythmias, and quinidine, verapamil, and amiodarone may significantly increase digoxin levels, requiring the decrease of the needed dose to maintain cardiac stability. Additive bradycardia may occur with beta blockers and other dysrhythmias; antacids and kaolin/pectin decrease digoxin absorption. Epinephrine, muscle relaxants, sympathomimetics, succinylcholine, and propranolol also potentiate digoxin's effects and increase the risk of cardiac dysrrythmias and metoclopramide decreases digoxin's effects by decreasing gastrointestinal (GI) absorption. In addition, thyroid replacement agents, sulfasalazine, and hypoglycemic agents decrease digoxin effects. The simultaneous use of German chamomile flower, ginseng, hawthorn, Iceland moss, ivy leaf, Indian snakeroot, licorice, rhubarb root, senna pod/leaf, sarsaparilla root, and marshmallow root potentiate digoxin's effects and increase the risk of toxicity. St. John's Wort decreases digoxin absorption by increasing its renal excretion. With *amiodarone HcL,* drug-to-drug interactions may occur with the simultaneous use of quinidine, procainamide, mexiletine, lidocaine, flecainide, cholesytramine, and cimetidine, which may alter amiodarone serum level. The simultaneous use with phenytoin decreases amiodarone blood level. Use with azithromycin increases the potential for prolonged QT intervals and dispersion. Beta-adrenergic blocking agents increase the risk of bradycardia and hypotension. Use with calcium channel blocking agents increases the risk of AV block when used with verapamil or diltiazem or hypotension with all calcium channel blockers. Cimetidine, indinavir, cholesytramine, and ritonavir decrease serum amiodarone HcL levels. If used with theophylline, amiodarone can increase theophylline levels and the risk of toxicity and if used concurrently with digoxin the risk of digoxin toxicity increases. If used with fluoroquinolones, there is an increased risk of life-threatening cardiac dysrhythmias. Use with pyridoxine increases the risk of amiodarone-induced photosensitivity. The concurrent use with warfarin sodium increases the activity of warfarin sodium, requiring the dose to be reduced. Drug-to-food interactions can occur with grapefruit juice, increasing serum amiodarone levels. Drug-to-herbal interactions are seen with the simultaneous use of echinacea, which may increase the risk for hepatotoxicity. Drug-to-drug interactions may occur with the simultaneous use of *diltiazem* and amiodarone, which may cause possible cardiotoxicity. The simultaneous use with amlodipine may cause increased plasma amlodipine levels and its use with anesthetics may depress the cardiac conduction system. The simultaneous use with buspirone may increase buspirone effects. Simultaneous use with carbamazepine may increase diltiazem effects. When used simultaneously with

cyclosporine, the effects of cyclosporine are increased, with risk for renal toxicity. The simultaneous use of diltiazem and digoxin results in increased risk of digoxin toxicity, and when used simultaneously with HMG-CoA reductase inhibitors, diltiazem increases the plasma levels of these drugs. Concurrent use with lithium increases the risk of neurotoxicity, and its use with methylprednisolone increases the risk of methyprednisolone toxicity. The simultaneous use of moricizine increases moricizine levels and decreases diltiazem levels, and ranitidine increases diltiazem bioavailability. If used simultaneously with quinidine, diltiazem, the risk of quinidine toxicity is increased. Diltiazem simultaneous use with tacrolimus increases tacrolimus levels, and when used with theophylline, it increases the risk of theophylline toxicity. Drug-to-drug interactions with *warfarin sodium* can occur with the simultaneous use of acetaminophen, amiodarone, androgen, beta-adrenergic, which increase anticoagulant effects, and the simultaneous use of aminoglutethimide and amiodarone decreases warfarin sodium levels. Drug-to-food interactions include avacado and vitamin K, both of which decrease warfarin's effects. Drug-to-herbal interactions include St. John's Wort, which decreases the effects of warfarin.

8. **Which modality is the definitive treatment of aortic stenosis for clients with complaints of dyspnea, fatigue, and chest pain?** The definitive treatment of aortic stenosis when clients complain of dyspnea, fatigue, and chest pain is valvular replacement. Valvular replacement is a surgical choice because with the stenosis, blood flow from the left ventricle into the aorta is obstructed during systole. The result is incomplete emptying of the left atrium, which causes back pressure through the pulmonary veins resulting in pulmonary hypertension. Eventually, right ventricular failure develops. As the stenosis progresses, there is reduction in left ventricular compliance and cardiac output fails, requiring surgery either to replace the diseased valve or to restore valve function, alleviate symptoms, and prevent complications and death.

9. **Identify the different types of valves used in valvular replacement procedures.** The different types of valves used in valvular replacement procedures are prosthetic (synthetic) and biologic (tissue) valves. Biologic valves may come from other species (xenograft), such as a porcine valve from a pig or a bovine valve from a cow. Biologic valves are not associated with high risk for clot formation; therefore, long-term anticoagulation is not needed. However, xenografts are not as durable as prosthetic valves and require replacement every seven to ten years. A client with aortic stenosis usually has valve replacement with a mechanical valve.

10. **What are the two post-surgery complications the nurse should monitor for when a client has valvular replacement?** The two post-surgery complications of concern are reduction in cardiac output (CO) and post-surgery bleeding. Prior to the surgery, the client's cardiac output is already reduced due to the significant hypertrophy of the left ventricular myocardium resulting in the inability to pump sufficient blood to achieve and maintain normal cardiac output. Decreased cardiac output could occur if there is valve failure post-surgery. Valve failure would lead to aortic regurgitation, resulting in blood flowing backward instead of forward, resulting in a decrease in cardiac output. Post-surgery bleeding could develop if a mechanical valve is inserted. Clients who receive mechanical valves are placed on anticoagulant medication to prevent clots from developing on the valve. Anticoagulant could result in subtle or overt bleeding, especially if client's bleeding and prothrombin times (PTs) are not closely monitored.

11. **Discuss client education for post-valvular surgery.** The client must comply with discharge orders, especially returning to the health care provider to have PT monitored to determine the effectiveness of anticoagulant therapy or the need for modification of prescription. The client should be shown how to plan work, activity, and rest to conserve energy. Even though a mechanical valve has replaced the native heart valve, the body needs time to heal. Therefore work, activity, and rest should be balanced. The client should be taught how to manage anticoagulant therapy, including dietary considerations, such as avoiding foods high in vitamin K to avoid interference with anticoagulants, such as bleeding. The client should be told to report any bleeding or unusual bruising to the primary health care provider promptly. Bleeding is the main complication of anticoagulation therapy, and the risk of bleeding also depends on the nature of the client's underlying clinical disorder or the intake of other drugs that impair platelet function. The client must inform any dentist that he or she has a prosthetic valve so that antibiotic therapy can be initiated prior to any procedures.

Carrying a wallet-sized card indicating the need for antibiotic therapy before invasive procedures should be recommended. The client must avoid procedures that use magnetic resonance imaging (MRI) techniques; implants such as heart valves cause artifacts in the image of the examination field. The client should follow all instructions for follow-up care. It is important to stress this so the client's health status can be monitored and modification to the discharge treatment can be made if necessary.

References

Broyles, B.E. (2005). *Medical-Surgical Nursing Clinical Companion.* Durham, NC: Carolina Academic Press.

Corbet, J.V. (2004). *Laboratory Tests and Diagnostic Procedures with Nursing Diagnoses* (6th ed.). Upper Saddle River, NJ: Prentice Hall.

Gahart, B.L. and Nazareno, A.R. (2005). *2005 Intravenous Medications.* St. Louis: Mosby.

Huether, S.E. and McCance, K.L. (2004). *Understanding Pathophysiology* (3rd ed.). St. Louis: Mosby.

Ignatavicius, D.D. and Workman, M.L. (2006). *Medical-Surgical Nursing across the Health Care Continuum* (5th ed.). Philadelphia: W.B. Saunders.

Lehne, R.A. (2004). *Pharmacology for Nursing Care* (5th ed.). Philadelphia: W. B. Saunders.

Phipps, W.J., Monahan, F.D., Sands, J.K., Marek, J.E., and Neighbors, M. (2004). *Medical-Surgical Nursing: Health and Illness Perspectives* (7th ed.). St. Louis: Mosby.

Spratto, G.R. and Woods, A.L. (2005). *2005 Edition: PDR Nurse's Drug Handbook.* Clifton Park, NY: Thomson Delmar Learning.

CASE STUDY 8

Hodgkin's Disease

GENDER
- M

AGE
- 54

SETTING
- Outpatient clinic of a medical center

ETHNICITY/CULTURE
- White Englishman

PREEXISTING CONDITIONS
- Enlarged, painless, freely movable mass in the neck

COEXISTING CONDITIONS
- History of viral infection

LIFESTYLE
- Worked as a subway worker before immigrating to the U.S.

COMMUNICATION

DISABILITY

SOCIOECONOMIC STATUS
- Middle

SPIRITUAL/RELIGIOUS
- Anglican

PHARMACOLOGIC
- Mechlorethamine HcL (Mustargen)
- Vincristine sulfate (Oncovin)
- Procarbazine HcL (Matulane)
- Prednisone (Deltasone)
- Ondansetron HcL (Zofran)

PSYCHOSOCIAL
- Anxiety

LEGAL
- Assistance with financial resource

ETHICAL
- Do recent immigrants to the U.S. have a right to optimum health care benefits in lieu of unemployment related to work status?

ALTERNATIVE THERAPY

PRIORITIZATION
- Physical assessment
- Prepare for staging of lymph node

DELEGATION
- RN
- Client education

MODERATE

THE CARDIOVASCULAR AND LYMPHATIC SYSTEMS

Level of difficulty: Moderate

Overview: This case study involves a thorough assessment of the client's condition with careful palpation for lymphadenopathic lesions. It also involves critical questioning pertaining to night sweats and weight loss of more than 10%, unusual headaches, dry cough, and neck or back pain.

Client Profile

Mr. O is a 54-year-old male who has been a resident of the United States for the past three years after relocating from London, England, where he worked as an underground railroad employee. He is 5'8" and weighs 165 pounds.

Case Study

Mr. O is seen in the outpatient clinic of a major medical center with complaints of gradual fatigue and weight loss over the past two months. He also reports fever of unknown cause, unusual pruritus on the trunk and chest of his body, headaches, and vertigo. After initial interview by the nurse, Mr. O is seen by a health care provider, who continues with the history and physical examination. Large, painless lymph nodes are found in the neck and axilla areas. Mr. O denies the use of medications or herbal supplements and denies past medical or surgical history. Vital signs on admission reveal:

> Blood pressure: 120/80
> Pulse: 78
> Respirations: 16
> Temperature: 98.4° F

Lab results reveal:

> White blood cell (WBC) differential:
>> Lymphocytes 22%
>> Segmented neutrophils: 60%
>> Monocytes: 6.2%
>> Eosinophils: 0.9%
>> Basophils: 1.1%
>> Bands: 5%
>
> Red blood cell (RBC) count: 4 million/mm^3
> Hematocrit (Hct): 42%
> Hemoglobin (Hgb): 13 g/dL
> Platelet count: 267,000/mm^3
> Granulocyte: 20.4%
> Sodium (Na): 138 mEq/L
> Potassium (K+): 3.9 mEq/L
> Calcium: 8.4 mg/dL
> Blood urea nitrogen (BUN): 15 mg/dL
> Creatinine: 0.7 mg/dL
> Magnesium: 2 mg/dL

After the labs and physical assessment findings are reviewed by the health care provider and a hematologist, Mr. O is admitted to a medical unit for further evaluation. A positron emission test (PET) shows cancer cells in the peripheral lymph node and peripheral lymph node enlargement. A chest X-ray and an abdominal computed tomography (CT) scan are done, but the findings for lymphadenopathy in the thoracic and abdominal areas are negative. Mr. O is advised of the need for lymph node biopsy, and he signs an informed witnessed consent. The biopsy is positive for Reed-Sternberg cells. Staging procedures reveal stage IIa lymphoma. After the health care provider and hematologist review the results of the labs and diagnostic reports, a diagnosis of stage IIa Hodgkin's disease is confirmed and discussed with the client, who agrees with the treatment plan.

Questions and Suggested Answers

1. **Discuss the prevalence, incidence, risk factors, and pathophysiology of Hodgkin's disease.** Hodgkin's disease is a relatively rare malignancy that has an impressive cure rate. It is somewhat more common in men than women and has two peaks of incidence: one in the early 20s and the other after age 50. Hodgkin's disease spreads by contiguous extension along the lymphatic system. The cause is not presently known. However, 20% of clients are also infected with *Epstein-Barr virus*, which occurs more commonly in the younger client population. There is a familial pattern associated with the disease: first-degree relatives have a higher-than-normal frequency of the disease. Mr. O's family might have been exposed to some form of chemical agents during his years of work in the underground railroad, enhancing the development of Hodgkin's disease.

2. **Discuss clinical manifestations of Hodgkin's disease.** Hodgkin's disease usually begins as a painless enlargement of one or more lymph node on one side of the neck. The individual nodes are painless and firm, but not hard. The most common sites for lymphadenopathy are the cervical, supraclavicular, and mediastinal nodes; involvement of the iliac or inguinal nodes or spleen is much less common. A mediastinal mass may be seen on chest X-ray; occasionally the mass is large enough to compress the trachea and induce dyspnea. Pruritus is common and can be extremely distressing, although the etiology is unclear. A fairly common finding (20%) is the development of brief but severe pain after drinking alcohol. The pain is usually at the site of the Hodgkin's disease, and the cause is unknown. Because all organs are vulnerable to invasion of Hodgkin's disease, symptoms result from the tumor compressing other organs, such as cough and pulmonary effusion; jaundice from hepatic involvement or bile duct obstruction; abdominal pain from splenomegaly or retroperitoneal adenopathy; or bone pain from skeletal involvement. Herpes zoster (i.e., shingles) infections are common. "B" symptoms are found in 40% of persons with Hodgkin's disease and are more common in the advanced stage of the disease. The symptoms include fever (without chills), drenching sweats (particular at night), and unintentional weight loss of more than 10%. A mild anemia is the most common hematologic finding. The WBC count may be elevated or decreased.

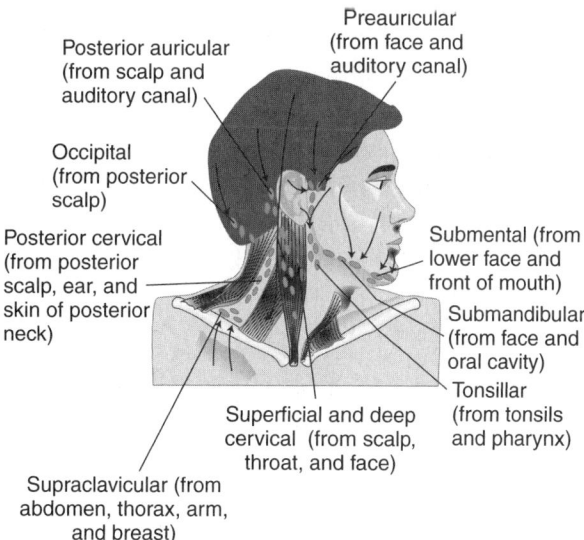

3. **Discuss diagnostic studies used to confirm Hodgkin's disease.** The diagnosis is made by means of an excisional lymph node biopsy and the presence of *Reed-Sternberg cells*. The malignant cell of Hodgkin's disease is the Reed-Sternberg cell, a gigantic tumor cell that is morphologically unique and is thought to be of immature lymphoid origin. It is the pathologic hallmark and essential diagnostic criterion for Hodgkin's disease. However, the tumor is very heterogeneous, and may actually contain only few Reed-Sternberg cells. Therefore, repeated biopsies are required to establish the diagnosis. Staging is done to assess the extent of

the disease, along with a chest X-ray and a CT scan of the chest, abdomen, and pelvis, all of which are crucial to identify the extent of lymph-adenopathy within these regions.

4. **Discuss medical management for Hodgkin's disease.** Treatment is determined primarily by the stage of the disease, not the histologic type; however, extensive research is ongoing to target treatment regimens to histologic subtypes or prognostic features. Current approach to treatment focuses on two to four months of chemotherapy followed by radiation therapy in early-stage disease (stages lA and IIA). Combination chemotherapy includes (adriamycin, bleomycin, vinblastine, and dacarbazine, referred to as ABVD) alone is now the standard treatment for more advanced disease (stages III and IV, and B stages). Radiation therapy is sometimes used for clients with extensive adenopathy (bulky disease).

5. **Discuss complications of Hodgkin's disease.** *Jaundice* due to obstruction of the bile duct as a result of liver damage, which causes bilirubin to accumulate in the blood and discolor the skin. *Renal failure* related to ureteral obstruction by enlarged lymph nodes. *Progressive anemia* accompanied by fatigue, malaise, and anorexia because erythrocyte life span is shortened, and erythropoiesis is unable to keep pace with erythrocyte destruction. *Edema* and *cyanosis* of the face and neck due to the enlarged lymph nodes placing pressure on veins, obstructing drainage of this area. *Pulmonary symptoms* such as cough, stridor, dyspnea, chest pain, cyanosis, and pleural effusion because of mediastinal lymph node enlargement, involvement of the lung parenchyma, and invasion of the pleura. *Bone pain* and *vertebral compression* due to dissemination of disease from lymph nodes to bones. *Paraplegia* because of compression of the spinal cord resulting from extradural involvement. *Nerve pain* caused by compression of nerve roots of brachial, lumbar, or sacral plexuses.

The following are prescribed:

MOPP combination therapy q4 weeks for six cycles:

- Mechlorethamine HcL (Mustargen) IV 6 mg/m^2 on day one and eight of a 28-day cycle
- Vincristine sulfate (Oncovin) IV 1.4 mg/m^2 weekly
- Procarbazine HcL (Matulane) PO 2 mg/kg/d for one week, then 6 mg/kg/d
- Prednisone (Deltasone) 30 mg PO daily
- Ondansetron HcL (Zofran) 32 mg IV 30 minutes before chemotherapy

6. **What are the purposes for the prescribed medications?** *Mechlorethamine HcL* is an alkylating nitrogen mustard antineoplastic agent that interferes with DNA replication and RNA protein synthesis, retards the growth of abnormal lymphoid cells and slows the disease process. It interferes with the replication and synthesis by forming highly reactive carbonium ion, which causes cross-linking and abnormal base-pairing in DNA, thereby slowing or halting the process of the disease. *Vincristine sulfate* is a mitotic inhibitor-vinca alkaloid antineoplastic that inhibits cell division and slows the abnormal process of the disease by arresting mitosis at the metaphase phase where cell division takes place. With this action, the disease process is slowed or stopped. *Procarbazine HcL* is an alkylating neoplastic that inhibits DNA, RNA, and cell protein synthesis. It also delays myelosuppression and aids in producing remission. It does this due to its highly toxic effects on rapidly proliferating tissue such as seen with Hodgkin's lymphoma. *Prednisone* is a glucocorticoid that decreases the antiinflammatory effect of the disease process. It is a glucocorticoid. Therefore; it has multiple effects on blood cells such as to maintain the blood cells within normal range. *Ondansetron HcL* is a 5HT-3 receptor antagonist antiemetic used to prevent nausea and vomiting following chemotherapy by blocking the effects of serotonin at 5-HT$_3$ receptor sites (selective antagonist) located in the vagal nerve terminals and the chemoreceptor trigger zone in the central nervous system (CNS).

7. **What are the most common adverse reactions, drug-to-drug, drug-to-food/herbal interactions for the prescribed medications?** The most common adverse reactions to *mechlorethamine HcL* are alopecia, bone marrow suppression resulting in thrombocytopenia and neutropenia, nausea, vomiting, rashes, hyperuricemia, anemia, and tissue necrosis if extravasation occurs. Drug-to-drug interactions may occur with the simultaneous use of mechlorethamine HcL and anti-gout agents, which may raise serum uric acid levels. Its simultaneous use with succinylcholine, a neuro-muscular blocking agent, may prolong the effects of the blocking

agent. Simultaneous use with salicylates, nonsteroidal anti-inflammatory agents (NSAIDs), amphotericin B, and platelet inhibitors may potentiate the bleeding effects. Use with other alkylating agents will increase the risk of bone marrow suppression. There are no clinically significant drug-to-food/herbal interactions established. The most common adverse reactions to *vincristine sulfate* are nausea, vomiting, ascending peripheral neuropathy, paresthesia (especially the hands and feet), immunosuppression, alopecia, phlebitis at IV site, severe constipation with upper-colon impaction, and paralytic ileus. With vincristine sulfate, drug-to-drug interactions may occur with the simultaneous use of mitomycin, which may cause acute shortness of breath and severe bronchospasm. Simultaneous use with digoxin and phenytoin may decrease serum digoxin and phenytoin levels, requiring increase in their dosages. L-asparaginase if used simultaneously with vincristine may decrease vincristine hepatic metabolism. Use with asparaginase inhibits the excretion of vincristine and increases its toxicity. Acute pulmonary reactions can occur with the concurrent use of mytomycin-C. Use with filgrastim may cause severe atypical neuropathy. Vincristine should be used with caution with fluconazole, itraconazole, ketoconazole, cimetidine, diltiazem, verapamil, macrolide antibiotics, omeprazole, and ranitidine. If used simultaneously with live-virus vaccine, it may increase the risk of adverse reactions. There are no clinically significant drug-to-food/herbal interactions established. The most common adverse reactions of *procarbazine HcL* are thrombocytopenia, anemia, leukopenia, epistaxis, severe nausea and vomiting, diarrhea, constipation, pleural effusion, and cough. Drug-to-drug interactions may occur with the simultaneous use of procarbazine and drugs containing alcohol, antihistamines, opioids, barbiturates, hypotensive agents, phenothiazines, and other CNS depressants as procarbazine may increase sedating effects of these depressant drugs. The simultaneous use of phenylpropanolamine, guanethidine, levodopa, methyldopa, and reserpine may precipitate hypertensive crisis. There is increased risk of hypoglycemia if used with insulin or oral hypoglycemics and the potential exists for life-threatening hypertension if used concurrently with sympathomimetics. Drug-to-food interactions may occur with the simultaneous use of foods containing tyramine, resulting in hypertensive crisis. There are no clinically significant drug-to-herbal interactions established. The most common adverse reactions of *prednisone* are depression, euphoria, hypertension, anorexia, nausea, acne, decreased wound healing, ecchymoses, fragility, hirsutism, petechiae, adrenal suppression, muscle wasting, osteoporosis, gastrointestinal (GI) disturbances, and cushingoid appearance. With prednisone, drug-to-drug interactions may occur with the simultaneous use of phenytoin and rifampin, which may increase steroid metabolism, requiring increase in doses of prednisone. The simultaneous use with amphotericin B and diuretics may increase potassium loss. There are no clinically significant drug-to-food/herbal interactions established. The most common adverse reactions to *ondansetron HcL* are headache, constipation, and diarrhea. Drug-to-drug interactions may occur with the simultaneous use of ondansetron HcL and drugs that alter the activity of liver enzymes. There are no clinically established drug-to-food/herbal interactions.

8. **Discuss staging classification for Hodgkin's disease.** Staging reflects the microscopic appearance of the involved lymph nodes, the extent and severity of the disorder and the prognosis. Accurate staging is important for determining treatment options. *Stage I:* Involvement of a single lymph node region or a lymphoid structure (e.g., spleen, thymus). *Stage II:* Involvement of two or more lymph node regions on the same side of the diaphragm (i.e., the mediastinum is a single site, hilar lymph nodes are lateralized). *Stage III:* Involvement of lymph node regions or structures on both sides of the diaphragm. *Stage IV:* Involvement of extranodal site(s) beyond that designated as E.

9. **Discuss management for vincristine infusion therapy.** Vincristine is a vesicant agent that can cause severe reaction such as extravasation. Signs and symptoms may be sudden with localized pain at the injection site, sudden redness or extreme pallor, or loss of blood return in an intravenous (IV) needle. If the condition is severe, tissue slough and necrosis may occur. Therefore, nurses assigned to administer vesicant such as vincristine should be vigilant during the therapy, such as monitoring the site for signs of extravasation. If leakage into the surrounding tissue occurs during intravenous administration of vincristine, the infusion should be immediately stopped. One protocol is that if the remaining portion of the dose should be introduced into another vein, and local injection of hyaluronidase with the application of heat is used to disperse the drug in order to minimize discomfort and the possibility of tissue damage. Nursing responsibilities include maintaining the

client's IV line without the medication for hydration purposes, elevating the affected area, applying ice packs, notifying the health care provider, and documenting the occurrence and actions taken.

10. **Discuss client education for Hodgkin's disease.** Teach the client the importance of follow-up care to monitor laboratory status and evaluate overall health status. Teach the client (and write down the information) the importance of reporting night sweats and unintentional weight loss, since these may be indication of pulmonary tuberculosis or the development of "B" symptoms indicating exacerbation of Hodgkin's disease. Because herpes zoster infections are common, the client should be made aware (document information) of the signs of the infection (e.g., onset of pain and itching at a site on the skin, followed by grouped vesicles one to two days afterward). Emphasize that herpes zoster of the facial or acoustic nerve (nerve that allows hearing) can result in the loss of sight and hearing, therefore any sign of vesicle (a small blister containing fluid) should be reported promptly to the health care provider.

References

Broyles, B.E. (2005). *Medical-Surgical Nursing Clinical Companion.* Durham, NC: Carolina Academic Press.

Corbett, J.V. (2004). *Laboratory Tests and Diagnostic Procedures with Nursing Diagnoses* (6th ed.). Upper Saddle River, NJ: Prentice Hall.

Gahart, B.L. and Nazareno, A.R. (2005). *2005 Intravenous Medications.* St. Louis: Mosby.

Guyton, A.C. and Hall, J.E. (2006). *Textbook of Medical Physiology* (11th ed.). Philadelphia: W.B. Saunders.

Huether, S.E. and McCance, K.L. (2004). *Understanding Pathophysiology* (3rd ed.). St. Louis: Mosby.

Ignatavicius, D.D. and Workman, M.L. (2006). *Medical-Surgical Nursing across the Health Care Continuum* (5th ed.). Philadelphia: W.B. Saunders.

Skidmore-Roth, L. (2006). *Mosby's Handbook of Herbs & Natural Supplements* (3rd ed.). St. Louis: Mosby.

Spratto, G.R. and Woods, A.L. (2005). *2005 Edition: PDR Nurse's Drug Handbook.* Clifton Park, NY: Thomson Delmar Learning.

CASE STUDY 9

Multiple Myeloma (Plasma Cell Myeloma)

GENDER
- F

AGE
- 64

SETTING
- Hospital

ETHNICITY/CULTURE
- Black American

PREEXISTING CONDITIONS

COEXISTING CONDITIONS
- Renal failure

LIFESTYLE
- Worked 15 years for a company that sells wood and soil for agricultural and building purposes

COMMUNICATION

DISABILITY
- Difficulty ambulating independently

SOCIOECONOMIC STATUS
- Middle

SPIRITUAL/RELIGIOUS
- Baptist

PHARMACOLOGIC
- Acetaminophen (Tylenol)
- Melphalan (Alkeran)
- Prednisone (Deltasone)
- Pamidronate disodium (Aredia)
- Cyclophosphamide (Cytoxan)
- Furosemide (Lasix)
- Palonosetron HcL (Aloxi)

PSYCHOSOCIAL
- Anxiety

LEGAL
- Supplemental resource to defray hospital expenses

ETHICAL
- The right to receive disability benefits if illness is job related

ALTERNATIVE THERAPY
- Fish oil

PRIORITIZATION
- Assess bone or joint pain
- Promote comfort
- Provide safety

DELEGATION
- RN
- CNA
- Client education

MODERATE

THE CARDIOVASCULAR AND LYMPHATIC SYSTEMS

Level of difficulty: Moderate

Overview: This case involves a thorough assessment of the client's condition with focus on bone and joint pain, easy bruising, and signs of renal insufficiency. It involves nursing measures to avoid exposure to infections. The certified nursing assistant (CNA) can be delegated the duty of observing for discoloration while assisting with hygiene care.

Client Profile

Mrs. R, a 64-year-old widow for the past ten years, is accompanied by her home health aide (HHA) via ambulance to the hospital's emergency department (ED) after falling at home. Mrs. R is 4'5" and weighs 120 pounds.

Case Study

On arrival in the triage area, she reports pain of the right upper extremity, which she said began after she fell at home. The nurse attempts to assess the upper extremity but is unable to do so because of the pain and the guarding of the extremity by Mrs. R. On initial interview, she reports being fatigued, weak, anorexic, and constipated for the past four days. She describes back and joint pain that is not related to her recent fall and explains that the pain is worse in the supine position and is not relieved by ibuprofen or acetaminophen. Mrs. R points to bluish discoloration on areas of her body, which she believes occur whenever she bumps on an object in her apartment. The HHA confirms the report of easy bruising, telling the nurse that Mrs. R bruises even with the slightest contact on soft furniture, and informs the nurse that Mrs. R has been showing signs of confusion and occasional disorientation for the past two weeks. Mrs. R denies significant past medical history but reports fracture of the left ankle that occurred six months ago due to a fall while ambulating in her apartment. Mrs. R is seen by the health care provider and a history and physical are done. She is then admitted to a medical unit for further evaluation and diagnosis. Serum lab reports reveal:

- Calcium: 16.5mg/dL
- Phosphorous: 2.5 mg/dL
- Neutrophils: 2,500%
- Lymphocytes: 2,000/mm^3
- Monocytes: 150/mm^3
- Eosinophils: 200/mm^3
- Basophils: 80/mm^3
- Red blood cell (RBC) count: 4.2 mm^3
- Platelet count: 140,000 cells/mm^3
- Creatinine 1.5 mg/dL
- Blood urea nitrogen (BUN): 9 mg/dL

A bone marrow biopsy is done, after an informed consent is signed, and shows significant presence of sheets of malignant plasma cells. A 24-hour urinalysis by protein electrophoresis is positive for Bence Jones protein, and X-ray studies of bones find thinning and signs of osteoporosis and osteopenia. A diagnosis of multiple myeloma is confirmed.

Questions and Suggested Answers

1. **Discuss the pathophysiology of multiple myeloma.** Multiple myeloma is a white blood cell (WBC) cancer that is manifested by an overgrowth of B-lymphocyte plasma cells in the bone marrow. These cells normally make antibodies. However, when they become cancerous, they overproduce both complete and incomplete antibodies or gamma globulins. Because of the overproduction of both complete and incomplete gamma globulins, the term gammopathy is also used. Multiple myeloma cells produces excess cytokines, which are small protein hormones that function like other types of hormones. In their actions, one cell produces a cytokine, which in turn exerts its effects on other cells of the immune system. Cytokines control many inflammatory and immune responses, yet some are capable of directly attacking membranes of cellular agents, causing rupture and destruction of cells. Neoplastic cells of multiple myeloma reside in the bone marrow and occasionally may spread to other tissues, with the basic effect being genetic with alterations in the tumor DNA, and more destruction of bones.

2. **Discuss clinical manifestations of multiple myeloma.** Bone pain is the most common presenting symptom (70%), and the most common causes for the pain are pathologic fractures and bone lesions, which occur on 93% of clients over the course of illness. Diffuse osteoporosis is common and manifests as multiple osteolytic lesions of the skull, sternum, rib cage, and spine. Hypercalcemia is present as seen with confusion, somnolence, bone pain, constipation, nausea, and thirst. Hyperuricemia is usually present and manifests as renal failure attributable to renal tubule obstruction and interstitial nephritis. Infections resulting from leukopenia, hyperviscosity caused by the high volume of monoclonal proteins, bleeding attributable to thrombocytopenia, and carpal tunnel syndrome may be present.

3. **Discuss assessment and diagnostic findings.** Elevated monoclonal protein spike in the serum (via serum protein electrophoresis) or urine (via protein electrophoresis) or light chain in the urine (sometimes referred to as *Bence Jones protein*), are considered major criteria in the diagnosis of multiple myeloma. Diagnosis of multiple myeloma rests on radiographic studies, bone marrow biopsy, and blood and urine examination. In Mr. R's case, radiographic studies reveal lytic bone lesions, and the presence of anemia or hypercalcemia, widespread demineralization, and osteoporosis. The bone marrow contains large numbers of immature plasma cells (a hallmark diagnostic criterion), and peripheral blood samples for electrophoresis reveal a large number of abnormal immunoglobulins.

4. **Discuss different steps of diagnostic staging used to guide and manage treatment of multiple myeloma.** *Stage I:* tests indicate a low tumor amount. Lab values fall in the following range: M protein IgG less than 5 gm/100 mL serum; IgA less than 3 gm/100 mL serum or urine Bence Jones protein less than 4 gm in 24 hours; normal serum calcium, normal bones and hemoglobin over 10 gm/100 mL serum. Stage I is divided into two groups: monoclonal gammopathy of undetermined significance (MGUS) and smoldering myeloma. *Stage II:* an intermediate tumor mass. Lab values are between stage I and stage III. *Stage III:* tests indicate a high tumor amount. Lab values fall in the following range: M protein IgG greater than 7 gm/100 mL serum; IgA greater than 5 gm/100 mL serum; urine Bence Jones protein over 12 gm in 24 hours; three or more bone lesions; hemoglobin less than 8.5 gm/100 mL serum, or calcium over 12.5 gm/100 mL serum.

5. **Discuss nursing diagnoses for multiple myeloma.**

    - Mobility impairment R/T pain or discomfort – Painful bony infiltrates and pathologic fractures may limit mobility. The nurse will observe the client's functional ability daily, document and report any changes using the functional mobility scale. Gently support extremities during movements to decrease pain and enhance mobility. The client is to be encouraged to verbalize pain and discomfort so that pain medication can be administered appropriately. Analgesics are usually most effective when they are administered before pain occurs or becomes severe. Medication alleviates pain so that client will maintain his or her functional activity level. Provide a trapeze to assist in repositioning. A trapeze provides better leverage, allowing the client to assist with repositioning and providing a degree of independence.
    - Risk for infection R/T disease process and immunocompromised status of the client – The nurse will promptly report manifestations of infection: fever, chills, throat pain, cough, burning on urination, and elevated or depressed WBC count (the inflammatory response may be impaired in the multiple myeloma). Maintain protective isolation as indicated, and ensure meticulous hand washing among all people in contact with the client. Restrict visitors with colds, flu, or infections. These precautions minimize exposure to bacterial, viral, and fungal pathogens.
    - Risk for injury R/T hypercalcemia – The nurse will place needed items close at hand, since straining for each object increases the risk of falling or the occurrence of pathologic fractures. Provide safety measures to prevent falls from bed. Place the bed in low position, use side rails as indicated, and place call bell within easy reach. A secure environment minimizes risks and helps prevent falls and fractures.
    - Knowledge deficit R/T understanding of disease process and its effect on self-care – Provide quiet, calm environment for learning to enable the client to process information without distraction from background noise or stress. Limit length of each teaching session to avoid information overload. Write instructions out for clients, if applicable. Set aside time during each session for answering questions and clarifying information.

6. **Discuss common complications of multiple myeloma.** *Osteoporosis* is a disorder characterized by abnormal loss of bone density and deterioration of bone tissue, with an increased fracture risk. In multiple myeloma, diffuse osteoporosis develops as the myeloma protein destroys bone. Loss of bone integrity develops and the client is at risk for fractures and other complications. If the client can ambulate, this is encouraged, since weight bearing helps the bones reabsorb some calcium. Fluids are encouraged to help dilute the calcium and prevent protein precipitates from causing renal tubular obstruction. Pharmacologic management includes the use of biphosphonates such as pamidronate disodium (Aredia), zoledronic acid (Zometa), and etidronate disodium (Didronel) to help inhibit bone breakdown. They are also used for the treatment of skeletal pain and hypercalcemia (to be discussed later). Calcium is an essential mineral in the process of bone formation and other significant body functions.

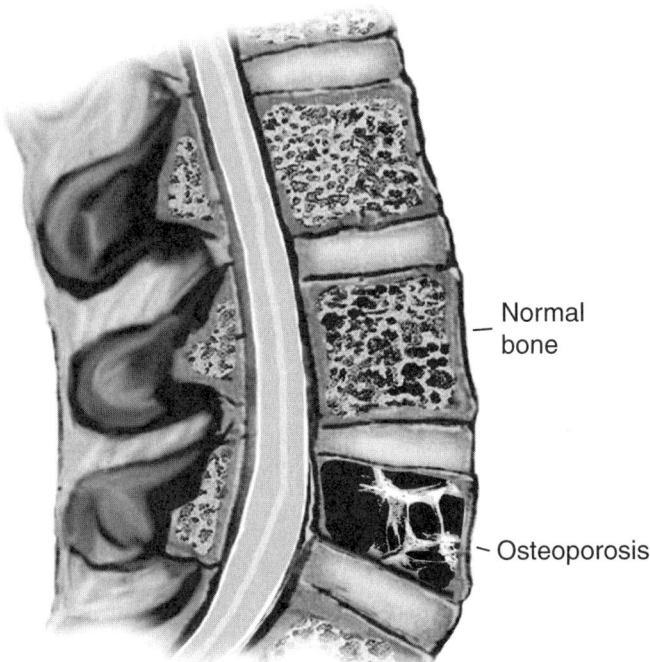

Hypercalcemia usually results from increased resorption of calcium from the bones, with hyperparathyroidism and malignancies being the two most common causes. Multiple myeloma is a malignant neoplasm of the bone marrow. The tumor is composed of plasma cells; it disrupts normal bone marrow functions and destroys osseous tissue, especially in flat bone, resulting in pain, fractures, and hypercalcemia. The client with hypercalcemia will complain of muscle weakness and fatigue dysrhythmias, confusion, constipation, polyuria, and lethargy. Complications of hypercalcemia can develop such as peptic ulcer disease due to an increased gastric acid secretion. Pancreatitis can occur as a result of calcium deposits in pancreatic ducts. Kidney stones can develop due to excess calcium precipitating and forming kidney stones. Cardiac arrest can develop from acute increase in serum calcium. Management of hypercalcemia includes administering calcitonin, which promotes the uptake of calcium into bones or to rapidly lower serum calcium levels. Fluid therapy and loop diuretics such as furosemide (Lasix) promote elimination of excess calcium. Rapid reversal of hypercalcemia in emergency situations may be accomplished by intravenous administration of sodium phosphate or potassium phosphate. The calcium will bind to the phosphate, resulting in decrease in serum calcium levels. Other drugs used to decrease serum calcium level are plicamycin (Mithramycin) to inhibit bone resorption, and glucocorticoid (cortisone) to compete with vitamin D. A low-calcium diet may be prescribed to decrease gastrointestinal (GI) absorption of calcium and to increase urinary calcium excretion. *Constipation* is difficulty in passing stools or incomplete or infrequent passage of stools. There are many causes for constipation, both organic and functional. Constipation that occurs with multiple myeloma is due to the high levels of serum calcium on the GI system, decreasing neuromuscular excitability and, in so doing, causing weakness of muscle tone and GI motility. The result is the normal expulsion of fecal material and the development of constipation. After doing a thorough history and physical, and determining the client's normal bowel pattern, high fiber, bulk formers, and stool softeners are usually prescribed to maintain stool consistency. A bowel program may be necessary every other day, approximately 45 minutes after the largest meal, to take advantage of the gastro-colic reflex.

The following are prescribed:

- Cyclophosphamide (Cytoxen) 10 mg/kg IV once daily × five days
- M combined with elphalan (Alkeran) 9 mg/ PO daily × four days; alternate with 6 mg PO daily × seven days
- Prednisone (Deltasone) 50 mg PO two times per day × four days; alternate with 100 mg PO daily × seven days
- Pamidronate disodium (Aredia) 30 mg once daily IV × three days
- Palonosetron HcL (Aloxi) 0.25 mg IV 30 minutes before administration of antineoplastic
- Monitor serum labs daily: WBC count, Hct, Hgb, leukocytes, PLT, calcium, creatinine, BUN, and phosphorous
- Monitor urine for blood each void
- Maintain fluid hydration 3,000 mL daily and monitor intake and output and urine specific gravity

7. **What are the purposes for the prescribed orders?** *Melphalan HcL* is an alkylating nitrogen mustard antineoplastic agent that interferes with DNA and RNA replication and protein synthesis by inhibiting mitosis by cross-linking of DNA strands. Cross-linking is very injurious to cells. Therefore, this property of melphalan prevents myeloma cells from reproducing. *Prednisone* is a glucocorticoid that is used for its anti-inflammatory and immunosuppressant effects. It is used in conjunction with melphalan to enhance the treatment of multiple myeloma. It is a glucocorticoid that exerts direct toxicity to lymphoid tissue, resulting in suppression of mitosis and eventually cell death. *Pamidronate* is a bone resorption inhibitor that decreases normal and normal bone resorption but does not interfere with bone formation and mineralization. It is believed to inhibit osteoclast activity, and in doing so absorbs calcium and phosphate crystals in bone, reducing bone turnover, thereby reducing serum calcium and phosphates concentrates. *Cyclophosphamide* is an alkylating nitrogen mustard antineoplastic agent that suppresses neoplastic growth, and although it is non-cell phase specific, it is most effective during the S phase of cell division. It is activated by hepatic microsomal enzymes causing malignant cell regression. Like ondansetron, *palonosetron* is a 5TH3 receptor antagonist that acts as an effective antiemetic when administered 30 minutes prior to emetogenic antineoplastic agents. It is a selective serotonin antagonist, having strong affinity for the 5TH3-serotonin receptors while not affecting other receptors. By this action, it prevents the nausea and vomiting associated with chemotherapy. *Ongoing evaluation* is critical because WBC count, Hct, Hgb, leukocytes, platelets, calcium, creatinine, blood urea nitrogen, and phosphorous may be affected by the disease process and medication regimen. Monitoring can avert complications. When using cyclophosphamide, the urine needs to be monitored for blood each void because of the risk for hemorrhagic cystitis characteristic of this antineoplastic agent. *Maintaining high levels of hydration* is important to maintain urinary hydration to prevent renal impairment and hemorrhagic cystitis from the negative effects of chemotherapy. *Closely monitoring intake and output* and urine specific gravity is done to determine renal status and hydration.

8. **What are the most common adverse reactions of the prescribed medications?** The most common adverse reactions of *melphalan* are neutropenia, thrombocytopenia, pancytopenia, pulmonary fibrosis, skin hypersensitivity, alopecia, diarrhea, and hepatic toxicity. The most common adverse reactions of *prednisone* are depression, euphoria, hypertension, anorexia, nausea, acne, decreased wound healing, ecchymoses, fragility, hirsutism, petechiae, adrenal suppression, muscle wasting, osteoporosis, and cushingcoid appearance. The most common adverse reactions of *pamidronate* are fever with or without rigors within 48 hours of the drug initiation, thrombophlebitis at injection site, hypocalcemia, hypomagnesemia, hypophosphatemia, leukopenia, nausea, epigastric discomfort, and generalized pain. The most common adverse effects of cyclophosphamide are hemorrhagic cystitis, alopecia, amenorrhea, asthenia, leukopenia, stomatitis, and nausea and vomiting. The most common adverse effects associated with *palonosetron* are abdominal pain, constipation, diarrhea, dizziness, fatigue, and headache.

9. **Discuss the drug-to-drug and drug-to-food/herbal interactions for the prescribed medications.** Drug-to-drug interactions may occur with the simultaneous use of *melphalan HcL* and antineoplastics, cyclosporine, or radiation therapy, which may increase bone marrow depression, cyclosporine, which may increase nephrotoxicity, and cimetidine and H_2 antagonists, which may increase gastric pH, decreasing the effect of melphalan. Its simultaneous use with live virus vaccines may decrease antibody response to adverse reactions, interferon alfa may decrease serum concentrations of melphalan HcL, and use with carmustine increases the risk of pulmonary toxicity. Use with nalidoxic acid may result in severe hemorrhagic necrotic enterocolitis in children. There are no clinically significant drug-to-food/herbal interactions established. With *prednisone* drug-to-drug interactions may occur with the simultaneous use of estrogen which may decrease clearance rate, digoxin may cause digitalis toxicity secondary to hypokalemia, phenobarbital, phenytoin, and rifampin may increase prednisone's metabolism, thiazide and loop diuretics, amphotericin B, piperacillin, and ticarcillin may cause hypokalemia, nonsteroidal anti-inflammatory agents (NSAIDs) increase the risk of adverse GI effects, use with live-virus vaccines increases the risk of adverse reactions from the vaccine, and antacids decrease the absorption of prednisone. There are no clinically significant drug-to-food/herbal interactions established. Drug-to-drug interactions may occur with the simultaneous use of *pamidronate disodium* and forcarnet, which may further decrease serum levels of ionized calcium. Pamidronate should be used with caution with aminoglycosides and cisplatin because of increased risk of nephrotoxicity. Fluid overload, hypokalemia, hypomagnesemia, and hypophosphatemia occur more frequently when pamidronate is used with increased volumes of fluids and with certain diuretics, however, use with furosemide does not interfere with the action of pamidronate. The simultaneous use with digoxin and vitamin D will antagonize the beneficial effects of pamidronate. There are no clinically significant drug-to-food/herbal interactions established. With *cyclophosphamide*, drug-to-drug interactions may occur with the simultaneous use of thiazide diuretics (may increase and prolong leukopenia), anticoagulants (increased bleeding potential), doxorubicin (may increase risk of cardiotoxicity characteristic of doxorubicin), and neuromuscular blockage agents (cyclophosphamide may increase their respiratory depression, particularly characteristic when used with succinylcholine). No significant drug-to-food/herbal interactions have been established. Clinically significant drug-to drug/food/herbal interactions are rare with *palonosetron*. It has been safely used with analgesics, antiemetics, antispasmodics, anticholinergics, and corticosteroids.

10. **Discuss client education for multiple myeloma.** Reinforce with the client the importance of complying with orders as prescribed to enhance quality of life, minimize pain, and prevent the development of complications. Because pain is a classic symptom of multiple myeloma, instruct the client on the use of noninvasive pain relief methods that are also effective in relieving different types of pain. The client's significant other (S/O) should be informed of the importance of ambulation, using assisted devices, if needed, to provide safety and help maintain bone strength. Teach the client and S/O signs of hypercalcemia that should be reported to a health care provider promptly. Remaining in a comfortable position outdoors for appropriate periods of time exposes the client to sunlight, which helps enhance vitamin D.

References

Broyles, B.E. (2005). *Medical-Surgical Nursing Clinical Companion.* Durham, NC: Carolina Academic Press.

Corbet, J.V. (2004). *Laboratory Tests and Diagnostic Procedures with Nursing Diagnoses* (6th ed.). Upper Saddle River, NJ: Prentice Hall.

Gahart, B.L. and Nazareno, A.R. (2005). *2005 Intravenous Medications.* St. Louis: Mosby.

Huether, S.E. and McCance, K.L. (2004). *Understanding Pathophysiology* (3rd ed.). St. Louis: Mosby.

Ignatavicius, D.D. and Workman, M.L. (2006). *Medical-Surgical Nursing across the Health Care Continuum* (5th ed.). Philadelphia: W.B. Saunders.

Lewis, S.M., Heitkemper, M.M., and Dirksen, S.R. (2004). *Medical-Surgical Nursing: Assessment and Management of Clinical Problems* (5th ed.). St. Louis: Mosby.

Spratto, G.R. and Woods, A.L. (2005). *2005 Edition: PDR Nurse's Drug Handbook.* Clifton Park, NY: Thomson Delmar Learning.

CASE STUDY 10

Chronic Myelogenous Leukemia

GENDER
- M

AGE
- 60

SETTING
- Hospital health clinic

ETHNICITY/CULTURE
- White/Portuguese

PREEXISTING CONDITIONS

COEXISTING CONDITIONS

LIFESTYLE
- Retired plastic factory employee

COMMUNICATION

DISABILITY
- Yes

SOCIOECONOMIC STATUS
- Middle

SPIRITUAL/RELIGIOUS
- Anglican

PHARMACOLOGIC
- Imatinib mesylate (Gleevec)
- Leucovorin calcium (Folinic acid)
- Hydroxyurea (Hydrea)
- Interferon alfa-2b (Intron-A)

PSYCHOSOCIAL
- Depression

LEGAL
- If work-related factors are the cause of CML, employers should help with treatment costs, and the client should receive lifelong compensation.

ETHICAL
- Clients should be informed of risk factors in the workplace and educated on how to prevent direct exposure to those risks.

ALTERNATIVE THERAPY
- Naturopathy
- Ginseng
- Soy foods

PRIORITIZATION
- Private room
- Monitor platelet function

DELEGATION
- RN
- Client education

MODERATE

THE CARDIOVASCULAR AND LYMPHATIC SYSTEMS

Level of difficulty: Moderate

Overview: This case involves a thorough history that should include questions pertaining to risk factors and causative factors, occupation, and hobbies to detect causative environmental factors that may have aggravated leukemic process. The case involves questioning the client about frequency and severity of infectious process during the preceding six months, because the risk for infection is increased in clients with leukemia. It requires asking about overt or hidden excessive bleeding episodes, because platelet function is usually diminished with leukemia. Aggressive treatment is needed with chronic myelogenous leukemia (CML), because it can and often does progress to acute leukemia.

Client Profile

Mr. K is a 60-year-old client who came to the hospital outpatient clinic complaining of increased sensitivity at his right side, unusual loss of appetite, and weight loss, which he believes is due to lack of appetite. He reports discomfort in the right and left upper quadrants and informs the nurse that he is concerned about his health because of a family history of leukemia. Mr. K is 5'6" and weighs 285 pounds. On initial discussion with a nurse, he remarks that he is wondering if his symptoms are early signs of recurring leukemia because he was diagnosed with "childhood leukemia" at the age of 12. However, "he had complete remission" after several treatments at a children's hospital in Portugal. Mr. K reports that he was employed for ten years in a factory that manufactures plastic covers for furniture and household items.

Case Study

Mr. K is known to the clinic and is a reliable historian. Mr. K informs the nurse he has been seeing a naturopathic practitioner, he is currently taking ginseng, and he has recently included soy foods in his diet. The nurse assesses Mr. K and, on physical exam, finds an enlarged spleen and liver and a palpable mass on palpation. Upon completion of the nursing history and assessment, the nurse informs the nurse practitioner (NP) of the findings. The NP continues with further physical assessment on Mr. K and elicits that he has been experiencing weakness, early satiety, and sweating more frequently over the past week. He also reports easy fatigability with minimal activities of daily living (ADLs) and occasional "gouty attacks." After the NP reviews the assessment findings with a medical doctor and a hematologist, the following serum labs are ordered: complete blood count (CBC) with peripheral blood smear, serum acid levels, and alkaline phosphatase. The CBC reveals:

>   High numbers of mature white blood cells (WBCs): $30,000/mm^3$
>   Decreased hematocrit (Hct): 33.2%
>   Hemoglobin (Hgb): 12.9%
>   Platelet counts: elevated at $480,000/mm^3$

The peripheral smear reflects the presence of granulocytes at all levels of maturation, serum uric acid level is elevated (9.2 mg/dL), and alkaline phosphatase (LAP score) is reduced (28 U/L). The multidisciplinary team reviews the recent serum lab data and determines that a bone marrow aspiration and biopsy would enhance the diagnosis. Mr. K is informed of the need for the procedures, agrees, and signs an informed witnessed consent. Mr. K is given two oxycodone/acetaminophen 5/325 mg tablets prior to the bone marrow aspiration and biopsy procedure. The bone marrow aspiration and biopsy reveal hypercellularity, megakaryocytosis, and B-cell proliferation. After reviewing the results and report from the hematologist, the oncologist assigns the diagnosis of CML. The health care provider discusses the diagnosis and chemotherapy treatment plan with Mr. K, and refers him to the dietitian, who, in collaboration with the health care team, plans a balanced diet with supplemental vitamins and iron.

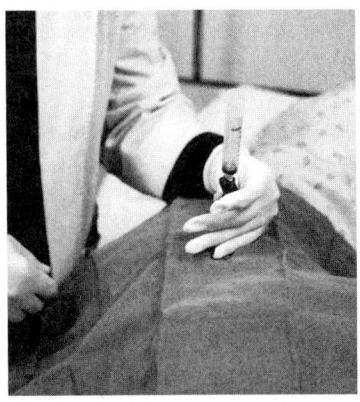

Bone marrow biopsy/aspiration

Questions and Suggested Answers

1. **Discuss the incidence and prevalence of CML.** CML constitutes about 20% of adult leukemias, occurring more often in people older than 50 years of age. Leukemia accounts for 2% of all new cases of cancer and for 4% of all deaths from cancer. The incidence depends on many factors, including the type of WBC affected, age, gender, race, and geographic locale.

2. **Discuss the pathophysiology of CML.** CML, also referred to as chronic granulocytic leukemia (CGL), is a malignant neoplasm of blood-forming tissues characterized by a proliferation of granular leukocytes and, often, of megakarocytes and excessive development of mature neoplastic granulocytes in the bone marrow. The excess neoplastic granulocytes move into the peripheral blood in massive numbers and ultimately infiltrate the liver and spleen. These granulocytic cells contain a distinct cytogenetic abnormality called the *Philadelphia chromosone*, which serves as a disease marker and results from translocation of genetic material between chromosones 9 and 22. The disease occurs most frequently in mature adults and begins insidiously. Its progress is marked by malaise, fatigue, heat intolerance, bleeding gums, purpura, skin lesions, weight loss, hyperuricemia, abdominal discomfort, and massive splenomegaly. Differential blood count and bone marrow biopsies are performed to aid in the diagnosis. The alkaline phosphatase activity of the leukocytes is low, and the Philadelphia chromosome is present in myeloblasts of most of the clients with CML. The chronic phase of the disease will eventually progress to the accelerated phase, ending in a blastic phase. Once it is transformed into an acute or blastic phase, it is often refractory to therapy, resulting in a decreased expected life span.

3. **Discuss diagnostic studies for CML.** Peripheral blood evaluation and bone marrow examination are the primary methods of diagnosing and classifying the subtypes of leukemia, such as CML. Peripheral blood evaluation or blood smear look for abnormal blood cells. The bone marrow examination (aspiration, biopsy) requires removal of a small sample of bone marrow either by aspiration, needle biopsy, or open surgical biopsy to identify types of cells that are present. Cells that are normally present in hematopoietic marrow include erythrocytes and granulocytes (neutrophils, basophils, and eosinophils) in all stages of maturation; megakaryocytes, from which platelets develop; small numbers of lymphocytes; and occasional plasma cells. Because bone marrow examination involves an invasive procedure with risk for infection, trauma, and bleeding, a signed consent is required. Contraindications for bone marrow examination include coagulation defects, although the test may be performed if its importance for information to be obtained outweighs the risks involved in carrying out the test. Positioning is dependent on the site used for biopsy. The prone, or side-lying, position is used if the spinous processes are the sites to be used, and are the preferred sites if more than one specimen is to be obtained. The client may also sit, supported by a pillow on an overbed table, for a spinous process site utilization. The side-lying position is used if the iliac crest or tibia is the site to be used. For sternal punctures, the supine position is used. Bed rest is provided for specific time as per the agency's protocol. Puncture sites are assessed for bleeding, and an ice bag may be applied to the site to alleviate discomfort and prevent bleeding. Non-narcotic analgesic may be prescribed to alleviate discomfort. Morphologic, histochemical, immunologic, and cytogenetic methods are used to identify cell subtypes and the stage of the development of leukemic cell populations. Other studies such as lumbar puncture and computed tomography (CT) scan can determine the presence of leukemic cells outside of the blood and bone marrow. The histologic cell found in CML is the Philadelphia chromosone, which is of diagnostic value.

4. **Discuss main prognostic indicators in CML.** Some of the main prognostic indicators in CML are lymphocyte count, hemoglobin level, and bone marrow histology. Lymphocytes are the principal components of the body's immune system, although only a small proportion of them circulate in the bloodstream. Those in the bloodstream are T lymphocytes. Lymphocyte count is a significant indicator in CML, because a common reason for marked lymphocytes is lymphocytic leukemia. Because the client with CML is usually fatigued, knowledge of the hemoglobin level will guide treatment appropriately. The bone marrow examination looks at the all stages of erythrocytes and granulocytes, which are predominant in the bone marrow, to aid in the diagnosis and treatment of CML.

5. **Discuss common nursing diagnoses and expected outcome criteria for adult clients with CML.**

   Nursing diagnosis: Activity intolerance R/T fatigue, ineffective tissue perfusion
   Expected outcome: The client will demonstrate gradual progression toward optimal level of physical activity tolerance based on improvement in bone marrow function and psychological readiness, as evidenced by the ability to pace activities and verbalize decreased fatigue.

   Nursing diagnosis: Risk for injury R/T alteration in bone marrow function, platelets abnormality
   Expected outcome: The client will identify safety measures to prevent falls. The client will avoid over-the-counter drugs such as nonsteroidal anti-inflammatory agents (NSAIDs), unless prescribed, to avoid increasing bleeding tendencies. The client will know the signs of bleeding (e.g., ecchymosis, easy bruising) and inform primary health care provider.

   Nursing diagnosis: High risk for infection R/T lack of mature leukocytes
   Expected outcome: The client will verbalize knowledge of how to self-protect from infection and be able to identify signs of infection in the early stages, when it can be treated minimally before the infection becomes life-threatening. The client will remain free of infection and maintain intact oral mucous membranes.

   Nursing diagnosis: Imbalanced nutrition R/T anorexia, nausea, and vomiting associated with disease process
   Expected outcome: The client will restore adequate nutritional balance, as evidenced by increase in appetite, no further nausea or vomiting, normal serum albumin level, and a positive nitrogen balance.

   Nursing diagnosis: Knowledge deficit R/T disease, treatment, and prognosis
   Expected outcome: The client will verbalize ways to decrease fatigue and maintain energy; will verbalize factors that can aggravate disease process, and avoid them appropriately; will comply with treatment regimen as prescribed; will communicate understanding of remission versus exacerbation.

The following are prescribed:

- Imatinib mesylate (Gleevec) 400 mg PO four times per day
- Leucovorin calcium (Folinic acid) 10 mg/M^2 IV q6h until serum methotrexate level is less than 0.05 micromolar
- Hydroxyurea (Hydrea) 30 mg/kg PO daily
- Interferon alfa-2b (Intron-A) 2 million U/m^2 three times per week

6. **What are the purposes for the prescribed medications?** *Imatinib mesylate* is a miscellaneous antineoplastic agent and protein-tyrosine inhibitor that prevents the cells from growing and dividing by blocking the signals within the leukemia cells that express the BCR-ABL protein. Blocking these prevents the series of chemical reactions from occurring that would cause the cell to grow and divide. *Leucovorin calcium* is a rescue agent for methotrexate by competing with methotrexate at the cellular level and causing methotrexate excretion to prevent damage from delayed excretion of methotrexate. *Hydroxyurea* is an antimetabolite antineoplastic agent that inhibits the synthesis but does not affect RNA or protein synthesis. It reduces the WBC count to a more normal level but does not alter cytogenetic changes. The use of its antimetabolite activity blocks the incorporation of thymidine, a single carbon-nitrogen ring that is necessary for metabolic process, into DNA. When this ring is blocked, replication of abnormal cell development is also stopped. *Interferon alfa-2b* is a biologic response modifier antineoplastic agent that causes hematologic remission to occur by adjusting the immune system so that it is better able to combat foreign invasion of antigens and viruses. "It binds to specific membrane receptors on the cell surface and initiates a complex sequence of intracellular events (e.g., induction of specific enzymes, suppression of cell proliferation, immunomodulating activities [enhancement of phagocytic activity of macrophages, augmentation of the specific cytotoxicity of lymphocytes for target cells, inhibition of virus replication in virus-infected cells])" (Gahart and Nazareno, 673).

7. **What are the most common adverse reactions of the prescribed medications?** The most common adverse reactions of *imatinib mesylate* are fluid retention, edema, fatigue, fever, headache, nausea, vomiting, diarrhea,

abdominal pain, constipation, anorexia, neutropenia, thrombocytopenia, petechiae, muscle cramps, pain, arthralgia, dyspnea, and rash. The most common adverse effects associated with *methotrexate* are bone marrow suppression, abdominal distress, chills, dizziness, fatigue, fever, malaise, nausea, increased uric acid levels, and stomatitis. Methotrexate toxicity is dose related but may include GI toxicity, bone marrow toxicity, hepatic toxicity, pulmonary toxicity, and severe skin reactions. Although rarely occurring, allergic reactions to *leucovorin calcium* have occurred. Most adverse effects are associated with methotrexate or fluorouracil. The most common adverse reactions of *hydroxyurea* are constipation, redness of the face, and leukopenia. The most common adverse reactions of *Interferon alfa-2b* are flu-like syndrome (fever, chills, myalgia, headache), alopecia, anemia, dyspnea, granulocytopenia, paresthesia, taste alteration, thrombocytopenia, fatigue, dizziness, nausea, diarrhea, anorexia, rash, and coughing.

8. **Discuss the drug-to-drug and drug-to-food/herbal interactions of the prescribed medications.** Drug-to-drug interactions may occur with the simultaneous use of *imatinib mesylate* and clarithromycin, erythromycin, ketoconazole, and itraconazole, which may increase imatinib levels and risk of toxicity. The simultaneous use of carbamazepine, dexamethasone, phenobarbital, pheyntoin, and rifampin may decrease imatinib levels. The simultaneous use of large doses of acetaminophen (Tylenol) may cause hepatotoxicity. If used concurrently with calcium channel-blocking agents, warfarin, triazolobenzodiazepines, or simvastatin, imatinib mesylate increases the plasma levels of these drugs. Drug-to-food interactions may occur with the simultaneous use of antacids and grapefruit juice. Drug-to-herbal interactions may occur with the simultaneous use of St. John's Wort, which may decrease imatinib mesylate levels. With *methotrexate*, drug-to-drug interactions may occur with simultaneous use of alcohol, amiodarone, antibacterials, cyclosporine, docycycline, hepatotoxic agents etretinate, acetylated salicylates, NSAIDs, omeprazole, penicillins, probenecid, salicylates, sulfonamides, para-aminobenzoic acid, phenylbutazone, phenytoin, pyrimethamine, trimethoprim, and vancomycin can enhance methotrexate toxicity even to the level of being life-threatening. It "may increase serum levels of mercaptopurine decreases phenytoin serum levels, causing SMZ-TMP (Bactrim)-induced megaloblastic anemia and decrease theophylline clearance and increase serum levels" (Gahart and Nazareno, 779). Vitamins with folic acid may decrease methotrexate's antifolate activity. Drug-to-drug interactions may occur with the simultaneous use of *leucovorin calcium* and hydantoins, phenobarbital, and primidone by inhibiting their actions and increasing the risk of seizures. When used as rescue for methotrexate, all agents that may interfere with methotrexate excretion should be avoided. These include NSAIDs, indomethacin, probenecid, procarbazine, salicylates, and sulfonamides. Treatment failure may result with concurrent use of sulfamethoxazole and trimethoprim, causing increased morbidity for clients with HIV-related *pneumocystis carinii* pneumonia. Currently, there are no clinically significant drug-to-drug or drug-to-food/herbal interactions established for *hydroxyurea*. Drug-to-drug interactions may occur with the simultaneous use of *interferon alfa-2b* and theophylline, increasing theophylline level; the simultaneous use of zidovudine may increase hematologic toxicity. The simultaneous use with doxorubicin and vincristine will increase toxicity and neurotoxicity. The simultaneous use of aldesleukin (IL-2) may potentiate the risk for renal failure. There are no clinically significant drug-to-food/herbal interactions established.

9. **Discuss health care resources that are usually needed by clients with CML.** The client with limited social support may need help at home until strength and energy return. A home care aide or a visiting nurse depending on the client's needs may be necessary at time of discharge for an indefinite period of time. The client may need durable equipment to assist with ADLs and ambulation. Transportation cost can be a burden depending on clients' income or support system; therefore, social service department should be included in the discharge planning at the time of admission and prior to discharge. Referral to the Leukemia Society of America and community and regional resources for support.

10. **Discuss client education for CML.** Encourage self-care, with focus on hygiene measures and energy conservation during self-care activities. Stress the use of a soft-bristle toothbrush several times daily. Flossing should be avoided, to prevent bleeding. Discuss the effects of chemotherapeutic agents, their purpose, and negative effects. Stress the importance of good hand washing and other measures to reduce exposure to pathogens.

Avoid over-the-counter prescription drugs that interfere with platelet function. Teach the importance of reporting any types of bleeding. Encourage eating several small, low-fat, high-calorie meals and increasing fluid intake. Stress the importance of follow-up care, especially to monitor serum laboratory values, which help to determine the client's need for aggressive therapy.

References

Broyles, B.E. (2005). *Medical-Surgical Nursing Clinical Companion.* Durham, NC: Carolina Academic Press.

Corbet, J.V. (2004). *Laboratory Tests and Diagnostic Procedures with Nursing Diagnoses* (6th ed.). Upper Saddle River, NJ: Prentice Hall.

Deglin, J.H. and Vallerand, A.H. (2005). *Davis's Drug Guide for Nurses* (9th ed.). Philadelphia: F. A. Davis.

Gahart, B.L. and Nazareno, A.R. (2005). *2005 Intravenous Medications.* St. Louis: Mosby.

Huether, S.E. and McCance, K.L. (2004). *Understanding Pathophysiology* (3rd ed.). St. Louis: Mosby.

Ignatavicius, D.D. and Workman, M.L. (2006). *Medical-Surgical Nursing across the Health Care Continuum* (5th ed.). Philadelphia: W.B. Saunders.

http://patientrecruitment.nhlbi.nih.gov/leukemia. "Imatinib for Chronic Myelogenous Leukemia (CML)." Leukemia Research Study, January 2005.

Spratto, G.R. and Woods, A.L. (2005). *2005 Edition: PDR Nurse's Drug Handbook.* Clifton Park, NY: Thomson Delmar Learning.

CASE STUDY 11

Femoral-Popliteal Bypass for Peripheral Vascular Disease

GENDER
- M

AGE
- 72

SETTING

ETHNICITY/CULTURE
- White/American

PREEXISTING CONDITIONS

COEXISTING CONDITIONS

LIFESTYLE
- Retired computer sales manager

COMMUNICATION

DISABILITY

SOCIOECONOMIC STATUS
- Middle

SPIRITUAL/RELIGIOUS
- Catholic

PHARMACOLOGIC
- Morphine sulfate (Duramorph)
- Dipyridamole (Persantine)
- Piperacillin sodium/tazobactam sodium (Zosyn)

PSYCHOSOCIAL
- Anxiety

LEGAL

ETHICAL

ALTERNATIVE THERAPY

PRIORITIZATION
- Assess and manage pain
- Peripheral vascular assessment
- Increase tissue perfusion

DELEGATION
- RN
- Client education

MODERATE

THE CARDIOVASCULAR AND LYMPHATIC SYSTEMS

Level of difficulty: Moderate

Overview: This case requires critical post-operative care for the client with peripheral vascular disease. The nurse must use critical decision making in pain management and be able to critically assess for signs or symptoms of reocclusion of the graft.

Client Profile

Mr. T is a 72-year-old male admitted to the surgical intensive care unit (SICU) following a femoral-popliteal bypass graft of the right lower extremity for peripheral vascular disease. Mr. T is initially admitted to the emergency department (ED) of the hospital with complaints of severe pain of the extremity even at rest (ischemic rest pain). He reports a long history of cigarette smoking and history of hypertension and coronary artery disease (atheroclesrosis) and denies surgical history in the past. A Doppler study is done; peripheral pulses of the right extremity are faint and are absent on palpation, peripheral pulses of the left lower extremity are weak, and bilateral extremities are cool to touch.

Case Study

During the history and physical in the ED by a health care provider, Mr. T's pain becomes so unbearable even at rest that he is transported to the operating room for emergency surgery. The surgery is completed, and Mr. T is transferred to the SICU. On arrival, Mr. T is alert but drowsy. However, he moves his head and responds to his name when called, and is responsive to tactile stimuli. He has an arterial line in place, intravenous catheter with Ringer's lactate infusing at 125 mL per hour via electronic pump. He is attached to telemetry, with normal sinus rhythm and occasional unifocal premature ventricular contractions (PVCs) noted. He has a face mask with 40% oxygen in place and a Foley catheter in situ with clear, amber-colored urine draining in a urometer. He has an arterial line in situ, and on arrival to the unit, his vital signs are:

Blood pressure: 140/82
Pulse: 98
Respirations: 18
Temperature: 99.4° F

His leg is wrapped with a light dressing and orders are written to keep the leg flat in bed. His chart reveals post-embolectomy. The receiving nurse completes the assessment, provides initial care to the client, and proceeds to document the data.

Questions and Suggested Answers

1. **Discuss the factors from Mr. T's past medical history that predispose him to the need for femoral-popliteal bypass.** *Aging* produces changes in the walls of the blood vessels that affect the transport of oxygen and nutrients to the tissues. The intima thickens as a result of cellular proliferation and fibrosis. Elastin fibers of the media become calcified, thin, and fragmented, and collagen accumulates in both the intima and the media. These changes cause the vessels to stiffen, which results in increased peripheral resistance, impaired blood flow, resulting in predisposition to vascular compromise affecting the lower extremities. Another factor is history of *cigarette smoking* because of the nicotine, which over a prolonged period of time decreases blood flow to the extremities and increases heart rate and blood pressure by stimulating the sympathetic nervous system, causing vasoconstriction. In addition, it increases the chances of clot formation by increasing the aggregation of platelets. The number of cigarettes smoked is directly related to the extent of injury to the vascular system in the extremities. History of *hypertension* often accompanies risk factors for atherosclerosis, such as dyslipidemia (abnormal fat levels). Hypertension contributes to the rate at which atherosclerotic plaque accumulates within arterial walls. It is a major contributing factor to death from peripheral vascular disease. Prolonged hypertension damages blood vessels throughout the body, requiring surgical interventions in some people. History of *atherosclerosis* results in fibrous plaque that is composed of smooth muscle cells, collagen fibers, plasma components, and lipids, all of which protrude in varying degrees into the arterial lumen, and at times completely obstruct it, requiring surgical intervention. Fatty streaks constitute one

of the earliest lesions of atherosclerosis. Although atherosclerosis can develop at any point in the body, there are sites that are more vulnerable, typically bifurcation or branch areas such as in the orifice of the superficial femoral artery.

2. **Discuss the femoral-popliteal bypass procedure.** Femoral-popliteal bypass is a procedure that is done to remove blockage in the main artery of an extremity. Various surgical approaches can be used to improve arterial blood flow beyond a stenotic or occluded artery. The most common is a peripheral arterial bypass operation with autogenous vein or synthetic graft material to bypass or carry blood around the lesion. Antiplatelet agents are used often to prevent thrombosis after arterial bypass surgery.

3. **Discuss a specific diagnostic test to determine that the bypass procedure is needed and how the test is performed.** An angiogram is done to confirm the need for the bypass. The angiogram allows X-ray visualization of the arteries or veins of the lower extremities after the injection of an iodinated contrast medium. The angiography is done to mark the level of inflow or areas of obstruction.

4. **Discuss important post-operative assessment findings to which a nurse should give critical attention.** A dramatic increase in the level of pain, loss of palpable pulse or pulses distal to the operative site, extremity pallor or cyanosis, numbness or tingling, or a cold extremity, necessitates immediate notification of the surgeon, since these signs may be due to clot formation or occlusion of the bypass graft.

5. **Discuss common nursing diagnoses, expected outcomes, and nursing interventions for the client with post-femoral-popliteal bypass.**

    Nursing diagnosis: Acute pain R/T surgical tissue trauma
    Expected outcome: Client verbalizes or demonstrates increased level of comfort.
    Nursing interventions: Assess location, duration, and intensity of pain, and promote comfort measures. Medicate with prescribed analgesics as needed, and evaluate the effectiveness of analgesics after each administration.

    Nursing diagnosis: Risk for ineffective tissue perfusion R/T graft thrombosis
    Expected outcome: Client will maintain adequate tissue perfusion to lower extremities will full pulses and capillary refill within three seconds; skin warm to touch, minimal or no swelling of extremity.
    Nursing interventions: Check pedal pulses every hour for 24 hours, then every shift and PRN. Check sensory and motor function of the affected extremity. Check capillary refill and temperature of extremities. Check leg for hematoma or unusual swelling. Observe extremity for change in color. Document observations.

    Nursing diagnosis: Impaired physical mobility R/T surgical procedure, pain
    Expected outcome: Client will maintain intact motor function, and demonstrate ability to move around in bed without assistance.
    Nursing interventions: Assess factors for immobility, and client's range of motion. Report and document client's inability to mobilize in bed without assistance. Encourage independence in activities of daily living (e.g., hygiene care to anterior upper torso). Collaborate with health care provider for request for physical therapy. Maintain pain medication regimen as prescribed.

    Nursing diagnosis: Risk for impaired skin integrity R/T altered circulation
    Expected outcome: Client will maintain adequate skin integrity.
    Nursing interventions: Inspect lower extremities PRN and during every shift. Protect lower extremities from trauma (e.g., on sheepskin, egg crate, bed cradle). Document condition during every shift.

    Nursing diagnosis: Deficient knowledge R/T post-operative prescriptions and home care
    Expected outcome: Client will describe post-surgery care, including signs of graft failure. Client will verbalize importance of follow-up care and when to promptly contact primary health care provider (e.g., intolerable pain at surgical incision site).
    Nursing interventions: Identify factors that may interfere with learning, such as perception of the surgical outcome, physical ability upon discharge, available support systems. Teach client about activity restrictions

(e.g., avoiding unusual bending of the extremity, long standing in one place). Stress the importance of smoking cessation, because of the effects of the nicotine in cigarette. Emphasize the importance of meticulous foot care to reduce the risk of infection and injury to feet.

6. **Discuss the potential complications post femoral-popliteal bypass graft.** *Compartment syndrome* (CS) is a condition in which elevated intracompartmental pressure within a confined myofascial compartment compromises the neurovascular function of tissues within that space. It causes capillary perfusion to be reduced below the level necessary for tissue viability. It is associated with fractures, soft tissue damage, crush injury, reperfusion syndrome, severe burns, and knee or leg surgery. CS may occur initially from the physiologic response of the body or may be delayed for several days from the original injury. Characteristics of CS are paresthesia (numbness and tingling); pain distal to the site of injury that is not relieved by narcotic analgesics and pain on passive stretch of muscle traveling through the compartment; pressure of the compartment rises; pallor, coolness, and loss of normal color of the extremity; paralysis or loss of function; and pulselessness or diminished/absent peripheral pulses. However, the client may have only one of the characteristic signs/symptoms. Ongoing neurovascular assessment is required, with accurate documentation, and notifying of the primary health care provider immediately of the change in the client's condition. The extremity should not be elevated above the level of the heart, since elevation may raise venous pressure and slow arterial perfusion. Cold compresses should not be used since they may cause vasoconstriction and exacerbate CS. *Venous thrombosis* may occur post-surgery because the lower extremities are highly susceptible to thrombus formation due to inactivity of the muscles of the extremities that usually assist in the pumping action of venous blood returning to the extremities.

The following are prescribed:

- Morphine sulfate (Duramorph) 2 mg IV q1–2h PRN
- Dipyridamole (Persantine) 100 mg PO four times per day
- Piperacillin sodium/tazobactam sodium (Zosyn) 3 g IV q6h
- Serum PTT, aPTT, CBC, and INR daily
- Bed rest with extremity straight

7. **What are the purposes for the prescribed orders?** *Morphine sulfate* is an opioid analgesic that relieves severe post-op pain by causing analgesia at the spinal level through its binding with the delta receptors. *Dipyridamole* is an anticoagulant, platelet adhesion inhibitor that prevents post-operative thromboembolic complications by inhibiting platelet aggregation, by preventing the release of substances that stimulate platelets to aggregate or form a clot. *Piperacillin sodium/tazobactam sodium* is an extended-spectrum penicillin and beta-lactamase inhibitor that is effective against gram-positive, gram-negative, and aerobes, anaerobes, and enterococci that may be resistant to other antibiotics. Given the site of the surgery, the risk of infection is present. This agent prevents or stops the infectious process by binding to bacterial cell wall membrane, causing cell death. *Serum PTT* and *aPTT* provide information on the body's coagulation system, and aid in guiding treatment. *Bed rest* and maintaining extremity in straight alignment prevents undue pressure on the extremity and avoids stasis of blood and pending complication (e.g., thrombus formation).

8. **What are the common adverse reactions, drug-to-drug, drug-to-food/herbal interactions of the prescribed drugs?** The most common adverse reactions of *morphine sulfate* are constipation and sedation. Drug-to-drug interactions may occur with the simultaneous use of alcohol, sedative/hypnotics, clomipramine, barbiturates, tricyclic antidepressants, histamine-2 antagonists, phenothiazines such as chlorpromazine, and antihistamines, which increase central nervous system (CNS) depression. The concurrent use with buprenorphine, nalbuphine, butorphanol, rifampin, or pentazocine may decrease analgesia. Hypotensive effects may increase with the concurrent use of furosemide, antihypertensives, antidepressants, benzodiazepines, adrenergic blocking agents, calcium channel blockers, calcium, nitroprusside, and nitroglycerin, and the risk of constipation increases with concomitant use of anticholinergics and antidiarrheals. The concurrent use with warfarin may increase the anticoagulant effect, and its use with cimetidine decreases the

metabolism and may increase the effects. If used with metoclopramide, morphine may antagonize its effect. Extended respiratory depression or prolonged neuromuscular blockage is a risk when morphine is used with mivacurium, succinylcholine, and tubocurarine. Use with zidovudine may cause toxicity of both agents so they should not be used simultaneously. The most common adverse reactions of *dipyridamole* are dizziness, headache, hypotension, and nausea. Drug-to-drug interactions may occur with the simultaneous use of aspirin, anticoagulants, thrombolytic agents, nonsteroidal anti-inflammatory agents (NSAIDs), cefamandole, cefoperazone, cefotetan, plicamycin, valproic acid, or sulfinpyrazone, which increase the risk of bleeding. The concurrent use of theophylline may negate the effects of *dipyridamole*. There are no clinically significant drug-to-food interactions established. However, evening primrose oil, feverfew, garlic, ginger, gingko biloba, ginseng, and grapeseed extract increase the antiplatelet effects of dipyridamole. The most common adverse reactions of *piperacillin/tazobactam* are rashes, hypokalemia, phlebitis, and hypersensitivity reactions. Drug-to-drug interactions may occur with the concurrent use of gentamycin and amikacin, having a synergistic effect. Use with probenicid decreases renal excretion and increases blood levels of piperacillin/tazobactam. Concomitant use with heparin, warfarin, alteplase, anistreplase, aspirin, NSAIDs, naproxen, dextran, dipyridamole, and plicamycin increases the risk of bleeding. Chloramphenicol, erythromycin, and tetracycline may antagonize its bacteriocidal effects. (Gahart and Nazareno, 951). It may inhibit the action of oral contraceptives, and increase the potential for toxicity of methotrexate and neuromuscular blocking agents. The concurrent use with other hepatotoxic drugs will increase the risk of hepatotoxicity. There are no clinically significant drug-to-food/herbal interactions established.

9. **Discuss client education for post-femoral-popliteal bypass.** Inform the client that it is normal for the legs to be swollen after surgery, but the swelling will gradually go down. Provide the client with instructions on how to care for the incisional site, and stress the importance of reporting unusual signs, redness, drainage, and odor (indicating infection) promptly to the primary health care provider. The extremity should be elevated to enhance comfort and improve circulation. Pain and coldness of the extremity should be reported immediately. Stress the importance of gradual exercise within limits. The client should stop smoking to help with the healing process. Eating healthily includes drinking plenty of fluids, eating a well-balanced diet, including high-fiber foods and fresh fruits and vegetables, foods high in protein, vitamins C and A, and zinc, avoiding excess fried and high-fat foods. The client should keep follow-up appointments with the primary health care provider, and should inform the provider if there is increased leg or foot pain or change in the color or temperature of the foot and leg.

References

Broyles, B.E. (2005). *Medical-Surgical Nursing Clinical Companion.* Durham, NC: Carolina Academic Press.
Corbett, J.V. (2004). *Laboratory Tests and Diagnostic Procedures with Nursing Diagnoses* (6th ed.). Upper Saddle River, NJ: Prentice Hall.
Gahart, B.L. and Nazareno, A.R. (2005). *2005 Intravenous Medications.* St. Louis: Mosby.
Harkreader, H. and Hogan, M.A. (2004). *Fundamentals of Nursing: Caring and Clinical Judgment* (2nd ed.). Philadelphia: W.B. Saunders.
Huether, S.E. and McCance, K.L. (2004). *Understanding Pathophysiology* (3rd ed.). St. Louis: Mosby.
Ignatavicius, D.D. and Workman, M.L. (2006). *Medical-Surgical Nursing across the Health Care Continuum* (5th ed.). Philadelphia: W.B. Saunders.
Lehne, R.A. (2004). *Pharmacology for Nursing Care* (5th ed.). St. Louis: Mosby.
Skidmore-Roth, L. (2006). *Mosby's Handbook of Herbs & Natural Supplements* (3rd ed.). St. Louis: Mosby.
Spratto, G.R. and Woods, A.L. (2005). *2005 Edition: PDR Nurse's Drug Handbook.* Clifton Park, NY: Thomson Delmar Learning.

CASE STUDY 12

Premature Ventricular Contractions

GENDER
- M

AGE
- 72

SETTING
- Adult home and hospital

ETHNICITY/CULTURE
- Black American/West Indian

PREEXISTING CONDITIONS
- Premature ventricular contractions and atrial fibrillation

COEXISTING CONDITIONS
- Left-sided heart failure

LIFESTYLE
- Retired farmer

COMMUNICATION

DISABILITY
- Reduced ability to perform ADL

SOCIOECONOMIC STATUS
- Low

SPIRITUAL/RELIGIOUS
- Anglican

PHARMACOLOGIC
- Atropine sulfate (Atropine)
- Amiodarone HcL (Cardarone)
- Lidocaine HcL (Xylocaine)
- Carvedilol (Coreg)

PSYCHOSOCIAL
- Anxiety

LEGAL

ETHICAL
- Availability of place of residence upon discharge

ALTERNATIVE THERAPY

PRIORITIZATION
- Stabilize heart rate and rhythm

DELEGATION
- RN
- Client education

CARDIOVASCULAR AND LYMPHATIC SYSTEMS

Level of difficulty: Difficult

Overview: This case involves a thorough assessment of the client's condition with focus on his cardiac status, including the drugs he is presently on and those brought to the hospital. The case involves prioritization in a triage situation and critical thinking to appropriately delegate and transfer the client to the appropriate unit for continued observation.

DIFFICULT

Client Profile

Mr. J, is a 72-year-old male admitted to the emergency department (ED) from an adult home where he has been living for the past two years. Vital signs on admission are:

- Blood pressure: 110/74
- Pulse: 54
- Respirations: 18
- Temperature: 98.4° F

Case Study

On admission, Mr. J is alert and oriented to person, date, and current year. He complains of occasional pressure in his chest, and reports feeling tired and dizzy when he keeps his head down for short periods of time. Past medical history (PMH) reveals myocardial infarction five years ago and current left-sided heart failure. The certified nurse's assistant (CNA) who accompanies him to the ED informs the triage nurse that he self medicates with digoxin (Lanoxin), docusate sodium (Colace), and furosemide (Lasix) daily, but the CNA does not know the dosages of the mentioned medications. A chest X-ray is done and reveals pulmonary congestion and a 12-lead EKG shows decrease tissue perfusion, but no signs of new injury to the myocardium. An IV line is inserted and atropine sulfate 0.5 mg IV administered × one, with a noted increase of heart rate of 68. Mr. J is placed on continuous telemetry that reveals unifocal premature ventricular contractions (PVCs) that developed into coupling then trigeminy. Mr. J complains of chest discomfort, the health care provider is informed and reviews the current serum levels:

- Serum digoxin: 2.6 ng/dL
- Sodium (Na): 135 mEq/L
- Potassium (K+): 3 mEq/L
- Blood urea nitrogen (BUN): 15 mg/dL
- Calcium 8.5 mg/dL
- Magnesium 2 mg/dL

The drugs brought to the hospital with the client are reviewed and digoxin and furosemide are held. Mr. J is transferred to the coronary care unit (CCU) with a diagnosis of PVCs.

Questions and Suggested Answers

1. **Discuss PVCs or complexes.** PVCs (premature ventricular beats) are the most common of all dysrhythmias, other than those of the sinus node. They are usually caused by an irritable focus in the ventricle. They result from enhanced ventricular automaticity. They are dangerous when they are frequent (more than six per minute), coupled with normal beats, multiform, occurring in pairs, and fall on the T wave (the most vulnerable period of the cardiac cycle, which if the heart is stimulated at this time, it often cannot respond to the stimulus in an organized fashion because the muscle fibers are in various stages of repolarization). Therefore, PVCs occurring during this vulnerable period can precipitate more life-threatening dysrhythmias such as ventricular tachycardia and ventricular fibrillation.

2. **Discuss some risk factors for the development of PVCs.** Risk factors for the development of PVCs include chronic hypoxemia, hypokalemia, hypocalcemia, hypomagnesemia, acute acidosis, hypermetabolic states (strenuous exercises), and digoxin toxicity. Chronic hypoxemia causes vasoconstriction, preventing cardiac muscle fibers and conductive fibers from maintaining normal electrolyte concentration differentials across

their membranes. If their excitability is severely affected, the conduction pathway may lose the automatic rhythmicity, resulting in the development of PVCs. Decrease in serum potassium (hypokalemia) affects the transmission of cardiac muscle and the regulation and transmission of cardiac impulses; the most serious effect is risk for ventricular dysrhythmias. Decrease in serum calcium affects neuromuscular cell membranes, increasing neuromuscular excitability. One of the overall results of the deficiency is the change in the cell membranes, which causes a decrease in the contractility of cardiac muscle fiber. The nervous system becomes more excitable, and muscle spasms develop, resulting in the development of dysrhythmias such as PVCs. Hypomagnesemia usually occurs along with low serum potassium and calcium levels. It causes increased muscular excitability. It is an essential ion for cardiovascular function and muscular excitability. When magnesium is deficient in the myocardium, muscle irritability occurs and PVCs may develop. Acute acidosis leads to a loss of potassium. The process is related to the increase in hydrogen ion concentration that inhibits potassium secretion by reducing the activity of the sodium-potassium pump. The reduction in potassium irritates the ventricular muscle, resulting in the development of PVCs. PVCs can occur in healthy people, especially with the use of caffeine, nicotine, or alcohol, all of which cause temporary irritability of the ventricles manifesting by PVCs. Strenuous exercises may cause hyperkalemia by releasing potassium from skeletal muscle. Hyperkalemia alters the cell membrane potential, affecting the heart. The cardiac conduction is affected first with slowing of the heart rate, prolonged PR interval and widening of the QRS complex, and the development of PVCs. Digitalis toxicity can cause ventricular bigeminy or trigeminy due to overstimulation of ventricular contractions, ventricular emptying, and irritation of the conduction pathway.

3. **Discuss the effects of atropine sulfate in treating bradycardia and the development of PVCs.** The drug of choice for bradycardia is atropine sulfate, which was administered to Mr. J on arrival in the ED. The sudden increase of his heart rate from 54 to 68 could have caused transient development of PVCs. Atropine increases the heart rate by accelerating impulse formation in the sinus and atrioventricular node (AV) by inhibiting the vagal response.

4. **Discuss clinical manifestations of PVCs.** Depending on the frequency, PVCs may cause reduction in cardiac output (CO), precipitating an anginal attack. If cardiac output is reduced, peripheral pulses may be diminished or difficult to palpate. Palpitations may occur due to sudden electrical stimulation of the heart muscle.

5. **Discuss the complications that can result from PVCs, especially in Mr. J's case.** *Angina pectoris* could develop due to transient reduction in cardiac output. It is a clinical syndrome characterized by episodes or paroxysms of pain or a feeling of pressure in the anterior chest. The cause is considered to be insufficient coronary blood flow, resulting in inadequate oxygen supply to the myocardium. Therefore, myocardial oxygen demand has exceeded the supply of oxygen. *Ventricular tachycardia and fibrillation* could also develop as complications of PVCs. *Ventricular tachycardia* is caused by increased myocardial irritability, as are PVCs. Ventricular tachycardia is extremely dangerous and should be considered an emergency, because it could progress to other lethal dysrhythmias, severe decrease in CO, and eventually death if not aggressively treated. Management of ventricular tachycardia (VT), requires identification of the cause of the irritability, and prompt correction. Antidysrhythmic medications may be implemented or cardioversion may be indicated if the reduction in CO is severe. *Ventricular fibrillation* is a rapid, ineffective quivering of the ventricles. With this dysrhythmia, there is no audible heart beat, no palpable pulse, and no respiration. The pattern is grossly irregular, and there is no coordinated cardiac activity. Therefore, without aggressive implementation, cardiac arrest and death are imminent. The immediate treatment is defibrillation.

6. **Discuss common nursing diagnoses for clients with dysrhythmias.**

   - Decreased CO R/T PVCs, digoxin toxicity
   - Ineffective tissue perfusion R/T decreased CO
   - Risk for or actual impaired gas exchange R/T alteration in oxygen supply and consumption
   - Risk for injury R/T adverse effects of cardiac medications
   - Anxiety R/T fear of the unknown

A

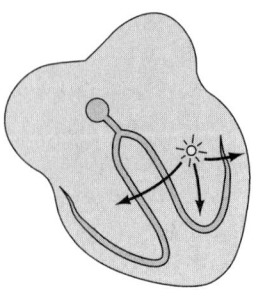

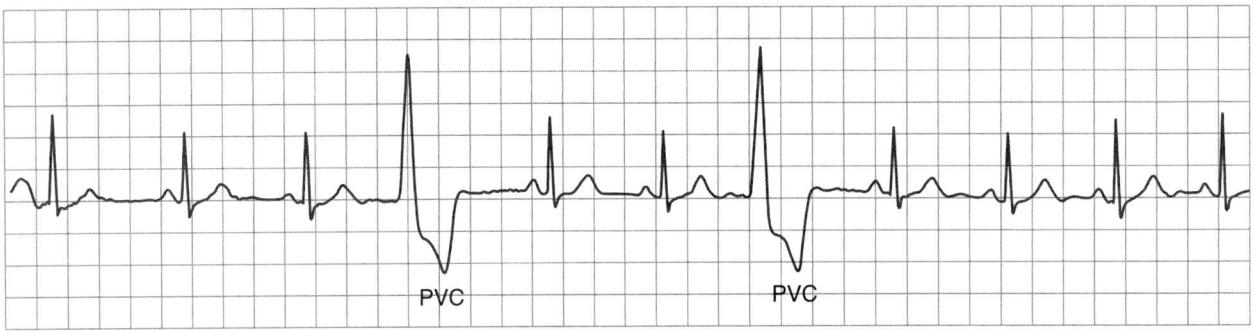

B

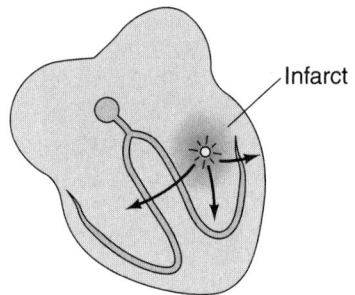

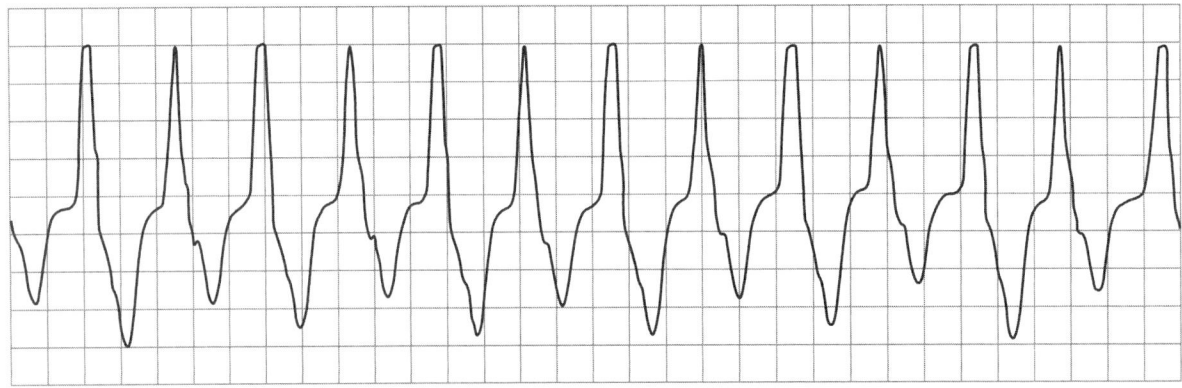

A. Unnatural pacemakers, created by an AMI, interrupt the normal sinus rhythm
B. Ventricular tachycardia robs the heart's coronary arteries of life-giving blood

- Disturbed sleep pattern R/T the activities of the CCU
- Deficient knowledge R/T condition, CCU environment and equipment, treatment, and home care on discharge

7. **Discuss the reasons why Mr. J's digoxin and furosemide are being held.** Mr. J's medical history includes myocardial infarction five years ago and left-sided heart failure. Persons with congested heart failure are usually placed on digoxin since it exerts a direct and beneficial effect on myocardial contraction in the failing heart, to strengthen the heart muscle, and improve cardiac output, so as to prevent the recurrence of myocardial infarction. Diuretic therapy is usually prescribed with digoxin because left ventricular failure causes pulmonary congestion, which could progress to pulmonary edema. The digoxin and furosemide were held because the heart rate was 54 on admission, and the serum digoxin level is 2.6 ng/dL due to digoxin toxicity. The furosemide is held because the serum potassium level is 3 mEq/L on admission, which is below normal. Both the elevated serum digoxin and the decreased serum potassium, if not treated, can cause other types of dysrhythmias and worsen the current cardiac status.

8. **Discuss the reason digoxin immune fab (Ovine) was not prescribed for Mr. J.** Digoxin immune fab was not administered as the reversal agent for digoxin-induced bradycardia because implementation of atropine sulfate increased the heart rate from 54 to 68 with only one intravenous dose of atropine sulfate.

The following are prescribed:

- Dextrose 5% and 0.45% sodium chloride with 20 mEq KcL IV infusion at 100 ml/hr
- Atropine sulfate (Atropine) 0.5 mg IV q1h PRN for a maximum of 2 mg
- Lidocaine HcL (Xylocaine) 50 mg IV bolus at 20 mg/min, repeat in five min, then start infusion of 20 mcg/kg/min immediately after first bolus
- Amiodarone HcL (Cardarone) 150 mg IV over 10 mg followed by 360 mg slow infusion over six hours followed by 540 mg at 0.5 mg/min over 18 hours
- Place client on continuous telemetry
- Monitor continuous oxygen saturation/pulse oximetry
- Oxygen to maintain oxygen saturation greater than 94%
- Serial arterial blood gas (ABG)
- Carvedilol 3.125 mg two times per day for two weeks
- Serum digoxin levels two times per day until stable
- Monitor serum sodium, potassium, and magnesium levels

9. **What are the purposes of the prescribed orders?** *The intravenous fluids* prescribed replace fluid losses and provide electrolytes including potassium depleted by furosemide contributing to the client's digoxin toxicity. *Atropine sulfate* is an anticholinergic agent that increases heart rate and cardiac output by blocking vagal impulses to the heart through inhibiting acetylcholine effects on the post-ganglionic cholinergic receptor in the cardiac muscle and the sinoatrial and atrioventricular nodes. *Lidocaine HcL* is a Class 1B antiarrhythmic agent that shortens the refractory period and suppresses the automaticity of ectopic foci in the atria, ventricles, Bundles of His and the Purkinje fibers of the ventricles. It controls PVCs as well as other arrhythmias and is the agent of choice to treat symptomatic PVCs. *Amiodarone HcL* is an antiarrhythmic agent used to decrease the number of ventricular tachycardia/ventricular fibrillation episodes that can occur as a result of bigeminal and trigeminal events by prolonging the action potentials in cardiac fibers, depressing conduction. Clients with cardiac dysrhythmias are placed on continuous *cardiac telemetry* to closely monitor their cardiac rhythms to detect current condition and to monitor therapeutic action of the medications used to treat their dysrrythmias. *Monitoring oxygen saturation/pulse oximetry* is necessary to detect both improving and worsening of the client's oxygen tissue perfusion so supplemental oxygen can be titrated to maintain oxygen saturation at the prescribed level to insure that the heart is receiving adequate oxygen. *Oxygen therapy* supplies needed oxygen to myocardial tissue and decreases its metabolic demand. *Serial ABG* readings are needed to evaluate the acid-base status of the client and any acid-base imbalance to determine if the client is acidotic, since acidosis can cause PVCs. ABG also looks at the oxygen saturation, which provides the need for supplemental oxygen. However, it is not as reliable a tool as pulse oximetry for titrating oxygen flow rates. *Carvedilol* is an alpha-beta adrenergic blocking agent that decreases myocardial oxygen demand and lowers cardiac workload

through vasodilation, which is beneficial for clients with congested heart failure. **Serum digoxin levels** guide management of the drug. If the blood level is bordering on high, the drug dosage is reduced and serum digoxin levels monitored. If the level is toxic, the drug is temporarily discontinued and the client closely monitored for effects of digoxin toxicity. If toxicity is evident, the client is treated with digoxin immune fab, the antidote for digoxin toxicity. **Serum sodium level** is monitored because Mr. J is on furosemide, a potent diuretic that aids in the excretion of sodium. If sodium level decreases from the effects of furosemide therapy replacement is required to avoid electrolyte imbalance. Monitoring of serum sodium prevents electrolyte imbalance. Sodium level can be decreased with prolonged use of furosemide. Deficits of sodium alter the cell's ability to depolarize and repolarize normally, and could irritate the myocardial cells resulting in an even faster heart rate. **Serum potassium** is monitored because the most recent value is 3 mEq/L, which is below the normal value. A deficit in potassium is a major contributing factor in the occurrence of PVCs, because low levels of potassium affects membrane excitability and alters contractility. **Serum magnesium** is monitored because an untreated deficit can contribute to electrolyte imbalance and the occurrence of PVCs. Because of Mr. J's age, there is a potential for decreased renal function, and digoxin therapy requires a healthy kidney to avoid toxicity since 80–90% of digoxin is excreted via the kidneys. Normal serum magnesium is important in the care of Mr. J, who has PVCs, because magnesium deficits prevents the movement of potassium into the cells. If potassium is not restored to the cells, other dysrhythmias may develop, and PVCs will progress to more serious dysrhythmias. **Serum calcium level** is monitored because calcium is needed to aid in the maintenance of myocardial contractility, and a deficiency would worsen the present occurring dysrhythmias.

10. **What are the most common adverse reactions, drug-to-drug, drug-food/herbal interactions for the prescribed medications?**

    The most common adverse reactions of *atropine sulfate* are drowsiness, dry mouth, blurred vision, tachycardia, and urinary hesitancy. The most common adverse reactions of *lidocaine HcL* are confusion, dizziness, hallucinations, lightheadedness, drowsiness, and euphoria, although these adverse effects are fleeting because of the short duration of lidocaine's action. They are more common in the presence of continuous infusion lidocaine. The most common adverse effects of *amiodarone HcL* include hypotension and irritation at the intravenous access site. The most common adverse reactions of *carvedilol* are bradycardia, postural hypotension, edema, dizziness, fatigue, weakness, diarrhea, impotence, and hyperglycemia. Drug-to-drug interactions may occur with the simultaneous use of *atropine sulfate* and other anticholinergics (amantadine, glycopyrrolate, phenothiazines, antihistamines, tricyclic antidepressants, quinidine, procainamide, and dysopyramide) which will increase atropine sulfate anticholinergic effects. The antipsychotic effects of phenothiazines may be decreased if used concurrently with atropine. The simultaneous use with methotrimeptrazine may precipitate extrapyramidal effects, and antacids decrease the absorption of and may increase mucosal lesions in clients taking oral potassium chloride. Atropine potentiates the effects of many oral preparations, including atenolol, digoxin, nitrofurantoin, and thiazide diuretics by delaying gastric emptying and increasing their absorption rate. It antagonizes cholinergic agents, such as pyridostigmine and edrophonium, which are used to treat myasthenia gravis. There are no clinically significant drug-to-food/herbal interactions established. With *lidocaine HcL*, drug-to-drug interactions may occur with the simultaneous use of procainamide or quinidine resulting in cross-sensitivity and increase in the pharmacologic effects of lidocaine HcL. Other agents whose concurrent use increases the action of lidocaine include amiodarone, beta-adrenergic blocking agents, and cimetidine. The simultaneous use with phenytoin increases cardiac depressant effects, and if used with tubocurarine, succinylcholine, and gentamicin (Gahart and Nazareno, 728), the action of these agents will increase. No clinically significant drug-to-food/herbal interactions have been established. Drug-to drug interactions may occur with the concurrent use of *amiodarone HcL* and other antiarrhythmic agents including disopyramide, mexiletine, procainamide, and quinidine increase the serum concentrations of these agents with risk of severe cardiac dysrhythmias resulting. Amiodarone should not be administered with ibutilide, pimozide, or sparfloxacin because of the increased risk of cardiotoxicity. Lidocaine may increase serum digoxin levels by decreasing its metabolism. If used with potassium-depleting diuretics, the risk of hypokalemia-induced dysrrythmias increases. Amiodarone increases the action of warfarin, cyclosporine, flecainide, phenytoin, lidocaine, methotrexate, procainamide, quinidine, and aminophylline and the risk of adverse effects of these agents. "Concomitant use with simvastatin (Zocor) has been associated with myopathy/rhabdomyolysis" (Gahart and Nazareno, 90). If used concurrently with fentanyl, bradycardia, hypotension, and decreased cardiac output may result. Agents that decrease the serum levels and action of amiodarone are cholestyramine, phenytoin, and rifampin. Increased plasma levels of amiodarone and potential adverse effects of both amiodarone and the other agents may occur with the simultaneous use cimetidine, protease inhibitors, beta-blocking agents, and calcium-channel blocking drugs. No specific drug-to-food interactions have been established, however St. John's Wort increases amiodarone clearance and decreases its serum levels and action. Drug-to-drug interactions may occur with the simultaneous use of **carvedilol** and rifampin and cimetidine may significantly reduce carvedilol levels; clonidine, reserpine, and MAO inhibitors may increase the risk of hypotension or bradycardia. The simultaneous use with intravenous phenytoin and verapamil may increase myocardial depression and increase risk for bradycardia if digoxin is also used simultaneously. The simultaneous use of carvedilol with insulin or oral hypoglycemic agents may alter the effectiveness of insulin and hypoglycemic agents, repuiring dose adjustments to maintain serum levels and prevent toxicity. Use with calcium-channel blockers and selective serotonin reuptake inhibitors (fluoxetine, paroxetine) increases the risk of conduction irregularities including bradycardia. Concurrent use with hydroxycholoroquine increases carvedilol plasma levels. Carvedilol increases the drug levels of disopyramide and cyclosporine. There are no clinically significant drug-to-food/herbal interactions established.

11. **Discuss the psychosocial impact of being in an intensive care unit (ICU).** The perception of the client that people in ICUs die, the numerous monitoring devices and alarms, as well as several intravenous infusion pumps, can increase the sick person's perception of his illness and increase his anxiety. Additional anxiety-producing factors are the constant activities of the environment, and the fact that his critical condition involves his heart, coupled with unasked questions about his treatment can generate a higher level of anxiety. People in ICU usually are subjected to serial laboratory tests either by venipuncture or the drawing of blood samples from arterial lines. Regardless of the route used to access these samples, there is a normal reaction of anxiety because of what the client may perceive as the uncertainty of his recovery.

12. **Discuss client education for a multiple diagnosis of left-sided heart failure and current episodes of PVCs.** The client should learn to regulate activity according to his response, so as to deter the progression of the disease and the development of complications. The client should be taught how to live within the limits of his cardiac reserve such as with adequate rest periods, avoiding emotional upsets, accepting the fact that taking digoxin daily and restricting sodium intake may be a permanent way of life. The client or significant other (S/O) should be taught the signs and symptoms indicating recurring heart failure, and to report weight gain of two or more pounds in a few days, loss of appetite, which could be an adverse effect of digoxin, shortness of breath with activity, swelling of the ankles, feet, or abdomen, persistent cough, or frequent urination at night, which could be signs of recurring failure. Teach the client how to take his radial pulse daily before taking digoxin, and if the pulse is below 60 or above 100 beats per minute, it should be held and the primary care provider made aware of the changes. The client should be taught signs of digoxin toxicity such as anorexia, nausea, vomiting, slow heart rate, headache, and fatigue. The client should avoid caffeine, nicotine, or alcohol intake because they stimulate the occurrence of PVCs. The client should have follow-up visits at least two times per year or more as per the primary health care provider's instructions.

References

Black, J.M. and Hawks, J.H. (2005). *Medical-Surgical Nursing: Clinical Management for Positive Outcomes* (7th ed.). Philadelphia: W.B. Saunders.

Broyles, B.E. (2005). *Medical-Surgical Nursing Clinical Companion.* Durham, NC: Carolina Academic Press.

Corbet, J.V. (2004). *Laboratory Tests and Diagnostic Procedures with Nursing Diagnoses* (6th ed.). Upper Saddle River, NJ: Prentice Hall.

Gahart, B.L. and Nazareno, A.R. (2005). *2005 Intravenous Medications.* St. Louis: Mosby.

Huether, S.E. and McCance, K.L. (2004). *Understanding Pathophysiology* (3rd ed.). St. Louis: Mosby.

Lewis, S.M., Heitkemper, M.M., and Dirksen, S.R. (2004). *Medical-Surgical Nursing* (5th ed.). St. Louis: Mosby.

Libster, M. (2002). *Delmar's Integrative Herb Guide for Nurses.* Albany, NY: Thomson Delmar Learning.

Spratto, G.R. and Woods, A.L. (2005). *2005 Edition: PDR Nurse's Drug Handbook.* Clifton Park, NY: Thomson Delmar Learning.

PART FOUR

The Nervous System

CASE STUDY 1

Unilateral Ménière's Disease

GENDER
- M

AGE
- 30

SETTING
- Clinic

ETHNICITY/CULTURE
- Hispanic American

PREEXISTING CONDITIONS

COEXISTING CONDITIONS
- Allergic reactions to sulfur, feathers

LIFESTYLE
- Licensed mechanic

COMMUNICATION
- Spanish and English

DISABILITY

SOCIOECONOMIC STATUS
- Middle

SPIRITUAL/RELIGIOUS
- Evangelical

PHARMACOLOGIC
- Meclizine HcL (Antivert)
- Diazepam (Valium)
- Hydrochlorothia-zide (HydroDIURIL)
- Nicotinic acid (Nicobid)
- Dimenhydrinate (Dramamine)

PSYCHOSOCIAL
- Anxiety
- Fear

LEGAL

ETHICAL
- Drugs that cause drowsiness will prohibit the client from working.

ALTERNATIVE THERAPY

PRIORITIZATION
- Maintain safety

DELEGATION
- RN
- Client education

EASY

THE NERVOUS SYSTEM

Level of difficulty: Easy

Overview: This case involves a thorough assessment of the client's condition including all drugs he may be currently taking. The case also involves a careful history for vertigo, the extent of disability, and implementing of measures to stabilize balance.

Client Profile

Mr. S is a 30-year-old single client who is employed by a major motor vehicle department as a licensed mechanic. Mr. S is seen in the clinic with complaints of imbalance, which he relates to a roaring sound and a feeling of fullness in his left ear for the past two weeks. On further history gathering by the nurse, Mr. S reports that periods of whirling infrequently last for a few minutes, but during the past two days, vertigo has lasted for 30 minutes.

Case Study

On further assessment, Mr. S complains of nausea, vomiting, diaphoresis, and a persistent feeling of imbalance, which occurred while he was on the job the previous day, causing him to request time off to seek medical assistance. History and physical are continued by a nurse practitioner (NP), who documents a normal physical examination, with the exception of evaluation of cranial nerve VIII, indicating impairment of the left ear. An audiogram is done, and reveals a sensorineural hearing loss in the left ear. An electronystagmogram is done and shows reduced vestibular response in the left ear. Physical examination findings and diagnostic results are discussed and a diagnosis of Ménière's disease is made in collaboration with a health care provider. Mr. S will be given prescriptions and instructions to return to the clinic in two weeks for follow-up evaluation. The registered dietitian discusses the need for a low sodium diet with Mr. S, and the RN provides him with a list of foods that are both high and low in sodium.

Questions and Suggested Answers

1. **Discuss the pathophysiology of Ménière's disease.** Ménière's disease is a disorder that affects both vestibular and auditory function. It is caused by excess endolymph (clear intracellular fluid in the membranous labyrinth of the inner ear) in the vestibular and semicircular canals. The right and left ears are affected with equal frequency; the disease occurs bilaterally in about 20% of clients, and about 20% of the clients have a positive family history for the disease. Regardless of the cause, endolymphatic hydrops, a dilatation in the *endolymphatic space*, develops. There are two subsets of the disease, known as atypical Ménière's disease: cochlear and vestibular. Cochlear Ménière's disease is recognized as a fluctuating, progressive sensorineural hearing loss associated with tinnitus and aural pressure in the absence of vestibular symptoms or findings. Vestibular Ménière's disease is characterized as the occurrence of episodic vertigo associated with aural pressure with no cochlear symptoms. Hearing loss is fluctuant and usually subtle and reversible in the early stages. Later, the hearing loss becomes permanent.

2. **Discuss the incidence and prevalence of Ménière's disease.** Ménière's disease affects more than 2.4 million people in the United States. More common in adults, it has an average age of onset in the 40s, with symptoms usually beginning between the ages of 20 and 60. It appears to be equally common in both genders.

3. **Discuss clinical manifestations of Ménière's disease.** Although it is associated with sensorineural hearing loss, the most prominent clinical manifestation is *vertigo* (feeling that the surrounding or one's own body is revolving), which is usually the most troublesome complaint. Typically, the client reports that vertigo lasts from minutes to hours, possibly accompanied by nausea and/or vomiting. There are complaints of diaphoresis and disequilibrium. The attacks can awaken the client at night but there is also one-sided sensorineural hearing loss and tinnitus (a roaring sound; a feeling of pressure or fullness in the ear).

4. **Discuss diagnostic studies for Ménière's disease.** The *electrocochleography* is used to evaluate the presence of Ménière's disease. It is designed to measure response of the cochlea and the eighth cranial nerve to acoustic stimulation. Electrodes are placed through the tympanic membrane onto the promontory near the round window or in the ear canal, and an acoustic stimulation is applied. The *Weber test* uses a tuning fork to elicit sound, which may lateralize to the ear opposite the hearing loss. An *audiogram* typically reveals a sensorineural

hearing loss in the affected ear. An *electronystagmogram* may be normal or may show reduced vestibular response. It provides graphic recording of vestibular system and its interaction to stimuli.

5. **Discuss common nursing diagnoses and goals for vertigo.**

   - Risk for injury R/T altered mobility because of gait disturbance and vertigo – The goal is that the client will be free of any injuries associated with imbalance of falls.
   - Risk for fluid volume imbalance R/T increased fluid output, and altered intake – The goal is to modify lifestyle to decrease disability and exert maximum control and independence within limits posed by vertigo.
   - Risk for trauma R/T balancing difficulties – The goal is to reduce the risk of trauma by adapting the home environment and by using rehabilitative devices as necessary.

   The following are prescribed:

   - Meclizine HcL (Antivert) 50 mg PO daily
   - Diazepam (Valium) 5 mg PO two times per day
   - Hydrochlorothiazide (HydroDIURIL) 50 mg PO daily
   - Nicotinic acid (Nicobid) 10 mg PO daily
   - Dimenhydrinate (Dramamine) 50 mg PO q6h

6. **What are the purposes for the prescribed medications?** *Meclizine HcL* is an antiemetic that suppresses the vestibular system by markedly depressing the labyrinthine excitability and conduction in the vestibular-cerebellar pathway. *Diazepam* is a benzodiazepine anxiolytic that helps to control mild anxiety, spasm, and spasticity that may occur with vertigo by enhancing the GABA-mediated presynaptic inhibition at the spinal level to relax the skeletal muscles. *Hydrochlorothiazide* is a thiazide diuretic that decreases endolymphatic volume. It does this by interfering with the absorption of sodium ions across the distal renal tubular segment of the nephron, which enhances excretion of sodium and water, and in doing so, decreases the endolymphatic fluid in the cochlear duct of the ear. *Nicotinic acid* is a B complex vitamin that vasodilates the cochlear duct by direct action on vascular smooth muscles. *Dimenhydrinate* is a cholinergic blocking agent and antiemetic that helps to reduce or stop an acute attack of vertigo by inhibiting cholinergic stimulation in the vestibular and associated neural pathways.

7. **What are the most common adverse reactions of the prescribed medications?** The most common adverse reactions of *meclizine HcL* are drowsiness, nervousness, restlessness, insomnia, nausea and vomiting, and diarrhea. The most common adverse reactions of *diazepam* are dizziness, drowsiness, lethargy, and the risk of physical and psychological dependence. The most common adverse reactions of *hydrochlorothiazide* are dizziness, weakness, lethargy, hypotension, hyperglycemia, hyperuricemia, and hypokalemia. The most common adverse reactions of *nicotinic acid* are gastrointestinal (GI) upset, flushing of the face and neck, and pruritus. The most common adverse reactions of *dimenhydrinate* are drowsiness and anorexia.

8. **Discuss drug-to-drug and drug-to-food/herbal interactions of the prescribed medications.** Drug-to-drug interactions may occur with the simultaneous use of *meclizine HcL* and alcohol-containing drugs, antihistamines, opioid analgesics, and sedatives/hypnotics, which may potentiate the sedating effects of meclizine. The simultaneous use with drugs containing anticholinergic properties, such as atropine, haloperidol, phenothiazines, quinidine, and disopyramide may cause additive anticholinergics effects. There are no clinically significant drug-to-food/herbal interactions established. With *diazepam*, drug-to-drug interactions may occur with the simultaneous use of alcohol, central nervous system (CNS) depressants, and anticonvulsants, which may potentiate CNS depression. The simultaneous use of hormonal contraceptives, disulfiram, fluoxetine, rifampin, isoniazid, ketoconazole, metoprolol, propoxyphene, propranolol, or valproic acid may decrease the metabolism of diazepam and increase diazepam plasma levels, increasing its toxicity. Ranitidine decreases the GI absorption of diazepam. Diazepam potentiates the antihypertensive effects of thiazide diuretics and also potentiates the action of muscle relaxants. The simultaneous use with Levodopa may decrease its effects. There are no clinically significant drug-to-food interactions established. Drug-to-herbal interactions may occur with the simultaneous use of kava-kava, skullcap, chamomile, and valerian,

which may potentiate sedation. With **hydrochlorothiazide**, drug-to-drug interactions may occur with the simultaneous use of amphotericin B, and corticosteroids, which increase hypokalemic effects. Cholestyramine and colestipol decrease thiazide absorption. As previously noted, diazepam potentiates the antihypertensive effects of hydrochlorothiazide, potentially causing hypotension. Drug-to-food/herbal interactions are seen with the simultaneous use of licorice and stimulant laxative herbs, which may increase risk of potassium depletion. When used simultaneously with gingko, it may increase antihypertensive effects. Drug-to-drug interactions may occur with the simultaneous use of **nicotinic acid** and HMG-CoA reductase inhibitors, which increase the risk of myopathy. Additive hypotension may occur with the simultaneous use of guanethidine. There are no clinically significant drug-to-food/herbal interactions established. With **dimenhydrinate**, drug-to-drug interactions may occur with the simultaneous use of antihistamines, alcohol, opioid analgesics, and sedative/hypnotics, which may increase CNS depression. The simultaneous use of ototoxic drugs (aminoglycosides, ethacrynic acid) may mask the signs of ototoxicity in clients taking ototoxic drugs. The simultaneous use with tricyclic antidepressants, quinidine, or disopyramide may increase anticholinergic effects. The simultaneous use of monoamine oxidase (MAO) inhibitors intensifies and prolongs the anticholinergic effects of antihistamines. There are no clinically established drug-to-food/herbal interactions.

9. **Surgical treatment of Ménière's disease is a last resort. When medical therapy is ineffective, discuss surgical procedures that may be performed.** Two surgical procedures that are usually done are labyrinthectomy and endolymphatic decompression. Labyrinthectomy is the surgical excision of the aural labyrinth (structure of the inner ear) to drain the normal fluid that causes normal vibration when sound waves from the stirrup bone strike against it. When the normal fluid and vibration are eliminated, vertigo will be minimized. Endolymphatic sac decompression, or shunting, equalizes the pressure in the endolymphatic space by the insertion of a shunt or drain through the endolymphatic sac via a postauricular incision.

10. **Discuss client education for Ménière's disease.** The client should comply with follow-up visits as per the health care provider's instructions. The client should practice moving the head slowly to prevent worsening of vertigo that may infrequently occur. The client should rest during episodes of vertigo to prevent falls and injuries, and should avoid bright lights such as watching television and reading during episodes of vertigo. During episodes of vertigo, the client may need assistance with ambulating, and should avoid climbing stairs and other hazardous activities if experiencing vertigo. The client should wear prescribed hearing aids, and should follow the instructions on the care of the aids. Written and verbal instructions on the use of prescribed medications should be emphasized, and side, adverse and toxic effects of prescribed medications should be included in the instructions. Adhering to a low sodium diet (2,000 mg/day) will help to regulate the balance of fluid within the body, because sodium and fluid retention disrupt the delicate balance between endolymph and perilymph in the inner ear.

References

Broyles, B.E. (2005). *Medical-Surgical Nursing Clinical Companion.* Durham, NC: Carolina Academic Press.

Corbet, J.V. (2004). *Laboratory Tests and Diagnostic Procedures with Nursing Diagnoses* (6th ed.). Upper Saddle River, NJ: Prentice Hall.

Deglin, J.H. and Vallerand, A.H. (2005). *Davis's Drug Guide for Nurses* (9th ed.). Philadelphia: F.A. Davis.

"FDA Approves Stavelo™ for treatment of Parkinson's Disease." (December 2005). From http://www.pharma.us.novartis.com.

Gahart, B.L. and Nazareno, A.R. (2005). *2005 Intravenous Medications.* St. Louis: Mosby.

Huether, S.E. and McCance, K.L. (2004). *Understanding Pathophysiology* (3rd ed.). St. Louis: Mosby.

Ignatavicius, D.D. and Workman, M.L. (2006). *Medical-Surgical Nursing across the Health Care Continuum* (5th ed.). Philadelphia: W. B. Saunders.

"Parkinson's Disease: Challenges, Progress, and Promise." (April 2005). Prepared by the Office of Communications and Public Liaison, National Institute of Neurological Disorders and Stroke, National Institutes of Health. Available at www.ninds.nih.gov/disorders/parkinsons_disease/parkinsons_research.htm.

Spratto, G.R. and Woods, A.L. (2005). *2005 Edition: PDR Nurse's Drug Handbook.* Clifton Park, NY: Thomson Delmar Learning.

CASE STUDY 2

Multiple Sclerosis

GENDER
- F

AGE
- 38

SETTING
- Hospital

ETHNICITY/CULTURE
- White American

PREEXISTING CONDITIONS

COEXISTING CONDITIONS

LIFESTYLE
- Accountant

COMMUNICATION

DISABILITY
- Impaired mobility

SOCIOECONOMIC STATUS
- Middle

SPIRITUAL/RELIGIOUS
- Baptist

PHARMACOLOGIC
- Interferon beta-1a (Avonex)
- Mitoxantrone HcL (Novantrone)
- Baclofen (Lioresal)
- Carbamazepine (Tegretol)
- Methylprednisolone (Medrol)
- Amantadine HcL (Symmetrel)

PSYCHOSOCIAL
- Anxiety
- Emotional instability
- Depression

LEGAL

ETHICAL
- Confidentiality
- Client and family involvement in decision making
- Disability issues
- Quality of life

ALTERNATIVE THERAPY
- Meditation

PRIORITIZATION
- Systems assessment
- Monitor temperature and serum calcium levels

DELEGATION
- RN
- Client education

MODERATE

THE NERVOUS SYSTEM

Level of difficulty: Moderate

Overview: This case uses systems assessment to detect features of multiple sclerosis (MS). It involves a thorough assessment of the client's condition including prescribed drugs and alternative therapy used to help relieve distressing symptoms. The nurse must use critical-thinking skills to prioritize and implement quality care, with the use of therapeutic management aimed at treating the disease process and providing symptomatic relief.

Client Profile

Mrs. N is a 38-year-old married woman with three children, ages 9, 11, and 13. She has been active with her family and community activities. She has worked as a certified accountant in a law firm for more than ten years. Her husband has been employed at a major bank in the city for 15 years. Mrs. N's husband accompanies her to the hospital's emergency department (ED) because of complaints of increased fatigue and stiffness in the lower extremities and double vision. She is 5′8″ and weighs 195 pounds. She is a good historian who responds to questions in a detailed manner. Mrs. N denies family history of neurological diseases and reports that her parents are alive and well.

Case Study

Ms. N's complaints on arrival to the ED include increased fatigue and stiffness of the lower extremities with unsteady gait and sudden fuzziness of the eyes followed by double vision (diplopia). She reports that similar symptoms were noticed two years ago, with brief periods of decreased visual acuity that disappeared after a while. Therefore, medical attention was not sought. Mrs. N is transferred to a medical unit of the hospital for continued assessment and evaluation. Her vital signs are:

Blood pressure: 130/78
Pulse: 78
Respirations: 16
Temperature: 98.6° F

The health care provider completes a thorough history and physical with focus on basic motor skills and sensory assessments which elicited positive indications for MS. A magnetic resonance imaging (MRI) is scheduled and the health care provider discusses ongoing plans with the primary nurse who continues with the nursing history and assessment. Further neurological assessment finds increased deep tendon reflexes, and the client's report of numbness, paresthesia, tingling, and burning in the lower extremities. Babinski reflex is positive, and abdominal reflexes are slow. Serum calcium level is drawn and sent to the lab, revealing a result of 9 mg/dL. The health care provider returns soon after the completion of the nursing assessment with a multidisciplinary team of a neurologist, medical doctor, pharmacist, a nurse practitioner, dietitian, and social worker. After further discussion with Mrs. N pertaining to the physical assessments, the following diagnostic studies are prescribed: Cerebrospinal fluid (CSF) analysis, CSF electrophoresis, MRI of the spine. The neurologist explains the need for a lumbar puncture to Mrs. N and how the procedure would be done. Mrs. N then signs an informed witnessed consent for the lumbar puncture. The social worker remains in the client's room after the rest of the team leaves to discuss the possible need for help at home while she remains in the hospital for continued evaluation. The diagnostic studies are completed and reviewed by the team, then discussed with Mrs. N and her husband as per her request. A diagnosis of MS is confirmed.

Questions and Suggested Answers

1. **Why is a lumbar puncture used as a diagnostic test for MS?** A lumbar puncture is done to identify agents that may have infiltrated the central nervous system (CNS) and have caused damage to the immune system, which may be a cause for damage to the myelin sheath, causing interruption of transmission impulses.

2. **Discuss the guideline for lumbar puncture.** A needle is inserted into the subarachnoid space through the third and fourth or fourth and fifth lumbar interspace to withdraw spinal fluid. The client is assured that insertion of the needle into the spine will not cause paralysis. The client's bowel and bladder should be emptied before the procedure. The client is positioned on one side with the back toward the health care provider

or nurse practitioner. The thighs and legs are flexed to increase the space between the spinous processes of the vertebrae, for easier entry into the subarachnoid space. A small pillow is placed under the client's head to maintain the spine in a horizontal position. A pillow may be placed between the legs to prevent the upper leg from rolling forward. The nurse assists the client to maintain the position to avoid sudden movement, which can produce a traumatic bloody tap. The client is instructed to breathe normally because hyperventilation may lower an elevated pressure. The health care provider inserts the needle into the subarachnoid space through the third and fourth or fourth and fifth lumbar interspace. After the procedure, the client is positioned in a prone position and instructed to remain in the position for two to three hours to separate the alignment of the dura and arachnoid needle punctures in the meninges, to reduce the leakage of CSF. The client is encouraged to increase fluid intake to reduce the risk of post-procedure headache.

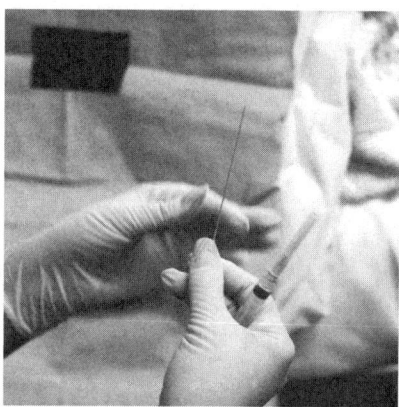

In a lumber puncture (also called a spinal tap), a needle is inserted into the subarachnoid space of the spinal column

3. **What are the expected findings of the diagnostic tests that aided in the confirmation of the diagnosis of MS?** The CSF fluid will have elevated protein level and a slight increase in the white blood cell (WBC) count, and the CSF electrophoresis will show an increase in the myelin basic protein and the presence of oligoclonal (IgG) bands, which are usually present in the CSF of clients with MS. The MRI will reveal the presence of plaques, which is considered diagnostic for MS. MRI is highly sensitive to areas of demyelination, and shows breakdown of the myelin and the beginning of the narrowing of the spinal cord.

4. **What are common nursing diagnoses related to clients with MS?**

   - Impaired physical mobility R/T weakness, muscle paresis, spasticity
   - Risk for injury R/T sensory and visual impairment
   - Altered urinary and bowel elimination R/T spinal cord dysfunction
   - Altered thought processes R/T cerebral dysfunction
   - Ineffective coping
   - Potential for sexual dysfunction R/T spinal cord involvement or psychological reactions to condition

   The following are prescribed:

   - Inteferon beta-1a (Avonex) 30 mcg IM every week
   - Mitoxantrone HcL (Novantrone) IV 12 mg/M² over 5–15 minutes
   - Baclofen (Lioresal) 5 mg PO three times per day
   - Methylprednisolone (Medrol) 40 mg PO daily
   - Amantadine HcL (Symmetrel) 100 mg PO q12h5

5. **What are the purposes for the prescribed medications?** *Inteferon beta-1a* is a biologic response modifier that decreases the number and severity of exacerbations by amplifying the immune system's ability to better

function as the body's defense, thus slowing physical disability. It works by binding to specific receptors on the surface of the human cells and stops the cells from losing their own antigenic markers, which would result in destruction of the myelin sheath, and worsening of the disease process. ***Mitoxantrone HcL*** is an antibiotic antineoplastic agent that reduces the relapse rate, reducing neurologic disability and the frequency of clinical relapses. It works by suppressing the immune system, reducing the number of new brain lesions by inhibiting cellular DNA synthesis, resulting in neurologic disability in MS. ***Baclofen*** is a centrally-acting skeletal muscle relaxant that relieves muscle spasticity and improves mobility. Baclofen works within the spinal cord and suppresses hyperactive reflexes that are involved in regulation of muscle movement. When these reflexes are suppressed, there is a decrease in flexor and extensor spasms. Baclofen also suppresses resistance to passive movement and in doing so, reduces the discomfort of spasticity, allowing improvement in performance. ***Methylprednisolone*** is a glucocorticoid that stabilizes the disease process because of its potent anti-inflammatory and immunosuppressive effects. Persons with MS usually exhibit evidence of immune-mediated inflammation, and methylprednisolone is effective in reducing edema and inflammatory response by inhibiting the synthesis of chemical prostaglandins, leukotrienes, and histamine that function to inhibited inflammatory responses. ***Amantadine HcL*** is an antiviral agent that decreases and controls the fatigue experience by the client. It works by triggering the release of dopamine from its storage sites to the ends of nerve cells that are still intact and have not yet been destroyed by the disease process, thus halting the progression.

6. **What are the most common adverse reactions of the prescribed medications?** The most common adverse effects associated with ***interferon beta-1a*** include headache, fever, pain, chills, malaise, flu-like symptoms, nausea, diarrhea, infection, gingivitis, and gastrointestinal (GI) bleeding. The most common adverse reactions of ***mitoxantrone Hcl*** are nausea, vomiting, and bone marrow suppression with manifestations of leukopenia and thrombocytopenia, abdominal pain, alopecia, altered liver function, fever, headache, stomatitis, and bleeding. The most common adverse reactions of ***baclofen*** are dizziness, drowsiness, weakness, and fatigue due to its CNS depressant effect. The most common adverse reactions of ***methylprednisolone*** are euphoria, edema, and delayed wound healing. The most common adverse reactions of ***amantadine HcL*** are dizziness, nervousness, insomnia, and difficulty concentrating.

7. **Discuss the drug-to-drug and drug-to-food/herbal interactions of the prescribed medications.** Drug-to-drug interactions may occur with the simultaneous use of ***interferon*** and any other potentially myelosuppressant agent including cisplatin and zidovudine. Further, it may increase aminophylline serum levels and may act synergistically with zidovudine to increase the risk of severe neutropenia. Drug-to-drug interactions may occur with the simultaneous use of ***mitozantrone HcL*** and influenzae and pneumoccocal vaccines, which may increase mitoxantrone serum levels and toxicity. When used with other bone-marrow depressing agents, additional suppression may occur with resulting increased risk of thrombocytopenia, anemia, and leukopenia. The simultaneous use of mitoxantrone Hcl with other anthracyclines, doxurubicin, epirubicin, and idarubicin increases risk of cardiotoxicity. Leukopenia and thrombocytopenia effects are increased with the concurrent use of drugs that cause blood dyscrasias, such as phenytoin, carbamazepine, and nonsteroidal anti-inflammatory agents (NSAIDs). There are no clinically significant drug-to-food/herbal interactions established. Drug-to-drug interactions may occur when ***baclofen*** is used simultaneously with other CNS depressants, antihistamines, and opioid analgesics that may increase sedating effects. The simultaneous use with monoamine oxidase (MAO) inhibitors may cause increased CNS depression or hypotension. Drug-to-food/herbal interactions may occur with the simultaneous use of kava, valerian, chamomile, or hops, which may increase CNS depression. Drug-to-drug interactions may occur with the simultaneous use of ***methypredisolone*** and amphotericin B, furosemide, thiazide diuretics, isoniazid, phenytoin, phenobarbital, and rifampin by decreasing the effectiveness of the drug and increasing its metabolism. Erythromycin increases methylprednisolone's effect due to decreased metabolism in the liver. Drug-to-food/herbal interactions include grapefruit, which increases the peak serum levels of methylprednisolone by decreasing liver metabolism. Drug-to-drug interactions may occur with simultaneous use of ***amantadine HcL*** and anticholinergic

drugs such as atropine sulfate or alcohol. Hydrochlorothiazide/triamterene combination, quinidine, and trimethoprim/sulfamethoxazole decrease amantadine excretion and increase plasma levels. Henbane leaf increases the anticholinergic effect of amantadine and pheasant's eye herb and scopolia root increase the overall effects of amantadine.

8. **What are some complementary and alternative therapies that may be included in the comprehensive treatment plan for the client with MS after the client has discussed his or her plans to include these therapies?** Some complementary and alternative therapies that may be included in the comprehensive treatment plan for the client with MS include nutrition with high protein and anti-inflammatory oils (nuts, seeds, and cold-water fish) and nutritional supplements such as Omega-6 oils (evening primrose; black currant oils; selenium; zinc; B-complex vitamins, especially B_{12} and B_6 and magnesium; vitamin C; vitamin E; and co-enzyme Q10). Herbs such as hawthorn (Crataegus monogyna) and gingko (Gingko biloba) are currently being used as alternative treatments for MS. Combination of the following herbs in equal parts are also used to nourish the nervous system and prevent constipation: oatstraw (Avena sativa), skullcap (Scutellaria laterifolia), lavender (Lavendula angustifolia), lemon balm (Melissa officinalis), passionflower (Passiflora incamata), and horsetail (Equisetum arvense). They may have therapeutic effects yet are not FDA approved for this use.

9. **Why is it important to discharge the client with MS to a rehabilitation center for a brief period after discharge from the hospital?** Discharging a client for a brief stay in a rehabilitation center is done to help the client regain and maintain maximum strength, function, and independence by providing a program to improve functional ability. The length of stay will depend on the client's response to the overall treatment plan.

10. **Explain a significant psychosocial problem for Mrs. N as it relates to discharge to a rehabilitation center briefly instead of to home.** A significant pyschosocial problem would be anxiety or depression because of her diagnosis with an illness that is one of the leading causes of neurological disabilities, and she has to be away from her immediate family, which includes her children, ages 9, 11, and 13. Her role as a mother is impacted. Her absence will not allow her to assist her children with their studies, which for most mothers of school-age and adolescent children is an important function. She will not be able to be the caregiver for her family and, with no mention of any external support systems, she will probably be very concerned about her family's needs being met during her absence from home. Because the client's concern may be magnified in light of her diagnosis, the discharge nurse, social worker, or case manager should become engaged in honest communication with the client, providing empathetic understanding to establish an atmosphere that allows the client to express her concerns freely. The discharge planning team needs to determine client's resources and significant others who will be available for support to her spouse and the children during her absence. Maximizing family potentials at this time will require one interdisciplinary method to guide the entire family to continue functioning in a healthy manner while the mother is rehabilitating. Maintaining intrafamily communication at the highest level will greatly help the temporary separation of the mother from the home.

11. **What should the client with MS do to help maintain a sense of well-being upon discharge to home?** The client should schedule work to accommodate energy level by spacing duties that place demands on body systems, prioritizing tasks, delegating, and discontinuing those that are not necessary but sufficient to deplete needed energy. The client should take frequent rest periods to decrease fatigue, and plan daily activities by using a chalkboard or paper to write things down instead of remembering them. Although the diagnosis may be difficult to accept, the client should love him/or herself like he/or she has never done before. The client should try to be a part of her family's daily plans, including helping her children with their homework which should not be overly energy consuming. Making microwave dinners instead of "homemade" meals would allow her to be involved in caring for her family's nutrition needs and conserve energy. She should delegate those home tasks to her children that at their ages they should be able to do, including doing laundry, washing dishes (if no dishwasher is available), cleaning their rooms, and taking care of other household chores. The MS client should use an air conditioner as often as necessary and stay out of direct sunlight.

References

Broyles, B.E. (2005). *Medical-Surgical Nursing Clinical Companion.* Durham, NC: Carolina Academic Press.

Corbet, J.V. (2004). *Laboratory Tests and Diagnostic Procedures with Nursing Diagnoses* (6th ed.). Upper Saddle River, NJ: Prentice Hall.

Gahart, B.L. and Nazareno, A.R. (2005). *2005 Intravenous Medications.* St. Louis: Mosby.

Huether, S.E. and McCance, K.L. (2004). *Understanding Pathophysiology* (3rd ed.). St. Louis: Mosby.

Ignatavicius, D.D. and Workman, M.L. (2006). *Medical-Surgical Nursing across the Health Care Continuum* (5th ed.). Philadelphia: W. B. Saunders.

Lewis, S.M., Heitkemper, M.M., and Dirksen, S.R. (2004). *Medical-Surgical Nursing Assessment and Management of Clinical Problems* (5th ed.). St. Louis: Mosby.

Smeltzer, S.C. and Bare, B.G. (2004). *Brunner and Suddarth's Textbook of Medical-Surgical Nursing* (10th ed.). Philadelphia: Lippincott Williams & Wilkins.

Spratto, G.R. and Woods, A.L. (2005). *2005 Edition: PDR Nurse's Drug Handbook.* Clifton Park, NY: Thomson Delmar Learning.

"Treatments for Multiple Sclerosis." (July 2005). Available at http://mscenter.ucsf.edu/treatments.htm.

CASE STUDY 3

Generalized Tonic-Clonic Seizure

GENDER
- F

AGE
- 24

SETTING
- Emergency department

ETHNICITY/CULTURE
- Black American/West Indian

PREEXISTING CONDITIONS
- Head injury two years ago

COEXISTING CONDITIONS

LIFESTYLE
- Nursing student

COMMUNICATION

DISABILITY

SOCIOECONOMIC STATUS
- Middle

SPIRITUAL/RELIGIOUS
- Baptist

PHARMACOLOGIC
- Phenytoin (Dilantin)
- Carbamazepine (Tegretol)
- Diazepam (Valium)

PSYCHOSOCIAL
- Anxiety

LEGAL
- If client injures a person while operating a moving vehicle due to a seizure attack, should the client be liable?

ETHICAL
- Does the client with history of seizure have the right to operate a moving vehicle?

ALTERNATIVE THERAPY

PRIORITIZATION
- Maintain safety
- Control seizure

DELEGATION
- RN
- Client education

THE NERVOUS SYSTEM

Level of difficulty: Difficult

Overview: This case involves a through assessment of the client's presenting symptoms and maintaining a patent airway. The case involves prioritization in a triage situation at a busy urban hospital emergency department (ED).

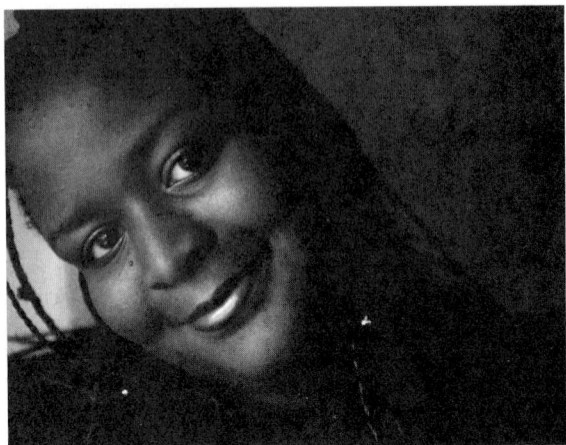

Client Profile

Ms. D is a 24-year-old nursing student who, after leaving the clinic for home via public transportation, complains to her classmates of an unusual feeling that she is not able to describe. A few minutes after her remarks, Ms. D starts to fall but is assisted to the ground by one of her classmates. Emergency medical service (EMS) is contacted, and Ms D's airway is maintained with the help of a passerby while waiting for EMS arrival. The EMS arrives in five minutes and, after a "quick assessment," applies a high-flow oxygen via a non-rebreather mask.

Case Study

Ms. D is taken to the emergency department (ED) of a hospital in a busy section of a large city. On arrival to the hospital triage area, the client is responsive to tactile and verbal stimuli, but not capable of giving an appropriate report of the occurrence. The report is given by a classmate, who describes a tonic phase seizure, with the client uttering a cry then slumping to the ground. The classmate describes Ms. D saying that she felt uneasy and saw unusually bright light, and a smell as though rubber was burning. There was an abrupt increase in muscle tone, loss of consciousness, and loss of postural control, and Ms. D began to fall to the ground but was assisted by her classmate and a passerby. The passerby dialed "911" as the classmate remained with Ms. D. Ongoing observation of Ms. D finds an opisthotonic posture (evidence of acute arching of the back, the head bent back on the neck, the heels bent back on the legs, and the arms and hands flexed rigidly at the joints due to prolonged and severe spasm of the muscles). Ms. D became unconscious, with urinary incontinence; pupils were fixed and dilated, lasting for approximately 45 seconds. Continued observation by the classmate describes alternating contraction and relaxation of the muscles in all the extremities along with hyperventilation. Ms. D is now in the ED, alert, and oriented to her name and place, but not to time of day. A triage nurse continues collection of additional data from the client and her classmate, while an ED clerk notifies the health care provider of Ms. D's arrival. She is placed in a single room, in a side-lying position, and a suction machine and apparatus are at the bedside. Vital signs are:

- Blood pressure: 130/80
- Pulse: 82
- Respirations: 20
- Temperature: 98.6° F

Serum labs are drawn: glucose, sodium, total calcium. The bed is placed in low position and side-rails are padded. A stat dose of diazepam (Valium) 10 mg IV is administered by the triage nurse while awaiting the arrival of the health care provider. Thirty minutes after the valium is administered, Ms. D responds appropriately to verbal and tactile stimuli. The health care provider arrives and orders a loading dose of phenytoin which is initiated by the triage nurse. The health care provider continues with a history and physical, history of seizures, psychosocial assessment and mental status examination, and a detailed neurologic examination. Ms. D denies history of seizure or prior episode before today. Upon completion of a neurological assessment, the health care provider orders an electroencephalogram (EEG), and a computed tomography (CT) scan. Result of an ECG shows brain wave abnormalities and the CT scan negative for congenital abnormalities or masses. Based on the documentation of the presenting symptoms on arrival to the ED, and the ECG brain wave abnormalities, a diagnosis of tonic-clonic seizure is confirmed.

Questions and Suggested Answers

1. **What is the incidence and prevalence of seizure (epilepsy) in the United States?** Approximately one in eleven people will experience at least one seizure during his/her lifetime. Epilepsy occurs in 1 in 100 persons. According to the Epilepsy Foundation of America, an estimated 2.5 million people in the United States have epilepsy and approximately two-thirds of the 125,000 people newly diagnosed with epilepsy each year are adults. The highest incidence is among older adults, most of whom have experienced a cerebrovascular accident which is noted as the etiology. Approximately 80% are able to control their seizures with medications. The prevalence of epilepsy in the United States is 0.5 to 1%.

2. **Discuss the pathophysiology of seizures.** When the integrity of the neuronal cell membrane is altered, the cell begins firing with increased frequency and amplitude. When the intensity of the discharge reaches a threshold, the neuronal firing spreads to adjacent normal neurons. Any process that disrupts the stability of the neuronal cell membrane can cause seizures to develop. One major causative factor is severe, penetrating head trauma, with the injury resulting in a long-lasting pathologic change in the central nervous system (CNS) that transforms a presumably normal neural network into one that is abnormally hyperexcitable. Some possible reasons for this mechanism when a severe head trauma occurs include neuronal structural impairment, abnormalities involving the sodium-potassium pump, and changes in various neuro-chemicals. Another possible cause is that an epileptogenic focus may develop at the location of increased cell membrane permeability, or may be limited to a specific area or encompass the entire cortical surface. Normally, excitatory messages from a single hypersensitive neuron in the cerebral cortex are modulated by deeper structures (e.g., thalamus and brain stem). When the normal, excitatory messages are altered, the electrical activity from the cortex is not controlled or modulated, and seizure activity develops.

3. **What is a tonic-clonic seizure?** A tonic-clonic seizure is a mixed seizure with uncontrolled activity that initially occurs with an abrupt increase in muscle tone, loss of consciousness, and loss of autonomic signs lasting from 30 seconds to several minutes. There is muscle contraction (generalized stiffness of the body) followed by relaxation of the muscles in all the extremities, accompanied by hyperventilation. The pattern of contraction and relaxation is manifested first with the clonic pattern that is rhythmic with jerking activities in all extremities. The client may bite the tongue and become incontinent of urine and feces. Following the contracting phase (clonic), the client remains unresponsive to stimuli, but is relaxed and breathes quietly, regaining consciousness gradually, but may be confused and disoriented upon waking.

4. **What are common nursing diagnoses for the client with seizure?**

    - Ineffective breathing pattern R/T neuromuscular impairment secondary to prolonged tonic phase or seizure or during postictal period
    - Risk for injury R/T seizure activity and subsequent impaired physical mobility secondary to postictal weakness or paralysis
    - Ineffective coping R/T perceived loss of control and denial of diagnosis

5. **What is the focus of documentation for a client having a seizure?**

    - How often seizures occur
    - Description of each seizure
    - Whether more than one type of seizure occurs

- Observations during the seizure
- How long the seizure lasts
- If seizure is preceded by an aura
- What client did after seizure
- How long it takes for the client to return to pre-seizure status

6. **What is included in the diagnostic assessment of seizures?** The client's history: prenatal birth and developmental history, family history, age of seizure onset, history of past and present illnesses, trauma, precipitating factors that cause seizures; psychosocial assessment; complete neurologic examination; skull radiographs, EEG, CT scan. The complete neurologic examination is performed to determine the focal neurologic deficit or the focus or origin of seizure activity. The skull radiographs are done to identify possible fractures, deformities in bone structures, or calcification, which may be triggers for seizure activity. The EEG helps to identify abnormalities, which aids in the confirming of the diagnosis. The CT helps to determine the presence of a tumor, congenital lesions, edema, infarct, hemorrhage, or structural deviation, all of which may trigger seizure activity.

The following are prescribed:

- Phenytoin (Dilantin) 100 mg three times per day × seven days then return to health care provider for evaluation
- Carbamazepine (Tegretol) 200 mg PO two times per day
- Complete blood count and serum electrolyte levels
- Carbamazepine and phenytoin levels in the morning

7. **What are the purposes for the prescribed orders, including diazepam administered in the ED?** *Phenytoin sodium* is a hydantoin anticonvulsant that acts on the motor cortex of the brain to decrease the spread of electrical impulses from rapidly firing in the multiple foci occurring in epilepsy. It is thought to accomplish this by stabilizing hyperexcitable cells by affecting sodium efflux. *Carbamazepine* is an anticonvulsant that controls tonic-clonic seizure. Its action is not completely understood, however it is thought to depress activity in the nucleus ventralis anterior of the thalamus, causing a reduction in polysynaptic responses by inhibiting the neurotransmitter sodium. Carbamazepine is effective because of its ability to reduce polysynaptic response and block post-tetanic potentiation. In blocking the potentiation, it reduces sustained high frequency repetitive neural firing and aborts seizure activities. *Diazepam* is a benzodiazepine antianxiety agent usually administered intravenously during epileptic seizures to decrease the risk of status epilepticus by enhancement of the GABA-mediated presynaptic inhibition at the brain stem reticular formation resulting in skeletal muscle relaxation. This further reduces the risk of physical injury during seizure activity. *Complete blood count* is ordered because an adverse effect of carbamazepine is transient leukopenia, and toxic effects are aplastic anemia, agraunlocytosis, and thrombocytopenia. *Serum electrolyte levels* are evaluated to determine the effects of carbazepine and phenytoin on serum sodium levels. *Carbamazepine and phenytoin drug levels* are prescribed to evaluate therapeutic and potential toxic levels of these two agents. Carbamazepine, although used for seizure control, can itself cause seizures if the serum level is greater than the therapeutic range. The therapeutic level is 5-12 microgram/mL, and the toxic level is 12 microgram/mL. The dosing objective of phenytoin is to produce levels between 10 and 20 microgram/mL. Levels below 10 microgram/mL are too low to control seizures; at levels above 20 microgram/mL, signs of toxicity begin to appear. Because phenytoin has a relatively narrow therapeutic range (between 10 and 20 mcg/mL), and because of the relationship between phenytoin dosage and phenytoin plasma levels, once a safe and effective dosage has been established, the client should adhere to it rigidly, because small deviations from the established dosage can cause toxicity or therapeutic failure. When treatment with phenytoin is discontinued, dosage should be reduced gradually. Abrupt withdrawal may precipitate seizures.

8. **What are the most common adverse reactions of the prescribed medications, including diazepam?** The most common adverse reactions of *carbamazepine* are nausea and vomiting, constipation, hyponatremia, and bone

marrow suppression. The most common adverse effects of *phenytoin sodium* are drowsiness, ataxia, dysarthria, confusion, insomnia, nervousness, irritability, depression, tremor, numbness, headache, and it may cause psychosis. Rapid parenteral administration may result in hypotension, dysrythmias, cardiovascular collapse, heart block, and severe central nervous system depression. Intravenous administration of *diazepam* may cause depressed respirations, apnea, bradycardia, cardiovascular collapse, and cardiac arrest. Other adverse effects include ataxia, blurred vision, confusion, coughing, diminished reflexes, drowsiness, dyspnea, headache, hiccups, hyperventilation, laryngospasm, somnolence, syncope, and vertigo. Phlebitis and venous thrombosis may occur at the injection site.

9. **Discuss the drug-to-drug and drug-to-food/herbal interactions for the prescribed medications, including diazepam.** With *carbazepine*, drug-to-drug interactions may occur with the simultaneous use of other anticonvulsants, which may decrease their effectiveness because of increased metabolism. The simultaneous use of cimetidine, danazol, diltiazem, fluoxetine, fluvoxamine, isoniazid, levetiracetam, macrolide antibiotics, propoxyphene, ticlopidine, and verapamil may increase carbamazepine levels, and toxicity. Barbiturates, charcoal, benzodiazepines, theophylline, lamotrigine, valproic acid, bupropion, and haloperidol may decrease carbamazepine levels and decrease its effectiveness. Concurrent use with isoniazid and acetaminophen may increase the levels of these agents and increase the risk of hepatotoxicity. Carbazepine may decrease the effects of cyclosporine doxycycline, felodipine, haloperidol, lamotrigine, methylphenidate, oral contraceptives, dertraline, thyroid hormone, tricyclic antidepressants, valproic acid, and warfarin sodium. Carbazepine increases the resistance to or reversal of the neuromuscular blocking agent effects. Drug-to-food interactions are seen with the simultaneous use of grapefruit juice, resulting in increased peak levels of carbazepine. Multiple drug-to-drug interactions can occur with *phenytoin sodium*, ethyl alcohol, antacids, carbazepine, charcoal, clonazepam, diazoxide, folic acid, loxapine, nitrofurantoin, pyridoxine, rifampin, theophylline, and sucralfate, which decrease phenytoin levels. Increased phenytoin levels occur with the simultaneous use of allopurinol, amiodarone, oral anticoagulants, tricyclic antidepressants, benxodiazepines, chloramphenicol, chlorpheniramine maleate, cimetidine, disulfiram, fluconazole, ibuprofen, isoniazid, metronicazole, miconazole, omeprazole, phenothiazines, salicylates, sulfonamides, trimethoprim, and valproic acid. Phenytoin decreases the effects of acetaminophen but may increase the risk of hepatotoxicity. It decreases the effects of oral contraceptives but also may precipitate seizures. The effects of corticosteroids, cyclosporine, dicumarol, digoxin, disopyramide, doxycycline, furosemide, haloperidol, irinotecan, levodopa, levonorgestrel, mebendazole, meperidine, methadone, metyrapone, mexiletine, mirtazapine, primidone, quetiapine, quinidine, dulfonylurea, and theophylline are decreased by concurrent use with phenytoin. There is an increased risk of lithium toxicity when used with phenytoin. There are no clinically significant drug-to-food interactions established. However, milk thistle may help prevent liver damage from phenytoin. Concurrent use of diazepam with other CNS depressants including antihistamines, alcohol, barbiturates, monoamine oxidase (MAO) inhibitors, phenothiazines, chlorpromazine, and tricyclic antidepressants may result in increased effects for up to 48 hours with intravenous use of diazepam. It may increase serum concentrations of digoxin and phenytoin. Ritonavir may prolong the CNS depressive effects of diazepam. Simultaneous use with beta-blocking agents, cimetidine, disulfiram, oral contraceptives, fluoxetine, isoniazid, itraconazole, ketoconazole, omeprazole probenecid, and valporic acid may increase plasma concentrations of diazepam because of decreased hepatic metabolism. Ranitidine decreases the absorption of diazepam if taken orally. Use with rifampin and theophyllines antagonizes the sedative effects of diazepam. Clozapine may result in respiratory depression and should be avoided when using parenteral diazepam. Drug-to-food interactions occur with the concurrent use of grapefruit juice, which may affect certain enzymes of the P_{450} system and should not be used with diazepam (Gahart and Nazareno, 385–386).

10. **What is a major complication of seizure activity?** Status epilepticus is a major complication and a *neurologic emergency*. It is a medical emergency because during the activity, the brain's metabolic needs increase dramatically, and the supply of glucose and oxygen to the brain becomes inadequate, and brain damage will occur if immediate and aggressive management is not implemented. Aggressive management is mandatory, because during the repetitive activities, the brain uses more energy than is supplied. Neurons become

exhausted and cease to function. If status epilepticus is a precursor of tonic-clonic seizure, it is most dangerous because it can cause ventilatory insufficiency, hypoxemia, cardiac arrhythmias, hyperthermia, and systemic acidosis.

11. **Discuss client education for seizures.** The client must take medications as prescribed, and should avoid alcohol consumption and excessive fatigue. The client should not take any unprescribed medications, unless instructed to do so by the primary health care provider. The client should know the name, dose, time of administrations, adverse effects and actions to take if they occur. The client's significant other (S/O) should be instructed on what to do if a seizure occurs. Significant others should be taught how to maintain a patent airway by positioning the client on the side to prevent aspiration and maintain airway, loosening constricting clothing such as ties or scarves. The client should not be restrained, and no object should be placed in the mouth. To prevent injury during a seizure, the S/O should ease the client to the floor, if the client is seated, while supporting and protecting the head. Signs and symptoms of worsening of seizure activity should be emphasized or written out for the S/O. These include repetitive and ongoing seizure with prolonged confusion or loss of consciousness. Significant others and the client should be informed that medical alert bracelets, necklaces, and identification cards are available through the Epilepsy Foundation (EF), local pharmacies, or companies specializing in identification devices (e.g., Medic Alert). The client and S/O should keep follow-up appointments, especially when scheduled for the monitoring of serum blood levels.

References

Beebe, R. and Funk, D. (2005). *Fundamentals of Basic Emergency Care.* Clifton Park, NY: Thompson Delmar Learning.

Broyles, B.E. (2005). *Medical-Surgical Nursing Clinical Companion.* Durham, NC: Carolina Academic Press.

Corbet, J.V. (2004). *Laboratory Tests and Diagnostic Procedures with Nursing Diagnoses* (6th ed.). Upper Saddle River, NJ: Prentice Hall.

Deglin, J.H. and Vallerand, A.H. (2005). *Davis's Drug Guide for Nurses* (9th ed.). Philadelphia: F. A. Davis.

Epilepsy Foundation of America. www.efa.org.

Gahart, B.L. and Nazareno, A.R. (2005). *2005 Intravenous Medications.* St. Louis: Mosby.

Huether, S.E. and McCance, K.L. (2004). *Understanding Pathophysiology* (3rd ed.). St. Louis: Mosby.

Ignatavicius, D.D. and Workman, M.L. (2006). *Medical-Surgical Nursing across the Health Care Continuum* (5th ed.). Philadelphia: W.B. Saunders.

Ko, D.Y. (October 2004). *Tonic Clonic Seizure.* Available at www.emedicine.com/NEURO/topic376.htm.

Lehne, R.A. (2004). *Pharmacology for Nursing Care* (5th ed.). St. Louis: Mosby.

Lewis, S.M., Heitkemper, M.M., and Dirksen, S.R. (2004). *Medical-Surgical Nursing: Assessment and Management of Clinical Problems* (5th ed.). St. Louis: Mosby.

Spratto, G.R. and Woods, A.L. (2005). *2005 Edition: PDR Nurse's Drug Handbook.* Clifton Park, NY: Thomson Delmar Learning.

CASE STUDY 4

Subarachnoid Hemorrhage – Grade II

GENDER
- F

AGE
- 42

SETTING
- Hospital

ETHNICITY/CULTURE
- Mixed race

PREEXISTING CONDITIONS
- Hypertension

COEXISTING CONDITIONS

LIFESTYLE
- Bank supervisor

COMMUNICATION

DISABILITY

SOCIOECONOMIC STATUS
- Middle

SPIRITUAL/RELIGIOUS
- Baptist

PHARMACOLOGIC
- Mannitol (Osmitrol)
- Nimodipine (Nimotop)
- Phenobarbital sodium (Luminal Sodium)
- Phenytoin (Dilantin)
- Valsartan (Diovan)
- Ducosate sodium (Colace)

PSYCHOSOCIAL
- Anxiety
- Denial

LEGAL

ETHICAL

ALTERNATIVE THERAPY

PRIORITIZATION
- Brief mental status exam
- Prevent increase in intracranial pressure

DELEGATION
- RN
- Client education

THE NERVOUS SYSTEM

Level of difficulty: Difficult

Overview: This case involves emergency management. The nurse must use critical-thinking skills to prioritize care in a busy triage area to prevent increase in intracranial pressure. The nurse must be skilled and competent at implementing care to maintain cerebral perfusion pressure, controlling intracranial pressure (ICP), managing cardiac dysrhythmias, and preventing rebleeding with ongoing neurologic assessment.

Client Profile

Mrs. M-W is a 43-year-old client who has been experiencing bouts of headache for the past two months. The headaches have become worse, increasing in severity and frequency over the past two weeks. Today, Mrs. M-W experienced a sudden onset of severe headache while preparing a meal for her family. She yells to her husband saying, "I just had a sudden headache that is so severe, I feel weak. It is the worst one I have had." The husband enters the kitchen to find Mrs. M-W projectile vomiting. Mr. W calls his brother-in-law (his neighbor) and they accompany Mrs. M-W to the emergency department (ED) in their community.

Case Study

On arrival at the ED, Mrs. M-W describes the pain as "awful" and sudden. She complains of nausea, and tells the nurse her eyes are blurred. The nurse examines the client, while the certified nursing technician requests that the ED health care provider be paged, then notifies the intensive care unit of the pending transfer. Mrs. M-W is awake, alert, and oriented to person, place, and time. Her conversation and response to questions are comprehensible and easily understood. Mrs. M-W reports a history of hypertension for ten years, and social drinking at dinner time. She is currently taking Valsartan 80 mg PO daily. She follows complex commands, her facial structure is normal, and she is able to move all extremities with equal strength. Her pupils are equal and reactive to light and accommodation. However, her neck is stiff and painful with positive Kernig's and Brudzinski's sign. Her vital signs are:

Blood pressure: 170/96
Pulse: 90
Respirations: 18
Temperature: 98.6° F

The health care provider orders a noncontrast computed tomography (CT) scan of the brain, which reveals blood in the subarachnoid space, intracerebral clots, and large clots surrounding an aneurysm. A transcranial doppler ultrasonography (TCD) is done with evidence of minimal vasospasms. The client is transferred to the medical intensive care unit (MICU) and is placed on complete bed rest, with the head of the bed elevated at 45 degrees, while the nursing team prepares her for possible surgery. An arterial line is inserted, and neurological assessment is ongoing, including blood pressure readings and monitoring of arterial pressure. An intravenous line of D 5.45% NS at 100 mL per hour is initiated. The client is instructed to avoid coughing, sneezing, or straining and is given reasons for these instructions. Bilateral pneumatic compression devices to lower extremities are applied as per protocol for subarachnoid hemorrhage (SAH). Seizure precautions are initiated as per protocol for SAH. After the interdisciplinary team reviews the history and physical and diagnostic studies, the neurologist decides that the diagnosis is grade II SAH secondary to cerebral aneurysm rupture. The treatment plan for a craniotomy is discussed with Mrs. M-W and her husband. An informed consent is signed by Mrs. M-W.

Questions and Suggested Answers

1. **Which factors in the case study indicate that Mrs. M-W has suffered an SAH?** One factor is the description of the headache as the client described to her husband. Literature indicates that the client experiences a sudden, severe headache, typically in the occipital area, often accompanied by vomiting. Mrs. M-W's description of her headache is that "it is sudden and so severe, I feel weak." She also had projectile-type vomiting. In the ED, she complains of more nausea and reports that her eyes are blurred, her neck is stiff and painful, and she has positive Kerning's and Brudzinski's sign. A CT scan reveals blood in the subarachnoid space, intracerebral clots, and large clots surrounding an aneurysm. SAH is commonly caused by rupture of a cerebral aneurysm, with blood coming into contact with the meninges, resulting in blurred vision, positive

Kernig's and Brudzinski's signs. Kernig's sign is a symptom of meningitis evidenced by reflex contraction and pain in the hamstring muscles when attempting to extend the leg after flexing the thigh upon the body. Brudzinski's sign is seen with flexion of the hips when the neck is flexed from a supine position.

2. **Discuss precautions that are important to avoid SAH.** *Complying with antihypertensive medications* is important because a history of hypertension increases arterial pressure (hemodynamic stress), which in turn increases intracranial pressure, increasing the risk of weakening of the vessel wall and the formation of an aneurysm that may rupture, resulting in hemorrhage. Antihypertensive medications vary in their actions. However, the primary purpose is to reduce blood pressure by promoting dilation of arterioles and veins, with vasodilation contributing most to reduction in blood pressure. *Smoking cessation* is another important factor in preventing SAH. Cigarette smoking has been frequently studied as a risk factor for SAH. It is believed that smoking increases the risk of SAH, because it causes smoking-induced hypertension, which promotes aneurysm formation, or it may even promote aneurysm rupture. Long-term cigarette smoking can weaken the vessel walls of cerebral arteries by releasing proteolytic enzymes into the systemic circulation, which could result in aneurysm formation. *Reducing heavy consumption of alcohol* is important because having a history of habitual heavy alcohol consumption, has shown to increase the risk of SAH by inducing hypertension. Since long-term, excessive consumption of alcohol reduces the size of the cerebrum and produces a dose-dependent increase in blood pressure, the formation of aneurysm and rupture can occur. *Avoiding stress* is another important means of preventing SAH. Physical and emotional stress cause transient elevations of blood pressure. However, frequent or continued stress can cause vascular smooth muscle hypertrophy or affect central integrative pathways of the brain, resulting in the weakening of cerebral arteries, increasing the risk of aneurysm formation or rupture.

3. **Discuss the incidence and socioeconomic impact of intracranial aneurysm and SAH.** SAH occurs in approximately 1 out of 10,000 people. About 5–10% of strokes are caused by SAH. The annual incidence of SAH caused by ruptured aneurysm is 6–16 per 100,000 persons, and the incidence increases with age and is higher in women than men. The highest incidence of SAH from a ruptured aneurysm occurs between the ages of 20–60 years, and it is slightly more common in women than men. Aneurysm-related SAH has a 50% pre-hospital mortality, indicating the significant nature of the hemorrhage. Looking at the risk factors of SAH, the socioeconomic impact is more critical among older persons of lower-socioeconomic status. For instance, recent documentation of research findings cites blood pressure management rates to be lowest in Mexican Americans and Native Americans/American Indians. However, the prevalence is significantly higher in blacks than in whites and Hispanics. Some reasons for the socioeconomic impact on these groups are related to lack of easier access to health care agencies, especially in rural areas. Another factor may be related to non-documented residents who have no access to health care or who do not know how to access such care; therefore, they live with health problems such as hypertension, high cholesterol, cigarette smoking, all of which are high risk factors for SAH. Cultural norms influence the management of the health issue of hypertension, such as diet and exercise, and a general lack of accurate understanding of the insidious nature of hypertension and the long-term complications that come with the disease. The cost of antihypertensive medications may be another factor for the predominance of hypertension among these groups. According to the American Heart Association, black American and Native American/American Indian men smoke the most of all ethnic groups. These ethnic groups are known to be in the lower socioeconomic status, with a history of cigarette smoking as part of their daily social activity. Current data document a strong relationship between serum norepinephrine levels (elevated by smoking), resulting in hypertension. Cigarette smoking lowers levels of high-density lipoprotein (HDL, the good cholesterol), and increases the progression of atherosclerosis, which increases the risk of hypertension, or has the long-term complication of hypertension, with risk for SAH. Although heavy alcohol consumption is a risk factor for SAH, it impacts all socioeconomic groups of people. History of alcohol consumption is found in all ethnic groups. However, it is probably more in the middle socioeconomic status, due to the cost of alcoholic beverages. Almost half of Americans ages 12 and older report current drinking of alcohol. Stress is everywhere, and among all socioeconomic groups. It is the intensity of the stress that is high risk for hypertension, which can eventually lead to SAH if not corrected.

4. **Discuss common nursing diagnoses and expected outcomes for the client with SAH.**

   Nursing diagnosis: Risk for injury R/T altered tissue perfusion from rebleeding or vasospasm
   Expected outcome: Following the interventions, the client should be free of secondary brain injury from rebleeding or vasospasm.

   Nursing diagnosis: Pain R/T headache or meningeal irritation
   Expected outcome: Following the interventions, the client will be free from pain and discomfort related to headache and meningeal irritation.

   Nursing diagnosis: Knowledge deficit R/T lack of education about the pathophysiology, diagnosis, treatment of aneurysms, and the need for compliance
   Expected outcome: Following instruction, the client and significant others should be able to explain the following:

   - The common causes of SAH
   - The reason presurgery precautions were necessary
   - The reason the surgery was performed
   - The importance of compliance with prescriptions after discharge
   - The need for follow-up care with a primary health care provider

5. **Discuss the conditions that occur after an aneurysm ruptures.** *Increased intracranial pressure* (ICP) is a life-threatening situation that is dependent on the balanced volumes of brain tissue, cerebrospinal fluid (CSF), and intracranial blood. Increased intracranial pressure is a major form of stress on the central nervous system. The normal intracranial pressure ranges from 0 to 15 mm Hg. When stressors such as rupture of an aneurysm occurs, intracranial pressure rises because the rupture also damages the blood-brain barrier, allowing fluid to enter the extracellular space, mainly in the white matter. Because the rupture causes a sudden increase in intracranial volume, CSF immediately shifts extracranially, vasoconstriction occurs causing cerebral blood to shift extracranially. The increase in intracranial volume and the shifting of cerebral blood extracranially results in increase in the venous system. However, since there are no valves in the cerebral veins, outflow of fluid is blocked, cerebral blood flow backs up, and volume increases, further increasing the ICP. The continued increase in ICP results in reduction in cerebral perfusion, leading to tissue hypoxia, a decrease in serum pH level, and an increase in the level of carbon dioxide. This process causes cerebral vasodilation, edema, and a further increase in ICP, and the continuing of the cycle. If the cycle of increasing ICP is not corrected promptly, the brain may herniate downward toward the brainstem or laterally from a unilateral lesion within one cerebral hemisphere, causing irreversible brain damage and possible death.

   > **Physical findings associated with a rise in intracranial pressure:**
   > Decrease in mental status
   > Persistent vomiting
   > Glasgow Coma Score less than eight
   > Unequal pupils
   > Seizure activity
   > Hypertension
   > Bradycardia
   > Altered respiratory pattern

   Cerebral vasospasm is a common but dangerous complication that usually occurs between 4 and 15 days after an SAH. It is associated with a large number of deaths and disability. The spasm narrows the lumen of one or more cerebral vessels, causing ischemia and infarction of tissue supplied by the affected vessels. It is believed to occur in blood vessels surrounded by thick blood clots, which suggests that there are substances in the clot that cause the spasm. ***Rebleeding*** is a common complication for the client with a ruptured aneurysm, and the greatest risk for rebleeding is within the first 24 hours, and again in 7 to 10 days (when the initial clot breaks down). It is manifested by sudden severe headache, nausea and vomiting, decreasing levels of consciousness, and new neurologic deficits. Because aneurysm rebleed can be fatal, aggressive monitoring of clients after an aneurysm ruptures is critical.

6. **Discuss specific factors that may cause hyponatremia and complications in clients with SAH.** Clients with continued *increased ICP (IICP)* may develop cellular edema, which commonly occurs from cerebral hypoxia, due to hyponatremia, which may be related to failure of the sodium pump. When the sodium pump fails, its normal function is reversed. The sodium-potassium pump is essential for healthy tissue survival. The pump normally transports sodium ions out of the cells, resulting in a lower sodium concentration in intracellular fluid than in the surrounding extracellular fluid. However, when the pump fails, its role reverses, and sodium ions back up into the cells, resulting in cellular edema. Because clients with SAH usually have history of hypertension, their medication regimen often includes *diuretics* and antihypertensive medications, which remove sodium out of the body, resulting in hyponatremia. At the time of hospitalization, an osmotic diuretic such as mannitol may be administered to reduce IICP and a loop diuretic such as furosemide (Lasix) is often used as an adjunctive therapy to reduce the incidence of rebound from the mannitol. Although mannitol produces selective diuresis, it can cause hyponatremia because its diuretic effects last for several hours (six to eight). Long-term effects of hyponatremia regardless of the cause result in deficits such as changes in cerebral function, muscle weakness, hypotension, and shock.

7. **Discuss the advantages and disadvantages of early or delayed surgery for SAH.** Advantages of early surgery (within the first two days after rupture) are the preventing of rebleeding and ischemic complications due to vasospasm. The disadvantages of early surgery are the risk of cerebral infarction, because blood pressure must be lowered during surgery to enable safe dissection of the aneurysm. Advantages of delayed surgery (10–14 days after rupture) allow time for rebleeding and vasospasm risk to be reduced. It also allows time for the person to recover from the rupture. Clients with grades IV and V SAH and those with vasospasm fall under "delay surgery" category, due to their high risk for morbidity and mortality.

8. **Discuss the types of surgeries that can be done for the client with SAH secondary to ruptured aneurysm.** One type is an *endovascular technique* known as *coiling*, by which a metal coil can be inserted into the lumen of the aneurysm via interventional neuroradiology. The result is thrombus formation around the coil, resulting in blockage of the aneurysmal sac. Another type is *surgical obliteration* of the aneurysm with a metal clip or suture to eliminate the risk of rebleeding. The clipping is performed through a craniotomy to expose the aneurysm. The aneurysm is isolated, and a clip is placed over the neck of the aneurysm.

The following are prescribed:

- Neurologic assessment and blood pressure q1h and PRN
- Mannitol (Osmitrol) IV 0.5–1 g/kg over five to ten minutes, may repeat 0.25–1 g/kg q4h per critical-care protocol
- Furosemide (Lasix) 40 mg IV prior to administration of mannitol
- Phenobarbital sodium (Luminal Sodium) 100 mg IV two times per day
- Phenytoin (Dilantin) 1 g loading dose IV, 100 mg q8h
- Nimodipine (Nimotop) 60 mg PO q4h for 21 days. Start in the morning
- Ducosate sodium (Colace) 100 mg PO three times per day
- Serum labs: sodium, platelet count
- Insert indwelling urinary catheter
- Hourly urine outputs

9. **What are the purposes for the prescribed orders?** *Mannitol* is an osmotic diuretic used to decrease intracranial pressure by its action as a sugar alcohol. Its primary action is in extracellular compartments and diuresis

occurs within one to three hours and a decrease in intracranial pressure occurs as early as 15 minutes following administration. ***Furosemide*** is a potent loop diuretic frequently used in conjunction with mannitol to decrease intracranial pressure by causing diuresis. ***Phenobarbital*** is a sedative-hypnotic, anticonvulsant barbiturate that provides mild sedation, raises the seizure threshold to prevent seizures, and helps control the headache. Pain from the headache can cause restlessness resulting in blood and intracranial pressures elevation. Mild sedation is appropriate because the client should be easily aroused for neurological and vital signs evaluation. It causes mild sedation by interfering with the impulse transmission of reticular activating system. ***Phenytoin*** is a hydantoin anticonvulsant that increases the seizure threshold, thus preventing seizures from occurring during SAH, since bleeding can irritate the brain cells, resulting in the occurrence of seizures. It reduces the voltage, frequency, and spread of electrical discharges within the cerebral cortex, averting seizures. ***Nimodipine*** is a calcium-channel blocker used to treat cerebral vasospasm either before or following aneurysm clipping or coiling. It improves neurologic deficits by reducing vascular spasms in the cerebral arteries because of its selectivity for cerebral arteries, and its specific binding ability to cerebral tissue. It has been found to reduce the incidence of ischemic deficits from arterial spasm without side effects. ***Docusate sodium*** is a stool softener used to prevent straining during defecation, because straining leads to the development of valsalva maneuvers, which increase intracranial pressure. It softens the stool, making it easier to expel during defecation. Monitoring ***serum sodium*** detects reduction in sodium, which can occur with covert rebleeding. The occurrence of rebleeding may cause excessive anti-diuretic hormone (ADH) secretion from the pituitary, fluid retention, and low serum sodium levels. Monitoring of ***platelet count*** provides early information for interventions to retard bleeding. ***Inserting an indwelling urinary catheter*** and ***monitoring hourly urine output*** provides an ongoing objective indicator of the effectiveness of mannitol and furosemide. Increased urine output is the first indicator of decreasing intracranial pressure, and neurological checks following surgical repair of the aneurysm will not be an accurate measure with the effects of premedications and general anesthesia required to perform the surgery.

10. **What are the most common adverse reactions of the prescribed medications?** The adverse effects of ***mannitol*** are rare but may include backache, blurred vision, chest pain, chills, convulsions, hypochloremia, hyponatremia, dehydration, hypotension, and dizziness (Gahart and Nazareno, 750). The most common adverse effects of intravenous ***furosemide*** include dehydration, hypokalemia, hyponatremia, hypotension, anorexia, and mental confusion, peripheral edema, nausea, vomiting, muscle cramps, and hypotension. The adverse reactions of ***phenobarbital*** administered via slow intravenous injection are rare. With an average dose, the client may experience dizziness, depression, facial edema, fever, headache, hypotension, nausea, vertigo, and somnolence. The most common adverse reactions of ***phenytoin*** are drowsiness, gingival hyperplasia, ataxia, diplopia, nystagmus, hypotension, nausea, hypertrichosis, and rashes. With peripheral intravenous administration, there is a high risk of phlebitis even with slow administration and a free-flowing sodium chloride infusion to buffer its action on the vein wall. The most common adverse reaction of ***ducosate sodium*** is diarrhea.

11. **Discuss the drug-to-drug and drug-to-food/herbal interactions of the prescribed medications.** Drug-to-drug interactions can occur with the simultaneous use of ***mannitol*** and lithium because mannitol increases the excretion of lithium, thus lowering its effects. As a result of mannitol-induced hypokalemia, there is an increased risk of digoxin toxicity. No clinically significant drug-to-food/herbal interactions have been established. This may in part be due to the fact that most clients receiving mannitol are in a critical care setting and NPO ("nothing by mouth"). Drug-to-drug interactions may occur with the simultaneous use of intravenous ***furosemide*** and corticosteroids, thiazide diuretics, and amphotericin B in terms of increased potassium depletion. It potentiates the actions of antihypertensives and may result in transient or permanent deafness if used with other ototoxic agents. The risk of nephrotoxicity is increased if furosemide is used concurrently with vancomycin, aminoglycosides, ciprofloxacin, and cyclosporine. Furosemide may increase the action of warfarin, heparin, and streptokinase requiring close monitoring of the prothrombin, partial thromboplastin times, and INR. An increased risk of cardiotoxicity exists with the simultaneous use of furosemide and amiodarone, digoxin, pimozide, and sparfloxacin. Furosemide may increase or decrease

the actions of mivacurium or theophyllines, and may cause hyperglycemia if used with insulin or sulfonylureas. The effects of furosemide may be decreased with concurrent use of angiotensin-converting enzyme (ACE) inhibitors, probenecid, and in clients with cirrhosis or ascites. Clofibrate may increase furosemide's diuresis activity and phenytoin may inhibit its action. Smoking may increase the secretion of ADH, thus decreasing the effects of furosemide. Drug-to-drug interactions may occur with the simultaneous use of **nimodipine** and beta blockers, calcium-channel blockers, digoxin, disopyramide or phenytoin may result in bradycardia, conduction defects, or congestive heart failure (CHF). Additive hypotension may develop with the simultaneous use of fentanyl, antihypertensives, nitrates, alcohol, or quinidine. Cimetidine and valproic acid may increase nimodipine serum levels. Drug-to-food interaction is seen with the use of grapefruit juice, which increases the serum levels and effect. There are no clinically significant drug/herbal interactions established. Drug-to-drug interactions may occur with the simultaneous use of CNS depressants, such as alcohol, opioid analgesics, anesthetics, antidepressants, antihistamines, hypnotics, MAO inhibitors, phenothiazines, sedatives, aminoglycosides antibiotics, or anxiolytics because of increased sedation when used with **phenobarbital**. Phenobarbital inhibits the effectiveness of propranolol, corticosteroids, doxycycline, oral anticoagulants, oral contraceptives, quinidine, and theophylline (Gahart and Nazareno, 930). It may increase furosemide-induced hypotension and with extended use may inhibit vitamin D metabolism. If used concurrently with phenytoin, febamate, carbamazepine, and barbiturates, the drug levels of these agents should be closely monitored. There are no clinically significant drug-to-food interactions established. Drug-to-herbal interactions may occur with the simultaneous use of kava-kava, valerian, skullcap, chamomile, or hops, which can increase CNS depression, and St. John's Wort may decrease effects of phenobarbital. With **phenytoin sodium**, drug-to-drug interactions are numerous and may be life threatening. Phenytoin drug levels may increase with the simultaneous use of phenylbutazone, disulfiram, acute ingestion of alcohol, amiodarone, antihistamines, antidepressants, fluorouracil, paroxetine, myocardial depressants, sulfonamides, tacrolimus, valproic acid, isoniazid, chloramphenicol, influenza vaccine, sulfonamides, fluoxetine, benzodiazepines, omeprazole, itraconazole, ketoconazole, fluconazole, miconazole, estrogens, halothane, methylphenidate, phenothiazines, salicylates, tolbutamide, trazodone, felbamate, cimetidine, and others. Barbiturates, antineoplastics, antitubercular agents, leucovorin, carbamazepine, reserpine, theophylline, and others may decrease phenytoin blood levels. Phenytoin may alter the effects of felbamate, corticosteroids, doxycycline, rifampin, quinidine, methadone, cyclosporine, digoxin, diuretics, itraconazole, quetiapine, quinidine, ranitidine, estrogens, and others. Phenytoin, if used simultaneously with dopamine and all other sympathomimetic antihypertensive agents will result in severe hypotension and bradycardia. Calcium and sucralfate decrease phenytoin absorption, and additive cardiac depression may occur with propranolol or lidocaine. Phenytoin, when used with warfarin simultaneously, will increase the effects of warfarin in clients already stabilized on warfarin. Drug-to-food interactions may occur with the use of folic acid, which may decrease phenytoin absorption. The concurrent use of enteral tube feedings may decrease phenytoin absorption. There are no clinically significant drug-to-herbal interactions established. With **docusate sodium**, drug-to-drug interaction may occur with the simultaneous use of mineral oil; it increases systemic absorption of the mineral oil. There are no clinically significant drug-food/herbal interactions established.

12. **Discharge instructions for the client with post-craniotomy related to SAH secondary to cerebral aneurysm.**
The client should comply with discharge instructions such as follow-up care. The client should continue to take prescribed anti-hypertensive medications, which will lower and stabilize blood pressure, preventing recurrence of increase intracranial pressure and SAH. The client should avoid foods high in sodium because excess sodium intake causes the body to retain water and sodium. Retention of sodium and water will increase blood pressure, resulting in a continuous cycle of SAH, which can eventually be fatal. The client should avoid unnecessary stress, with the use of stress management strategies or biofeedback. These stress reduction measures can be discussed with the nurse or social worker, so referrals can be initiated. The client should report unusual types of headaches immediately to the primary health care provider, because headaches can be indicators of elevated blood pressure.

References

Black, J.M. and Hawks, J.H. (2005). *Medical-Surgical Nursing: Clinical Management for Positive Outcomes* (7th ed.). Philadelphia: W.B. Saunders.
Broyles, B.E. (2005). *Medical-Surgical Nursing Clinical Companion.* Durham, NC: Carolina Academic Press.
Gahart, B.L. and Nazareno, A.R. (2005). *2005 Intravenous Medications.* St. Louis: Mosby.
"Guidelines for the Management of Aneurysmal Subarachnoid Hemorrhage." (January 2005). Available at www.americanheart.org/presenter.
Ignatavicius, D.D. and Workman, M.L. (2006). *Medical-Surgical Nursing across the Health Care Continuum* (5th ed.). Philadelphia: W.B. Saunders.
Lehne, R.A. (2004). *Pharmacology for Nursing Care* (5th ed.). St. Louis: Mosby.
Libster, M. (2002). *Delmar's Integrative Herb Guide for Nurses.* Albany, NY: Thomson Delmar Learning.
Lilley, L.L., Harrington, S., and Synder, J.S. (2005). *Pharmacology and the Nursing Process* (4th ed.). St. Louis: Mosby.
Smeltzer, S.C. and Bare, B.G. (2004). *Textbook of Medical-Surgical Nursing* (10th ed.). Philadelphia: Lippincott Williams & Wilkins.
Spratto, G.R. and Woods, A.L. (2005). *2005 Edition: PDR Nurse's Drug Handbook.* Clifton Park, NY: Thomson Delmar Learning.
Whyte, J.J. and Winchell, B. (July 2004). "Diagnosing and Managing Headaches." *Continuing Medical Education* 119 (11): 1–34.

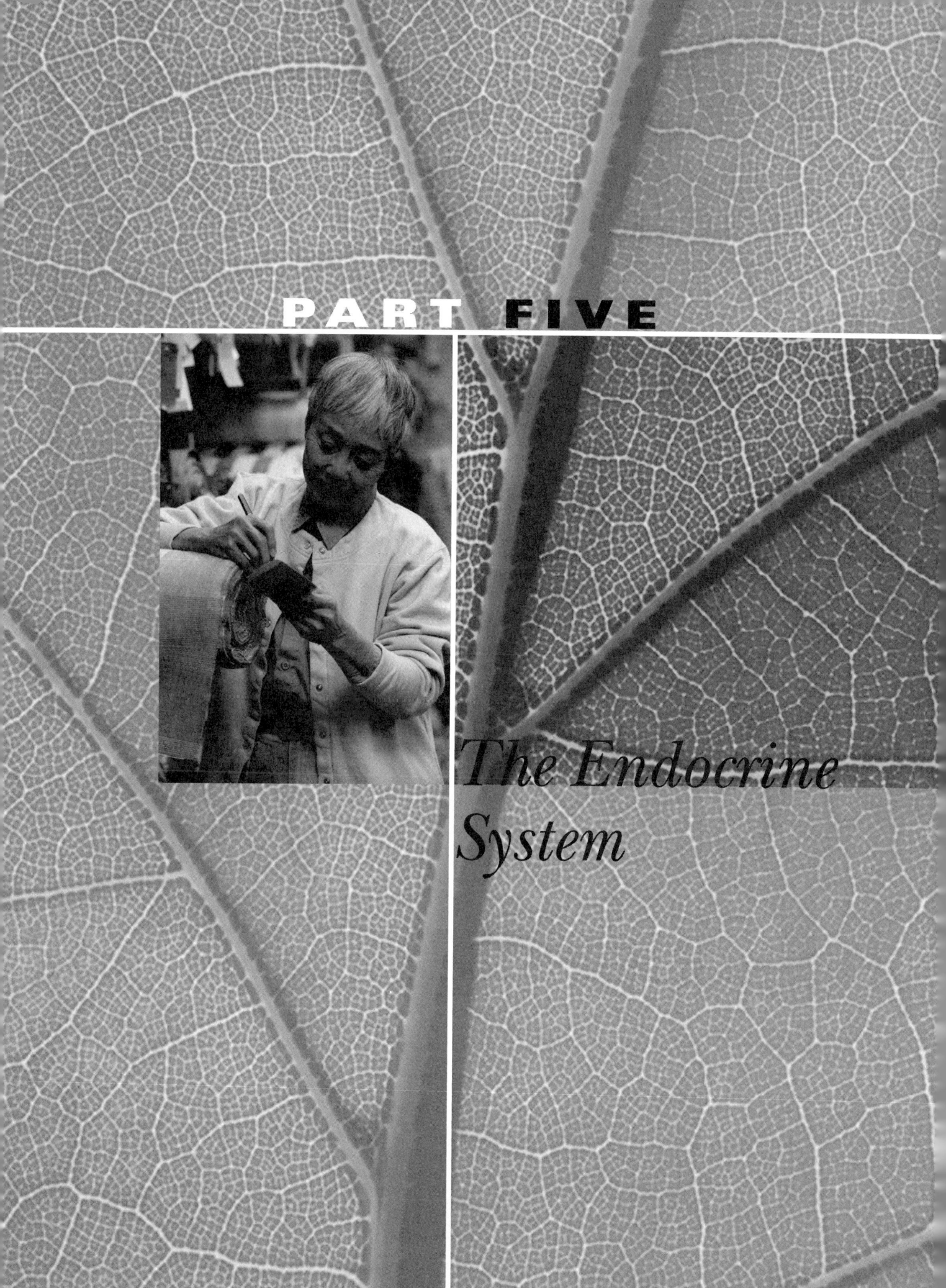

PART FIVE

The Endocrine System

CASE STUDY 1

Hyperthyroidism

GENDER
- F

AGE
- 30

SETTING
- Family health care provider's office

ETHNICITY/CULTURE
- Black American/West Indian descent

PREEXISTING CONDITIONS

COEXISTING CONDITIONS

LIFESTYLE
- Telephone installer, graduate student

COMMUNICATION
- English

DISABILITY

SOCIOECONOMIC STATUS
- Middle

SPIRITUAL/RELIGIOUS
- Believes in God

PHARMACOLOGIC
- Propylthiouracil (PTU)
- Propranolol HcL (Inderal)

PSYCHOSOCIAL
- Anxiety

LEGAL

ETHICAL

ALTERNATIVE THERAPY

PRIORITIZATION
- Avoid post-operative complication (thyroid storm)
- Maintain cardiac reserve

DELEGATION
- RN
- Client education

THE ENDOCRINE SYSTEM

Level of difficulty: Easy

Overview: This case involves thorough assessment of the client's condition including health history. Physical assessment should focus on testing muscle strength, vital signs, size of thyroid, and presence of bruits over the thyroid gland. The nurse must use critical thinking to prioritize care in a busy triage area in the event the client goes into thyroid crisis.

Client Profile

Ms. C is a 30-year-old female who is employed as a telephone installer for a major cable company. She is 5'7" with previous weight of 200 pounds. She is presently pursuing a masters degree in telecommunication. Ms. C lives with her parents, but reports that she pays rent for a one-bedroom apartment in her parent's home.

Case Study

Ms. C is seen at her family health care provider's office for follow-up review of observed patterns of behavior and changes in health status over the past month. On interview by the nurse, Ms. C reports unusual hunger, even after having a large meal. She has noted unusual weight loss that is not related to exercise or stress, diarrhea, and inability to tolerate normal heat that she would have not responded to in the past. On assessment, her vital signs are:

> Blood pressure: 150/92
> Pulse: 120
> Respirations: 22
> Temperature 101.6° F

She has visible tremors of the hands and her eyeballs are beginning to protrude. Current diagnostic studies reveal abnormal T_3, T_4, and TSH results.

> Serum calcium level: 11.2 mg/dL
> Red blood cell (RBC) count: 7/mm^3
> White blood cell (WBC) count: 4,000/mm^3
> Platelet count (PLT): 250,000 /mm^3
> Hematocrit (Hct): 34%
> Hemoglobin (Hgb): 14 g/100 mL

A thyroid scan with the use of radioactive tracers reveals an enlarged thyroid goiter with increased iodine uptake. Ms. C denies difficulty swallowing or pain upon swallowing. A diagnosis of hyperthyroidism is made by the health care provider, and is discussed with Ms. C, and the possibility for surgery is explained.

Questions and Suggested Answers

1. **Discuss the risk factors and pathophysiology of hyperthyroidism.** Hyperthyroidism may be due to overfunctioning of the entire thyroid gland or, less commonly, to a single or multiple functioning adenomas of thyroid cancer. Overtreatment of myxedema with thyroid hormones may also result in hyperthyroidism. The most common form of hyperthyroidism is Grave's disease (toxic, diffuse goiter), which has three principal hallmarks: hyperthyroidism, thyroid gland enlargement (goiter), and exopthalmus (abnormal protrusion of the eyes).

    Graves disease is an autoimmune disorder mediated by immunoglobulin G (IgG) antibody that binds to and activates TSH receptors on the surface of the thyroid cells. It is predominantly seen in women between the ages of 20 and 40 years, although 12% of the cases are found in men. Hyperthyroidism occurs because of loss of the normal regulatory controls of thyroid hormone (TH) secretion. Because the action of TH on the body is stimulatory, hypermetabolism results, with increased sympathetic nervous system activity. Excessive amounts of TH stimulate the cardiac system and increase the number of beta-adrenergic receptors, leading to tachycardia and increased cardiac output, stroke volume, adrenergic responses, and peripheral blood flow. Metabolism increases greatly, leading to a negative nitrogen balance, lipid depletion, and a state of nutritional deficiency and weight loss.

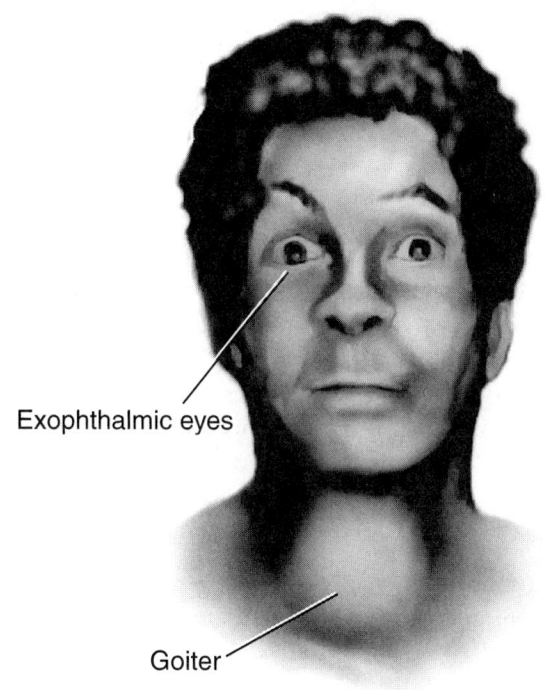

Hyperthyroidism

2. **Discuss clinical manifestations of hyperthyroidism.** Because of the excessive thyroid secretion, the client is extremely agitated and irritable, with hand tremor at rest. Despite a ravenous appetite, *weight loss* occurs as a result of the quickened metabolism. Because of the high levels of circulating TH, the body processes "speed up," resulting in loose bowel movements, *heat intolerance*, profuse diaphoresis (perspiration), tachycardia, and incoordination related to tremor. The skin is moist, warm, and smooth because of accelerated circulation to the tissues. The client's emotions may range from euphoria to extreme hyperactivity to delirium. There is fatigue due to the excessive hyperactivity and depression is also present. The ability to communicate effectively is altered which further worsens the emotional state. *Goiter* develops due to hyperplasia and hypertrophy of the thyroid cells, with the gland growing three to four times its normal size. The cellular growth results in the release of excessive amounts of TH into the blood. *Exopthalmus* is believed to be autoimmunity against retro-orbital tissues. The protruding eyes and a fixed stare caused by accumulation of fluid in the fat pads and muscles that lie behind the eyeballs. Because the eyes are surrounded by unyielding bone, edema forces them forward out of their sockets, producing the typical facies of exopthalmos.

3. **Discuss diagnostic findings of hyperthyroidism.** The two primary laboratory findings used to confirm the diagnosis of hyperthyroidism are decreased TSH levels and elevated free thyroxine (FT_4) levels. Total T_3 and T_4 may also be assessed, but they are not as useful in the confirmation of the disease. The radioactive iodine uptake (RAIU) test is indicated to differentiate Graves' disease from other forms of thyroid disorders.

4. **Discuss gerontologic considerations of hyperthyroidism.** Genetic considerations identify no specific gene or gene mutation as a cause of hyperthyroidism, but its high incidence among family members suggests a genetic component for risk. Gerontologic considerations require that elderly clients get periodic follow-up monitoring of serum TSH levels because poor compliance with therapy. If antithyroid agents are used in elderly clients, they must be monitored closely because elderly persons are more likely to develop granulocytopenia. The use of propranolol must be done with extreme caution in elderly persons to minimize adverse effects on cardiac function. Adverse effects may occur if clients take the medications erratically.

The following are prescribed:

- Weekly monitoring of WBC after initiation of PTU
- Propylthiouracil (PTU) 450 mg PO daily
- Strong iodine solution 4 drops three times per day × ten days
- Propranolol HcL (Inderal) 80 mg PO q6h

5. **What are the purposes for the prescribed orders?** *Weekly monitoring* of WBC count after the initiation of *propylthiouracil* is done because the drug causes agranulocytosis and the client's WBC count at present is only borderline normal. Agranulocytosis can predispose the client to infection, which would worsen the disease process. Propylthiouracil is an antithyroid agent that decreases the hyperthyroid state by inhibiting thyroid hormone synthesis by preventing the incorporation of iodine molecules into the amino acid tyrosine, a process required to make monoiodotyrosine and diiodotyrosine, the precursors of T_3 and T_4. *Strong iodine solution* decreases the thyroid state by blocking thyroid hormone production and release, and in doing so, prevents thyrotoxicosis. *Propranolol HcL* suppresses sinus tachycardia that usually occurs with hyperthyroidism due to increased sensitivity to catecholamines or to changes in neurotransmitter turnover. It does this by blocking beta$_1$-receptors, thereby preventing catecholamine-mediated stimulation to the heart.

6. **What are the most common adverse reactions, drug-to-drug, drug-to-food/herbal interactions of the prescribed medications?** The most common adverse reactions to *propylthiouracil* include hypothyroidism symptoms (bradycardia, constipation, fatigue, anorexia, weight gain, depression), agranulocytosis, aplastic anemia, nausea and vomiting, and rash. The most common adverse reactions to *strong iodine solution* are hypersensitivity reactions, diarrhea, and hypothyroidism. The most common adverse reactions to *propranolol HcL* are confusion, fatigue, drowsiness, bradycardia, and impotence. Drug-to-drug interactions may occur with the simultaneous use of propylthiouracil and amiodarone, potassium iodide and sodium iodide, ethionamide, isoniazid, rifampin, or nicotinic acid, which may alter the serum level of propylthiouracil. The simultaneous use with warfarin and heparin may increase anticoagulant effects. There are no clinically significant drug-to-food/herbal interactions established. With *strong iodine solution*, drug-to-drug interactions may occur with the simultaneous use of lithium, which may increase hypothyroidism effects, and the simultaneous use with methimazole, PTU, potassium-sparing diuretics, ACE inhibitors, angiotensin II receptor antagonists, or potassium supplements, which may increase serum potassium levels. There are no drug-to-food/herbal interactions clinically established. Drug-to-drug interactions may occur with the simultaneous use of propranolol HcL and albuterol, theophylline, atropine, beta-adrenergic bronchodilators, and nicotine from smoking may antagonize the effects of propranolol; phenobarbital and tricyclic depressants may increase side effects, ingestion of alcohol, nitrates, and diuretics may increase hypotensive effects. Use with rizatriptan decreases rizatriptan metabolism. Methimazole and propylthiouracil and methimazole may increase propranolol's effects and the simultaneous use of general anesthesia, IV phenytoin, and verapamil may cause additive myocardial depression. Additive bradycardia may occur with the concurrent use of digoxin. The simultaneous use of cimetidine may increase blood levels and toxicity. There are no clinically significant drug-to-food/herbal interactions established.

7. **Discuss complications of hyperthyroidism.** The three major complications of Graves' disease are exopthalmus, heart disease, and thyroid storm (thyroid crisis, thyrotoxicosis). *Exopthalmus* develops as a result of proptosis, lid retraction, muscle swelling, and tissue edema from prolonged hyperthyroid condition. The client may complain of a gritty sensation in the eye, photophobia, lacrimation, inflammatory changes, and *dyslogia* (difficulty in expressing ideas). Diuretics are usually prescribed to alleviate some of the periorbital edema. Prednisone, a glucocorticoid, may be prescribed to reduce the inflammation of the peri-orbital tissues. Methylcelluose eye drops, 14%, may be prescribed to help reduce irritation of the eyes. If the retro-orbital area is severely altered, radiation therapy may be implemented. Surgical decompression of the eyes is a last resort when all other measures fail in normalizing vision. *Heart disease* as seen with tachycardia and atrial fibrillation poses a serious threat to the client. Heart failure may also occur with older clients. The drug of choice used in stabilizing the dysrhythmias seen in hyperthyroidism is propranolol HcL (Inderal).

Propranolol works to reverse the dysrhythmias by depressing cardiac function including contractility and arrhythmias. When cardiac function is normally depressed, and the rate and rhythm is normalized, blood flow becomes normalized and clot formation is alleviated. ***Thyroid storm (Thyrotoxicosis)*** is a potentially fatal and acute episode of thyroid overactivity characterized by high fever, severe tachycardia, delirium, dehydration, and extreme irritability. Factors that may precipitate thyroid storm include underdiagnosed or untreated hyperthyroidism, infection, thyroid ablation, and metabolic dysfunction, surgery, trauma, myocardial infarction, pulmonary embolus, and medication overdose. Because thyroid storm is an emergency, nurses must be vigilant in monitoring for the signs of thyroid storm. The high fever is treated with hypothermia blankets; dehydration is managed with the use of intravenous fluid. However, the primary goal is to suppress thyroid hormone release, so as to inhibit hormone synthesis, and in doing so, inhibits the effects of TH on body tissues. Blockade of TH is usually achieved by oral administration of iodides, such as potassium iodide, and beta blockers are usually given to decrease the effects of sympathetic nervous system stimulation and to treat tachycardia.

8. **Discuss surgical management for hyperthyroidism.** Subtotal thyroidectomy involves removal of about five-sixths of the thyroid tissue, and total thyroidectomy is the removal of the entire thyroid tissue. However, surgeries are reserved for persons with large goiters, and known allergies to antithyroid agents. The client must be euthyroid (normalized thyroid hormones) before surgery. Antithyroid drugs are given to suppress secretion of thyroid hormones and iodide preparations are given to reduce the size and vascularity of the organs, which diminishes the chance of hemorrhage during and after surgery.

9. **Discuss relapse rate and risk for hyperthyroidism after treatment for thyroid storm.** None of the treatments for thyroid storm are without side effects, and all three forms of treatment (i.e., radioactive iodine therapy, antithyroid medications, and surgery) share the same complications: relapse or recurrent hyperthyroidism and permanent hypothyroidism. The relapse rate after radioactive iodine therapy is dependent on the dose used in treatment. Clients receiving a lower dose of radioactive iodine are more likely to require subsequent treatment than those being treated with a higher dose. Hypothyroidism occurs in almost 80% of clients at one year after treatment and 90–100% by five years for both the multiple low-dose and singly high-dose methods.

10. **Discuss client education for hyperthyroidism.** Regular exercise helps to stimulate the thyroid gland and should be done within tolerance. The client should avoid high environmental temperature, because high temperature inhibits thyroid regeneration. The client should have regular follow-up care with the heath care provider so that monitoring for the development of hypothyroidism can be ongoing. If total thyroidectomy is done, the client will need lifelong thyroid hormone replacement, and ongoing monitoring of thyroid hormone values. The client should be taught the signs and symptoms of progressive thyroid failure and instructed on the importance of seeking medical care if these signs or symptoms develop. Compliance with medication regimen should be stressed including reasons for the medications.

References

Broyles, B.E. (2005). *Medical-Surgical Nursing Clinical Companion.* Durham, NC: Carolina Academic Press.

Corbet, J.V. (2004). *Laboratory Tests and Diagnostic Procedures with Nursing Diagnoses* (6th ed.). Upper Saddle River, NJ: Prentice Hall.

Gahart, B.L. and Nazareno, A.R. (2005). *2005 Intravenous Medications.* St. Louis: Mosby.

Huether, S.E. and McCance, K.L. (2004). *Understanding Pathophysiology* (3rd ed.). St. Louis: Mosby.

Ignatavicius, D.D. and Workman, M.L. (2006). *Medical-Surgical Nursing across the Health Care Continuum* (5th ed.). Philadelphia: W.B. Saunders.

Lewis, S.M., Heitkemper, M.M., and Dirksen, S.R. (2004). *Medical-Surgical Nursing Assessment and Management of Clinical Problems* (5th ed.). St. Louis: Mosby.

Spratto, G.R. and Woods, A.L. (2005). *2005 Edition: PDR Nurse's Drug Handbook.* Clifton Park, NY: Thomson Delmar Learning.

CASE STUDY 2

Hypercortisolism (Cushing's Syndrome)

GENDER
- F

AGE
- 42

SETTING
- Hospital

ETHNICITY/CULTURE
- Native American/Argentina

PREEXISTING CONDITIONS
- Hypertension

COEXISTING CONDITIONS
- History of alcohol abuse

LIFESTYLE
- Self employed, Indian art antique shop

COMMUNICATION
- Spanish and English

DISABILITY

SOCIOECONOMIC STATUS
- Middle

SPIRITUAL/RELIGIOUS
- Roman Catholic

PHARMACOLOGIC
- Mitotane (Lysodren)

PSYCHOSOCIAL
- Emotional instability
- Irritability
- Depression

LEGAL
- Does the client have the right to bring charges against health care providers if necessary treatment is withheld?

ETHICAL
- Will the client have equitable access to essential health care benefits compared to clients with major medical health coverage?

ALTERNATIVE THERAPY
- Prayer

PRIORITIZATION
- Decrease cortisol levels
- Decrease blood glucose levels
- Provide safety

DELEGATION
- RN
- Client education

MODERATE

THE ENDOCRINE SYSTEM

Level of difficulty: Moderate

Overview: This case involves a thorough assessment of the client's condition, including questions related to recent onset of weakness, increase in weight or abdominal girth, bone pain or history of fractures, and history of frequent infections and easy bruising. It involves questioning the client about gastrointestinal (GI) discomfort and the use of steroid drugs and herbals. The nurse must use critical-thinking skills to prioritize care in the event of signs and symptoms indicating the development of adrenal crisis.

Client Profile

Mrs. V is a 42-year-old widow whose husband and only child, who was three years old, died in a motor vehicle accident three years ago, the day before Christmas. Prior to their deaths, Mrs. V and her husband of 12 years had wine as a social appetizer during meal times. Mrs. V is 5'4" and weighs 208 pounds.

Case Study

Mrs. V reports that since her husband's death, she has continued with the practice of having wine with her evening meals. However, she reports that as the years went by, she became lonely, missing her husband and child, especially at holidays, which led to an increase in the amount of wine consumed at meal times. The client reports social drinking with her friends who frequently visit her at the "shop" at which she worked as manager. The client's husband was a real estate broker for a progressive brokerage firm. Mrs. V finds out she had no health insurance when she goes to a community health center for elevated blood pressure and ongoing headaches. Her blood pressure at the time of arrival was 194/98 and she complained of nausea. A history is taken by a nurse practitioner (NP) at the clinic and Mrs. V is referred to the community hospital emergency department (ED), and transported from the clinic to the community hospital. On arrival at the ED, she informs the triage nurse that the headache is less severe in comparison to when she was at the clinic. Mrs. V believes the headache is directly related to her history of hypertension. The NP does the history and physical in the ED, during which time Mrs. V reports periods of emotional instability, with mood swings and depression. She informs the nurse that at times she is unusually irritable for no specific reasons, and experiences frequent urination, muscle weakness, and easy bruising. Physical assessment findings reveal hirsutism and a male pattern type balding of the head, abdominal striae, and dependent edema of the lower extremities. Mrs. V is admitted to a medical unit and will be seen by an endocrinologist for further evaluation. The primary nurse assigned to Mrs. V completes additional nursing history and assessment, after which Mrs. V is seen by an endocrinologist. The following tests are ordered: 24-hour urine for free cortisol and 17-hydroxycorticosteroids and 17-ketosteroids, plasma cortisol, ACTH level, erythro-sedimentation rate (ESR), white blood cell (WBC) count, lymphocyte count, sodium, potassium, and calcium, urine calcium, potassium, and glucose. A computed tomography (CT) of the adrenal gland is ordered, and a high-dose (8 mg) dexamethasone suppression test is ordered for the next day. The nurse instructs Mrs. V on how to collect the 24-hour urine and received verbal feedback that was positive. The results of the diagnostic studies reveal 24-hour urine for 17-hydroxycorticosteroids and 17-ketosteroids elevated (12 mg/24 h), and:

- Plasma cortisol: 30 ug/dL
- ACTH in AM: 100 pg/mL, and in PM: 75 pg/mL
- Erythro-sedimentation rate (ESR): elevated
- White blood cell (WBC) count: 12,000/mm^3
- Lymphocyte count: 700/mm^3
- Sodium (Na): 150 mEq/L
- Decrease potassium (K+): 2.8 mEq/L
- Calcium: 7 mg/dL
- Increase glucose: 140 mg/dL
- Urine calcium: 310 mg/24 h, elevated
- Urine potassium: 150 mEq/24 h
- Urine glucose: 300 mg/24 h

The high dose dexamethasone suppression test reveals reduction in plasma cortisol level less than 50% of the baseline, indicating positive finding for Cushing's syndrome. The CT scan reveals an inoperable adrenal tumor. An endocrinologist reviews the labs and diagnostic reports with the multidisciplinary team; a diagnosis of

Cushing's syndrome is confirmed. The multidisciplinary team discusses the plan of care with Mrs. V, and she agrees with the plan.

Questions and Suggested Answers

1. **Discuss the prevalence and pathophysiology of Cushing's syndrome.** The prevalence of Cushing's syndrome is rare, affecting 5–25 of every 1 million people annually. The gender incidence depends on the cause, with women ages 20–40 years having five times the incidence of men in developing pituitary adenomas. However, men are three times as likely to develop ectopic adrenocorticoid hormone (ACTH) syndrome, which results in Cushing's syndrome. Pituitary adenomas cause most cases of Cushing's syndrome. They are benign, but secrete increased amounts of ACTH. Oat-cell and small-cell lung tumors and long-term use of glucocorticoids also are responsible for some of the cases. All of these result in overproduction of endogenous corticosteroids by stimulating the adrenal cortex to increase its hormone secretion, although adequate amounts are being produced.

2. **Discuss clinical manifestations of Cushing's syndrome.** Central-type obesity with a fatty "buffalo hump" in the neck and supraclavicular areas, a heavy trunk, and thin extremities. The skin is thin and fragile, and easily traumatized. There is ecchymoses and deep striae. The client complains of weakness and disturbed sleep pattern due to altered diurnal secretion of cortisol. There is muscle wasting and osteoporosis, and "moon-faced" appearance. Distress and depression are common, and are increased by the severity of the physical changes that occur with the syndrome.

3. **Discuss assessment and diagnostic findings of Cushing's syndrome.** The 24-hour urinary free cortisol level is the most definitive diagnostic test. The client's urine is collected over a 24-hour period and tested for the amount of cortisol. Levels higher than 50–100 micrograms a day for an adult suggests Cushing's syndrome. Once Cushing's syndrome has been diagnosed, other tests are used to find the exact location of the abnormality that leads to the excess cortisol production. CT and magnetic resonance imaging are used to identify tumors. Serum potassium, sodium, calcium, and glucose levels add more confirmation to the diagnosis. An overnight dexamethasone suppression test is the most widely used screening test for diagnosing pituitary and adrenal causes of Cushing's syndrome. Radiography and bone density tests reveal the extent of bone involvement in the disease.

4. **Discuss common nursing diagnoses for Cushing's syndrome.**

   - Risk for injury R/T weakness secondary to excessive protein catabolism – The client needs a protective environment to prevent falls, fractures, and other injuries to bones and soft tissues. The client who is very weak may require assistance for ambulating to prevent falls or bumping into objects. Foods high in protein, calcium, and vitamin D are essential to minimize muscle wasting and osteoporosis. The client needs to be referred to a certified dietitian for the selection of the appropriate foods to consume while at home.
   - Risk for infection R/T altered protein metabolism and inflammatory response – The client should avoid others with infections. Health care providers directly assigned to the client should assess frequently for subtle signs of infection, because the anti-inflammatory effects of corticosteroids may mask the common signs of inflammation and infection. Health care providers and significant others who come in contact with the client during illness should maintain strict hand washing protocol.
   - Knowledge deficit R/T insufficient knowledge of the disease, processes, and management – The nurse should reinforce information given to the client by the health care provider or nurse practitioner, clarifying misconceptions. The nurse should emphasize the importance of avoiding all persons with infections due to the client's immune status. The client should be given clear explanation of the disease of the immune system, and the importance of adhering to client teaching during hospitalization and upon discharge.

5. **Discuss a potential complication of Cushing's syndrome.** A potential complication of Cushing's syndrome is Addisonian crisis. It is an acute, life threatening state of profound adrenocortical insufficiency, in which immediate therapy is required. It is characterized by glucocorticoid deficiency, a drop in extracellular fluid, hyperkalemia, and hyponatremia. Because of the acute state of the illness, intravenous isotonic solution of sodium chloride containing a water-soluble glucorticoid is administered rapidly. Vasopressor agents may be necessary to combat hypotension. If the client is vomiting, a nasogastric (NG) tube is inserted to prevent aspiration and relieve hyperemesis. If the condition is identified and treated promptly, the prognosis is good. Discharge instructions include a reminder to the client to seek medical attention in times of undue stress, to prevent recurrence of crisis. Because failure to comply with prescribed dosage of glucocorticoid, and exposure to infections are common causes of crisis, the client should be advised to adhere to these instructions at all times and to seek medical attention promptly in the event an infection develops.

The following is prescribed:

- Mitotane (Lysodren) 3 g PO three times per day

6. **What is the purpose for the prescribed medication?** *Mitotane* is an antineoplastic, adrenal cytoxic agent that is effective in suppressing cortisol production and lowering plasma and urine hormone levels. Its adrenal cytotoxic ability makes it effective in suppressing pituitary tumor and retarding the growth progress. Pharmacologic report cites that treatment with *mitotane* alone has proven successful in 30–40% of clients.

7. **What are the most common adverse reactions, drug-to-drug, drug-to-food/herbal interactions of the prescribed medications?** The most common adverse reactions of *mitotane* are anorexia, nausea, vomiting, diarrhea, hypouricemia, and hypercholesterolemia. Drug-to-drug interactions may occur with the simultaneous use of mitotane and alcohol containing medications. The simultaneous use with corticosteroids, phenytoin, phenobarbital, and warfarin may decrease the effectiveness of these agents, requiring increased dosages. There are no clinically significant drug-to-food/herbal interactions established.

8. **Discuss adrenalectomy for primary adrenal hypertrophy in Cushing's syndrome.** An adrenalectomy is the partial or total surgical resection of one or both adrenal glands. It is performed to reduce the excessive secretion of adrenal hormones caused by an adrenal tumor or a malignancy. A unilateral adrenalectomy is performed when one gland is involved. A bilateral adrenalectomy is needed when ectopic ACTH-producing tumors cannot be treated by other means, or when both glands are diseased. General anesthesia is used for surgery, and an incision is made under the twelfth rib in the rear flank area. Preoperatively, hemodynamic monitoring and steroid replacement are needed. Intraoperatively, careful positioning is necessary for this client because of the likelihood of osteoporosis, fragile bones, and muscle wasting. Postoperative care focuses on maintaining blood pressure with vasopressors or vasodilators as needed, giving replacement doses of corticosteroids and monitoring fluid and electrolyte status. When both glands are removed, the maintenance dose of steroids continues for life.

9. **Discuss management of adrenal insufficiency post adrenalectomy.** Corticosteroids are used extensively for adrenal insufficiency. Commonly used corticosteroids include hydrocortisone (Cortisol) and prednisone (Deltasone). High doses may be administered to help clients tolerate high degrees of stress. The anti-stress action of these medications is believed to be caused by the ability of corticosteroids to aid circulating vasopressor substances in keeping the blood pressure elevated, or the ability to maintain serum glucose levels. Corticosteroids are beneficial for their anti-inflammatory effects since the client with Cushing's syndrome is at high risk for infection. Cortisol can block the inflammatory process or even reverse many of its negative effects. Cortisol decreases both migration of WBCs into the inflamed area and phagocytosis of the damaged cells by diminishing the formation of prostaglandins and leukotrienes that would increase vasodilation, capillary permeability, and mobility of WBCs. It helps stabilize and improve the immune status by decreasing of the number of eosinophils and lymphocytes in the blood. It achieves these actions by causing atrophy of the lymphoid tissue throughout the body, which in turn decreases the output of both T cells and antibodies from the lymphoid tissue, which then decreases the level of immunity for almost all foreign invaders of the body.

10. **Discuss client education after bilateral adrenalectomy.** The client will need life-long replacement hormone. Medications must be taken as prescribed with meals or snacks to prevent gastrointestinal upset. The client should weigh daily, and report excess weight gain to the health care provider. The client must always wear a medical alert bracelet, and should make regular visits to the primary health care provider. The client should have prescribed hydrocortisone injections available, and should learn how to self-administer intramuscular injection in the event hydrocortisone injection is needed in an emergency.

References

Broyles, B.E. (2005). *Medical-Surgical Nursing Clinical Companion.* Durham, NC: Carolina Academic Press.

Corbet, J.V. (2004). *Laboratory Tests and Diagnostic Procedures with Nursing Diagnoses* (6th ed.). Upper Saddle River, NJ: Prentice Hall.

Gahart, B L. and Nazareno, A.R. (2005). *2005 Intravenous Medications.* St. Louis: Mosby.

Heitz, U. and Horne, M.M. (2005). *Mosby's Pocket Guide Series: Fluid, Electrolyte and Acid-Base Balance* (5th ed.). St. Louis: Mosby.

Huether, S.E. and McCance, K.L. (2004). *Understanding Pathophysiology* (3rd ed.). St. Louis: Mosby.

Ignatavicius, D.D. and Workman, M.L. (2006). *Medical-Surgical Nursing across the Health Care Continuum* (5th ed.). Philadelphia: W.B. Saunders.

Lehne, R.A. (2004). *Pharmacology for Nursing Care* (5th ed.). St. Louis: Mosby.

Lewis, S.M., Heitkemper, M.M., and Dirksen, S.R. (2004). *Medical-Surgical Nursing Assessment and Management of Clinical Problems* (5th ed.). St. Louis: Mosby.

Spratto, G.R. and Woods, A.L. (2005). *2005 Edition: PDR Nurse's Drug Handbook.* Clifton Park, NY: Thomson Delmar Learning.

CASE STUDY 3

Diabetes Mellitus Type 1

GENDER
- M

AGE
- 20

SETTING
- Hospital

ETHNICITY CULTURE
- Hispanic American

PREEXISTING CONDITIONS
- Viral infection

COEXISTING CONDITIONS
- Father and grandmother have history of diabetes

LIFESTYLE
- College student
- Basketball team member
- Lives with family

COMMUNICATION
- Spanish and English

DISABILITY

SOCIOECONOMIC STATUS
- Middle

SPIRITUAL/RELIGIOUS
- Evangelical

PHARMACOLOGIC
- Human regular (Novolin-R)
- Sodium bicarbonate
- Insulin aspart (NovoLog)

PSYCHOSOCIAL
- Anxiety
- Depression

LEGAL

ETHICAL

ALTERNATIVE THERAPY

PRIORITIZATION
- Assessment for signs and symptoms of pending complications
- Administering prescribed medications

DELEGATION
- RN
- LPN
- Client education

MODERATE

THE ENDOCRINE SYSTEM

Level of difficulty: Moderate

Overview: This case involves a thorough assessment of the presenting symptoms on arrival to triage, including all medications the client is currently taking. It involves critical thinking to appropriately delegate assignment to nurses highly competent in applying decision-making skills to clients requiring immediate medical and nursing interventions. The nurse must be capable of identifying pending signs of diabetic complications and able to collaborate with the team to prevent occurrences.

Client Profile

Mr. J is a 20-year-old college student with a history of diabetes mellitus type 1 for the past six years. Mr. J lives at home with his extended family. Mr. J's father and grandmother have a history of diabetes mellitus type 1. Mr. J is the only other member of the family diagnosed with the disease.

Case Study

Mr. J is a respiratory therapist major at a community college and is a member of the basketball team. Mr. J is brought to the emergency department (ED) by emergency medical services after Mr. J collapsed during basketball practice at the college. A member of the basketball team accompanies Mr. J in the ambulance. Mr. J is 6'3" and weighs 220 pounds. His family is notified by college authorities and arrives at the ED while Mr. J is being triaged. On arrival at the ED, he is responsive to verbal and tactile stimuli, is very diaphoretic, mildly lethargic, and is complaining of abdominal pain and nausea. He hyperventilates, manifesting acetone breath. Stat serum glucose, arterial blood gas (ABG), and serum electrolytes for sodium and potassium are done and reveal:

- Blood glucose: 450 mg/dL
- pH: 6.9
- pCO_2: 20 mm Hg
- HCO_3: 12 mEq/L
- Sodium (Na): 128 mEq/L
- Potassium (K+): 3.0 mEq/L

His vital signs on admission are:

- Blood pressure: 100/70
- Pulse: 88, rapid but regular
- Respirations: 22
- Temperature: 98.1°F

Mr. J is seen by the ED health care provider, and a diagnosis of diabetic ketoacidosis (DKA) is made. Mr. J is transferred to the medical intensive care unit (MICU).

Questions and Suggested Answers

1. **What are specific cultural considerations of diabetes mellitus?** Diabetes is a significant health problem for African Americans, Native Americans/American Indians, and Mexican Americans. The prevalence of diabetes varies with race and ethnicity, is slightly greater in women, and increases significantly with age. Each year approximately 1.3 million new cases are diagnosed, 95% of which are type 2 diabetes mellitus. The Pima Indians of Arizona have the highest rate of diabetes mellitus in the world: 50% of individuals 30–64 years of age.

2. **What is an extremely critical indicator of diabetes mellitus?** An extremely critical indicator of diabetes mellitus is body mass index (BMI). Among clients with diabetes, 68% have a BMI of at least 27 kg/m^2, and 46% have a BMI of at least 30 kg/m^3. The risk of diabetes increases dramatically as the degree of overweight increases.

3. **What are common nursing diagnoses for clients with diabetes?**
    - Ineffective health maintenance R/T exercise and increased need for insulin
    - Imbalanced nutrition: less than body requirements R/T exercise
    - Risk for injury R/T to hyperglycemia and disturbed sensory perception (visual)

- Risk for injury R/T sensory alterations (diabetic neuropathy)
- Chronic pain R/T peripheral nerve dysfunction (diabetic neuropathy)
- Deficient knowledge R/T condition, treatment, home care

4. **What is a primary collaborative problem for Mr. J because of the elevated blood glucose level on arrival to the ED?** The primary collaborative problem for Mr. J is potential for DKA. The reason this is a primary problem of concern is that hyperglycemia that is not effectively managed can progress to a serious complication such as DKA. DKA is a serious complication related to a deficiency of insulin and an increase in insulin counterregulatory hormones such as catecholamines, cortisol, glucagon, and growth hormone. DKA causes osmotic diuresis with loss of fluid and electrolytes which can further compound the symptom of hyperglycemia.

5. **What are the defining characteristics of DKA?** The defining characteristics of DKA are serum glucose greater than 300 mg/dL, osmolarity that varies, positive serum ketones, serum pH less than 7.35, serum HCO_3 <15 mEq/L, serum Na low, normal, or high, serum K normal, elevated with acidosis, low following dehydration, blood urea nitrogen greater than 20 mg/dL; elevated because of dehydration, creatinine greater than 1.5 mg/dL; elevated because of dehydration and urine ketones positive.

6. **What are the priorities of management for a client experiencing DKA?** The client experiencing DKA will be hyperglycemic. The priority intervention is to administer bolus of regular human insulin followed by regular human insulin in 0.9% sodium chloride. Human regular insulin is given bolus initially because it is quick-acting and therefore pulls the glucose back into the cells, stabilizing the serum glucose level. The 0.9% sodium chloride is the fluid of choice initially because osmotic diuresis is present due to the high glucose level. The sodium chloride role is to increase fluid volume and correct volume depletion. Because polyuria usually results in potassium loss, K+ therapy will be initiated. The client is placed on telemetry to monitor for dysrhythmias that may develop due to loss of fluid volume and K+. If acidosis is severe, sodium bicarbonate ($NaHCO_3$) is administered, but the health care provider must avoid early use of sodium bicarbonate, because early use can cause rebound metabolic alkalosis and severe hypokalemia, resulting in cardiac dysrhythmias. Monitoring of the glucose level is done during care and when the glucose levels approach 250 mg/dL, the insulin infusion should be reduced and 5% dextrose added to the infusion so that blood glucose can be maintained at about 250 mg/dL for the first 12–24 hours. A more rapid correction of hyperglycemia can lead to cerebral edema. Blood glucose levels should be monitored every one to two hours after reaching 250 mg/dL until the client is stable.

The following are prescribed:

- 0.9% NaCL at 1 liter per hour × two hours
- Human regular (Novolin-R) initial bolus 0.4 units/kg, followed by 2.4 u/hr continuous infusion
- Sodium bicarbonate ($NaHCO_3$) 5 mEq/kg infusion over four hours and low dose insulin at a continuous rate (five units per hour) at 25 mL per hour.
- Monitor serum glucose and potassium level; if stable, change infusion to 0.45% sodium chloride at 125 mL/hr
- Insulin aspart (NovoLog) insulin 100 U/mL inj four units and NPH ten units in combination SC three times per day, before meals

7. **What are the purposes for the prescribed orders?** *Isotonic solution (0.9% NaCl) infusion* is used to rapidly rehydrate the client due to diaphoresis, diuresis, and insensible fluid loss and to replace sodium loss, and prevent hypovolemic shock. ***Human regular insulin*** therapy is used to reverse the hyperglycemic state and prevent osmotic diuresis, which would worsen electrolyte imbalance. Regular insulin initial bolus 0.4 units/kg, followed by 2.4 u/hr continuous infusion is prescribed to quickly reduce glucose levels and then provide a basal rate for insulin to prevent to rapid a drop in the serum glucose resulting in hypoglycemia. ***Sodium bicarbonate*** therapy corrects metabolic acidosis, and the low-dose insulin inhibits fat breakdown, thereby stopping acid buildup. It is the systemic alkalinizing effect of sodium bicarbonate that effectively corrects metabolic

acidosis. ***Monitoring serum glucose levels*** is done to detect hyperglycemia and the need for insulin. Monitoring potassium levels is a major concern in DKA, because of the major loss of potassium from body stores, and the cellular shift of potassium that occurs in DKA. Serum potassium is also monitored because potassium levels usually decrease during the course of treatment for DKA. If left untreated, cardiac dysrhythmias could develop, resulting in other complications. ***Subcutaneous regular insulin*** given a half-hour before the infusion of regular insulin is completed is prescribed because regular insulin has a very short half-life. ***Combining insulin aspart and NPH insulin*** provides basal glycemic control between meals and during the night and, therefore, prevents episodes of hyperglycemia that could result in DKA.

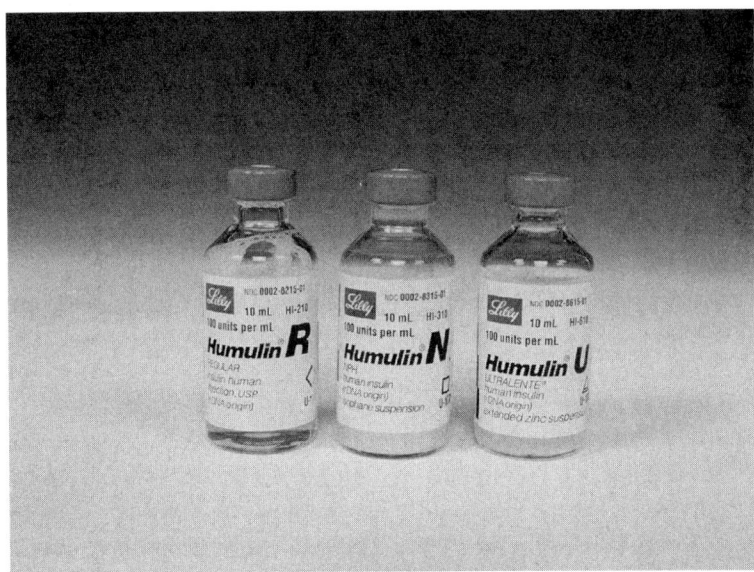

Human insulin

8. **What are the most common adverse reactions of the prescribed medications?** The most common adverse reactions of ***human regular insulin*** are hypoglycemia (profuse sweating, nausea, tremulousness, and palpitations). The most common adverse reaction to ***sodium bicarbonate infusion*** is metabolic alkalosis. The most significant common adverse reaction of ***insulin aspart*** is hypoglycemia. The most common adverse reactions and drug-to-drug interactions of ***isophane insulin*** are the same as with other insulins.

9. **Discuss the drug-to-drug and drug-to-food/herbal interactions for the prescribed medications.** With any type of ***insulin***, including ***aspart insulin, regular insulin,*** and ***isophane insulin***, drug-to-drug interactions may occur with the simultaneous use of alcohol, monoamine oxidase (MAO) inhibitors, angiotensin-converting enzyme (ACE) inhibitors, fluoxetine, octreatide, propoxyphene, sulfonamides, and salicylates that may potentiate hypoglycemic effects. The simultaneous use of danazol, dextrothyroxine, corticosteroids, somatropin, isoniazid, niacin, and epinephrine may antagonize hypoglycemic effects. Furosemide and thiazide diuretics may increase serum glucose levels, and propranolol and other beta blockers' simultaneous use with regular insulin may mask symptoms of hypoglycemic reaction. Drug-to-food/herbal interactions may occur with garlic and ginseng, which may potentiate hypoglycemic effects. Drug-to-drug interactions that may occur with the simultaneous use of ***sodium bicarbonate infusion*** and ketoconazole may result in a decrease of ketoconazole absorption. The simultaneous use of dextroamphetamine, ephedrine, pseudoepinephrine, and quinidine may decrease their elimination and increase toxicity. The simultaneous use of sodium bicarbonate with chlorpropamide, lithium, methotrexate, salicylates, and tetracyclines may increase the elimination, which may require an increase in dosage, but an increase in the dose will increase the risk of toxicity. Because sodium is incompatible with so many drugs, it should be infused without additives. There are no clinically significant drug-to-food/herbal interactions established.

10. **Explain the difference between Dawn phenomenon and Somagyi's phenomenon.** Dawn phenomenon results from a nighttime release of growth hormone that causes blood glucose elevations at about 5 to 6 AM. Dawn phenomenon is treated by providing more insulin for the overnight period (i.e., giving the evening dose of intermediate-acting insulin at 10 PM. Somagyi's phenomenon is morning hyperglycemia from the effective counterregulatory response to nighttime hypoglycemia. Somogyi phenomenon is prevented by ensuring adequate dietary intake at bedtime and evaluating the insulin dose and exercise programs to prevent conditions that lead to hypoglycemia. However, both phenomena are diagnosed by blood glucose monitoring during the night.

11. **What are the critical areas that should be included in client education for type 1 diabetes mellitus?** Insulin therapy is needed for type 1 diabetes, and there are many types of insulin and regimens, all aimed at achieving normal blood glucose levels. The client should be taught the importance of storing insulin, injection sites, rotating sites, injection depth, time of injection, dose preparation, standard syringes, mixing of insulin, and self blood glucose monitoring (SMBG). Further, the client should be provided with and encouraged to follow Centers for Disease Control and Prevention (CDC) guidelines for infection control during SMBG, emphasizing the importance of hand washing, and refraining from sharing the lancet to avoid spread of infection such as Hepatitis B. The principles of nutrition and how to use the American Diabetic Association guidelines should be addressed. Explain how the meal exchange system works and how to appropriately select foods for balanced meals. Clients with type 1 diabetes should consistently have three main meals and any between-meal or bedtime snacks, and should monitor blood glucose before and within one to two hours after meals. Special considerations for type 1 diabetes that should be stressed in education is that restricting calories may treat hyperglycemia better than increasing insulin. Special considerations for type 2 diabetes that should be stressed include weight loss of more than 10% of body weight can result in significant improvement in glycosylated hemoglobin (hemoglobin $A1_c$). Regular exercise is an essential part of the diabetic treatment plan. However, exercise in clients with uncontrolled diabetes causes further hyperglycemia and the formation of ketone bodies, and exercise also may cause hypoglycemia during exercise and up to 24 hours after exercise. Therefore, clients with type 1 and 2 diabetes mellitus should discuss exercise with their primary health care provider before starting an exercise program. Clients with diabetes should be taught how to manage hypoglycemia during exercise and the importance of daily foot care. Nurses should use monofilaments for testing of protective sensation on the sole of clients with diabetes. Clients should be taught about "sick day rules," management strategies that a client should use if sick, or has had surgery. In "sick day rules," blood glucose levels increase even though food intake decreases. "Sick day rules" include monitoring blood glucose at least four times a day throughout an illness. Urine for ketones is tested if blood glucose is greater than 240 mg/dL. The client continues to take the usual insulin dose prescribed. Sipping 8–12 ounces of fluid each hour, and substituting easily digested liquids or soft foods if solid foods are not tolerated are important components of the "sick day rules." The client should also call the health care provider if the client is unable to eat for more than 24 hours or if vomiting and diarrhea last for more than six hours. Stress the importance of notifying the health care provider immediately regarding persistent nausea and vomiting, moderate to large ketones, blood glucose elevation after two supplemental doses of insulin are administered, and temperature of 101.5°F or if increasing fever occurs for more than 24 hours. Teach the client with type 1 diabetes how to prevent DKA by reducing the risk of dehydration consistently, and to take liquids containing both glucose and electrolytes, such as Gatorade, if nausea is present. The client should be taught survival skills so as to understand what to eat, how much to eat and when to eat, and how to maintain food intake during illness. Clients with diabetes mellitus should be provided with information about resources.

12. **What are the nursing implications as they relate to diabetes mellitus?** If costs related to diabetes are to be reduced, attention must be directed to the prevention and treatment of chronic complications of diabetes. Therapies are available to reduce the incidence of blindness, medications are available to reduce the incidence of kidney and coronary artery disease, and regular sensory evaluation of the feet can reduce the incidence of amputation. The challenge for the nurse is to assist the diabetic client in achieving and maintaining

meticulous blood glucose control so that long-term complications are prevented. Long-term complications of clients with diabetes mellitus include hypertension, retinopathy, nephropathy, and neuropathy. Nursing care of clients with *hypertension* includes assessing *knowledge* of the disease and prescribed management. **Rationale** – Clients need to understand that hypertension is a chronic, lifelong disease in which they have a vital role in effective management. The family or significant others should be included in the *plan of care*. **Rationale** – When family or significant others are involved in the plan of care, they can effectively provide support designed in the treatment regimen. Family members may also need to be screened for hypertension because of its familial tendency. Teach clients and significant others how to accurately *measure blood pressure* at home, and inform them what constitutes a normal blood pressure. **Rationale** – Clients and significant others who have a sense of control over illness are more willing to effectively participate in the treatment regimen, and will more readily seek medical attention if blood pressure deviates from the normal. The degree of personal motivation is a prime factor in compliance with treatment regimen. Teach the risk factors of hypertension, and explain factors that can be modified, and stress the importance of working toward achieving and maintaining a normal balance. **Rationale** – Modifiable risk factors of hypertension include obesity, diet high in sodium, saturated fat and cholesterol, smoking, and stress. Studies have shown that *weight reduction* lowers blood pressure at all ages and in both genders. However, individualizing components of a weight loss program can increase initial and maintenance weight loss. Factors associated with maintenance of weight loss include continuation of regular exercise, which promotes circulatory health. However, to be beneficial, exercise should be done regularly and energetically. Establishing new eating habits and social support also helps with weight reduction. Maintaining a desirable lean weight is a continuing goal for clients with diabetes mellitus. A diet high in sodium contributes to fluid retention, which further increases blood volume and blood pressure. If blood pressure is sustained, heart disease, renal insufficiency, central nervous system dysfunction, impaired vision, impaired mobility, vascular occlusion, or edema can occur. A *diet low in sodium* will decrease fluid retention, and help to lower the blood pressure. Foods high in *saturated fats* and *cholesterol* should be avoided. **Rationale** – Saturated fats and cholesterol have been increasingly implicated in vascular disease, and as large risks in the development of atherosclerosis. Diabetes mellitus is a complex disease with a long-term complication of atherosclerosis. Continued increase in saturated fats and cholesterol will enhance this complication and increase the risk of coronary syndromes such as angina pectoris or myocardial infarction, because of the buildup of fatty plaques in the major arteries serving the heart muscle. *Smoking and stress* result in the development of hypertension. **Rationale** – They both potentiate the risk of hypertension or worsen current hypertensive problem, because both have potent vasoconstricting effects on arteries and veins. The constricting effects contribute to reduction in tissue oxygenation by reducing oxygen availability. To maximize client's success with smoking cessation and stress reduction, health care providers should have information about range of available options and support groups. There are two major forms of *diabetic retinopathy*: nonproliferative or background retinopathy and proliferative retinopathy. Nonproliferative retinopathy is the initial form, and proliferative retinopathy is marked by large areas of retinal ischemia and the formation of new blood vessels spreading over the inner surface of the retina and into the vitreous body. Nursing care focuses on questioning clients about the need to wear glasses for reading and distance, documenting and communicating all collected information to the health care provider or a nurse practitioner. However, the primary and significant nursing care is education. Clients should be taught the importance of regular eye examination, beginning five years after the onset of type 1 diabetes mellitus. Teach clients to promptly report any new visual manifestations, including blurred vision, black spots (floaters), or flashing lights in the visual fields. Emphasize that careful blood glucose control may help prevent diabetic retinopathy. **Rationale** – Questioning clients about the need to wear glasses for reading or distance vision will guide the nurse with effective management of care. Initial ophthalmology examination by a health care provider or nurse practitioner usually confirms the presence of diabetic retinopathy, which will guide appropriate treatment. Clients are instructed on the importance of careful blood glucose control, to help prevent or delay the process of retinopathy. Since much of the burden for the management of eye care falls on the client, good client teaching is the cornerstone to prevent vision loss related diabetes mellitus. Nursing care for clients with *diabetic nephropathy* is a critical component of care, because diabetic nephropathy is the single most common cause of end-stage renal disease (ESRD).

Primary nursing care focuses on the monitoring of urine to determine if albumin is present. ***Rationale*** – The first indication of diabetic nephropathy is abnormal level of albumin in the urine. Clients who are on antihypertensive medications should be taught the importance of strict adherence to prescribed medications. ***Rationale*** – Hypertension accelerates the progress of diabetic nephropathy; aggressive antihypertensive management should be maintained. Nursing care for clients with *diabetic neuropathy* involves understanding the various neuropathies and their effects on client's overall body systems. ***Rationale*** – Diabetic clients with polyneuropathies manifest bilateral sensory disorders, which appear first in the toes and feet and progress upward. Nursing will focus on eliciting from the client any change in sensation in the extremities such as numbness or tingling, pain described as aching, burning or shooting, and feelings of cold feet. The focus of nursing care after identification of these symptoms includes foot care and education to prevent trauma and ulcers. ***Rationale*** – Sensory neuropathy is a major factor in injuries to the legs.

References

Broyles, B.E. (2005). *Medical-Surgical Nursing Clinical Companion.* Durham, NC: Carolina Academic Press.

Corbet, J.V. (2004). *Laboratory Tests and Diagnostic Procedures with Nursing Diagnoses* (6th ed.). Upper Saddle River, NJ: Prentice Hall.

Gahart, B.L. and Nazareno, A.R. (2005). *2005 Intravenous Medications.* St. Louis: Mosby.

Huether, S.E. and McCance, K.L. (2004). *Understanding Pathophysiology* (3rd ed.). St. Louis: Mosby.

Ignatavicius, D.D. and Workman, M.L. (2006). *Medical-Surgical Nursing across the Health Care Continuum* (5th ed.). Philadelphia: W.B. Saunders.

Smeltzer, S.C. and Bare, B.G. (2004). *Texbook of Medical-Surgical Nursing* (10th ed.). Philadelphia: Lippincott Williams & Wilkins.

Spratto, G.R. and Woods, A.L. (2005). *2005 Edition: PDR Nurse's Drug Handbook.* Clifton Park, NY: Thomson Delmar Learning.

CASE STUDY 4

Addison's Disease (Acute-Primary Hypocortisolism)

GENDER
- F

AGE
- 50

SETTING
- Hospital

ETHNICITY/CULTURE
- White American

PREEXISTING CONDITIONS
- History of pulmonary TB

COEXISTING CONDITIONS
- Pernicious anemia

LIFESTYLE
- Clothing designer

COMMUNICATION

DISABILITY

SOCIOECONOMIC STATUS
- Middle

SPIRITUAL/RELIGIOUS
- Methodist

PHARMACOLOGIC
- Hydrocortisone (Hydrocortone)
- Fludrocortisone acetate (Florinef)

PSYCHOSOCIAL
- Depression

LEGAL

ETHICAL

ALTERNATIVE THERAPY
- Vegetarian

PRIORITIZATION
- Prevent Addisonian Crisis
- Maintain safety

DELEGATION
- RN
- Client education

MODERATE

THE ENDOCRINE SYSTEM

Level of difficulty: Moderate

Overview: This case involves a thorough assessment of the client's condition, including current medications and dietary regimen. It involves prioritization in a triage situation at a busy hospital emergency department (ED) to avoid Ms. X developing Addisonian Crisis.

Client Profile

Ms. X is a 50-year-old client who is seen in a hospital's outpatient clinic as follow-up to her primary health care provider's referral for diagnostic tests to rule out diagnosis of Addison's disease. During an interview by a registered nurse (RN), she reveals past history of pulmonary tuberculosis and fungal lesions of the skin. She reports currently taking oral vitamin B_{12} for history of pernicious anemia. On further collection of data, Ms. X reports weakness, fatigue, anorexia, nausea, vomiting, and weight loss during the past month. Ms. X visited her primary health care provider a month ago because of dizziness and weakness, when rising from bed in the mornings or when standing from a sitting position for an extended period of time. Initial vital signs on arrival to the clinic are:

Blood pressure: 90/64
Pulse: 126
Respirations: 14
Temperature: 98.9°F

Case Study

Physical assessment of Ms. X reveals hyperpigmentation of the hands and lower extremities. Ms. X is later seen by a physician assistant (PA) who completes the history and physical, and informs Ms. X she will be admitted to the hospital for short-term stay. Serum cortisol, fasting blood glucose, sodium, potassium, blood urea nitrogen (BUN), adrenocortical thyroid hormone (ACTH), and eosinophil count are sent to the lab. The results are:

Serum cortisol: 12 ug/dL
Fasting blood glucose: 50 mg/100 mL
Sodium (Na): 128 mEq/L
Potassium (K+): 6 mEq/dL
Blood urea nitrogen (BUN): 26 mg/100 mL

The ACTH stimulation test reveals 100 pg/mL at 6 to 8 AM (after the patient followed a low-carbohydrate diet for 48 hours and fasted from foods for 12 hours before the test). A computed tomography (CT) with contrast reveals beginning atrophy of the adrenal gland, and magnetic resonance imaging (MRI) is negative for tumors or infections. Urinary 17-hydroxycorticosteroids and 17-ketosteroid levels urinary free cortisol are explained to Ms. X and the procedures are appropriately completed. The result reveals low normal levels. After laboratory data and diagnostic tests are reviewed by an endocrinologist and a medical and nursing staff, the diagnosis of Addison's disease is confirmed. The findings, confirmation of the disease, and treatment plan are discussed with Ms. X.

Questions and Suggested Answers

1. **Discuss the incidence, prevalence, and pathophysiology of Addison's disease.** Addison's disease is rare, occurring in one out of every 100,000 persons in the United States. It affects all age groups and both sexes. It can occur at any age, although it is more common in adults under the age of 60, and is more common in women. The pathophysiology results as adrenocorticoid destruction initiates a decrease in adrenal glucocorticoid reserve, basal glucorticoid secretion is normal, and does not increase in response to stress and surgery. However, as the destruction of the adrenal cortex continues, even basal secretion of glucocorticoids and mineralocorticoids is deficient. There is decreasing plasma cortisol, which reduces the feedback inhibition of pituitary ACTH and plasma ACTH rises.

2. **Discuss risk factors of Addison's disease.** Autoimmune destruction of the adrenal glands is the most common cause, because the adrenal glands secrete glucocorticoid (cortisol, hydrocortisone), resulting in their

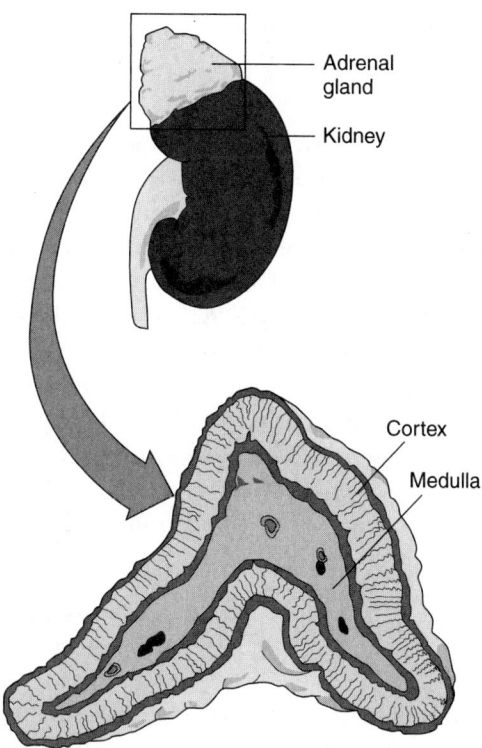

The adrenal or suprarenal glands are found on top of each kidney

deficiency. Addison's disease may also occur due to pituitary tumors, tuberculosis, or acquired immunodeficiency syndrome (AIDS), in which the pathogens have infiltrated and destroyed the adrenal gland.

3. **Discuss clinical manifestations of Addison's disease.** Hyponatremia and hyperkalemia occur because the deficiency of aldosterone affects the ability of the distal tubules of the nephron to conserve sodium. Therefore, sodium is lost and potassium is retained. There is depletion of extracellular volume and blood volume is decreased because of the alteration in sodium concentration, resulting in postural hypotension, dizziness, confusion, neuromuscular irritability, tachycardia, and dysrhythmias. There is hypoglycemia due to deficiency in cortisol resulting in hepatic glyconeogenesis, There is increased hyperpigmentation in about 90% of clients with Addison's disease due to increased levels of ACTH that stimulates the occurrence of hyperpigmentation.

4. **Discuss nursing diagnoses for Addison's disease.**

   - Fluid volume deficit R/T sodium wasting by the kidneys – Interventions involve monitoring of intake and output, vital signs, and daily weights, as well as assessing of skin turgor and mucous membranes to determine hydration status, and to implement changes to prevent complications. Monitoring the client for signs of hypovolemia, hypoglycemia, and hyponatremia, documenting and reporting alterations.
   - Risk for injury R/T weakness and fatigue, secondary to cortisol deficiency – Interventions involve assessment of gait and balance, and maintainance of safety. Administering glucocorticoids or mineralocorticoids as prescribed, and evaluating the effectiveness, reporting outcomes as appropriate. Monitoring for signs of Addisonian crisis, preparing for appropriate interventions.
   - Knowledge deficit R/T condition, treatment, and health maintenance – The client should be provided with information on normal adrenal functioning, the causes, signs, and complications of the disease, emphasizing the importance of reporting them promptly.

5. **Discuss diagnostic findings of Addison's disease.** The diagnosis of Addison's disease is confirmed by laboratory test results. These include low levels of adrenocortical hormones in the blood or urine, decreased serum

cortisol level, decreased blood glucose, serum sodium, increased serum potassium, and white blood cell (WBC) count. If the adrenal cortex is destroyed, urinary 17-hydroxycorticosteroids and 17-ketosteroids (17-KS) are decreased.

6. **Discuss urinary 17-hydroxycorticosteroids.** All glucocorticoids are degraded by the liver to metabolites, which as a group are called 17-hydroxycorticosterioids (17-OCHS). These steroid metabolities also are called Porter-Silber chromogens because of the method used to measure them in urine. Because 80% of urinary 17-OHCS are metabolities of cortisol, those disorders that are associated with elevated cortisol levels also associated with elevated 17-OCHS. Excessive exercise and stressful situations during the testing period may falsely elevate levels. Blood in the specimen may alter test results, therefore, the test should be postponed if the female client is menstruating. The test is performed with the use of a 24-hour urine sample. Medications that may interfere with the test should be temporarily discontinued. The client will initially urinate on arising in the morning, and afterward, collect all urine in a special container for the next 24 hours. The container is to be capped after each specimen is poured into the container, and placed in a refrigerator or a cool place during the collection period. Upon 24-hour completion, the container is labeled with the client's name, date, time of completion, and returned to the lab as instructed.

   The following are prescribed:

   - Hydrocortisone (Cortisol) 30 mg IV three times per day
   - Fludrocortisone acetate (Florinef) 0.1 mg PO daily

7. **What are the purposes for the prescribed medications?** *Hydrocortisone* is an adrenocorticoid, glucocorticoid hormone that corrects glucocorticoid deficiency. It does this by stimulating gluconeogenesis, and promotes glucose storage. *Fludrocortisone* is a mineralocorticoid prescribed to correct and maintain electrolyte balance, especially sodium and potassium. It does this by working on the distal renal tubule to promote sodium resorption from the nephron into the blood. When this activity occurs, it pulls sodium along with and increases the serum sodium level.

8. **What are the most common adverse reactions, drug-to-drug and drug-to-food/herbal interactions for the prescribed medications?** The most common adverse reactions of **hydrocortisone** are depression, euphoria, hypertension, anorexia, nausea, sodium and fluid retention, immunosuppression, peptic ulcer, acne, decreased wound healing, ecchymosis, fragility, hirsutism, petechiae, adrenal suppression, muscle wasting, osteoporosis, and cushingoid appearance. Drug-to-drug interactions may occur with the simultaneous use of alcohol, barbiturates, phenytoin, and rifampin, which may increase hepatic metabolism, and decrease cortisone levels, The simultaneous use with cholestyramine and colestipol decreases hydrocortisone absorption and the simultaneous use of amphotericin B or potassium-depleting diuretics exacerbates hypokalemia which increases the risk of digoxin toxicity. Concurrent use with anticholinesterases, isoniazid, salicylates, and somatrem may antagonize the effects of these agents, requiring dose adjustments. It may potentiate or inhibit the actions of anticoagulants, nondepolarizing muscle relaxants, or theophyllines. Use with ritodrine may increase pulmonary edema and simultaneous use with neostigmine may produce severe weakness. The use of grapefruit may increase the serum levels. There are no clinically established drug-to-herbal interactions established. The most common adverse reactions of *fludrocortisone acetate* are sodium and fluid retention, nausea, acne, and impaired wound healing. Drug-to-drug interactions may occur with the simultaneous use of insulin and sulfonylureas, which may diminish the effects of both of them, resulting in risk for hyperglycemia. The simultaneous use of amphotericin B, piperacillin, mezlocillin, and diuretics may increase potassium loss, and use with warfarin may decrease prothrombin time. Simultaneous use of fludrocortisone acetate with rifampin, barbiturates, and phenytoin may increase hepatic metabolism of fludrocortisone acetate, resulting in decreased action of this agent. The simultaneous use of indomethacin and ibuprofen may potentiate the pressor effect of fludrocortisone acetate. If used concurrently with aloe, buckthorn, cascara sagrada, or senna, there is an increased risk of potassium deficiency.

9. **Discuss management of hyponatremia and hyperkalemia found in Addison's disease.** Several factors can cause hyponatremia, but in Addison's disease hyponatremia results from decreased secretion of the hormone aldosterone, that impairs the ability of the kidneys to reabsorb sodium. The key to managing hyponatremia is assessment that includes the rate at which hyponatremia is occurring, instead of the patient's actual serum sodium value. After the primary cause is determined, and clinical manifestations are identified and categorized, careful administration of sodium either by mouth, nasogastric tube, or the parenteral route is implemented. If the client cannot consume sodium orally, lactated Ringer's solution or iso-tonic saline (0.9% sodium chloride) solution may be prescribed. However, serum sodium must not be increased by greater than 12 mEq/L in 24 hours, to avoid neurologic damage due to osmotic demyelination (destruction or removal of the myelin sheath of nerve tissue). Demyelination may occur when the serum sodium concentration is overcorrected (above 140 mEq/L) too rapidly. Administer hydrocortisone and fludrocortisone as prescribed, and evaluate and document effectiveness of prescriptions. Hyperkalemia is often due to iatrogenic (treatment-induced) causes, and is usually more dangerous than hypokalemia because cardiac arrest is more frequently associated with high serum potassium levels. As the plasma potassium level rises, disturbances in cardiac conduction occur, with the earliest changes often occurring at a serum potassium level greater than 6 mEq/L, are peaked, narrow T waves; ST segment depression; and a shortened QT interval, therefore, an immediate electrocardiogram (EKG) should be obtained, and the patient placed on telemetry. If the serum potassium levels are dangerously elevated, it may be necessary to administer intravenous calcium gluconate. Calcium antagonizes the action of hyperkalemia on the heart, does not reduce the serum potassium concentration, but immediately antagonizes the adverse cardiac conduction abnormalities. The client's blood pressure should be monitored to detect hypotension, which may result from rapid IV administration of calcium gluconate. The EKG should be continuously monitored during administration, because the appearance of bradycardia is an indication to stop the infusion. The administration of regular insulin and hypertonic dextrose solution causes a temporary shift of potassium into the cells, resulting in decrease in the potassium level.

10. **Discuss client education for Addison's disease.** Provide the client with verbal and written instructions on medication therapy, and the importance of contacting the health care provider with questions as needed. Emphasize the importance of seeking medical attention for the development of infections, vomiting, diarrhea, or fever. Stress the importance of frequent hand washing to decrease the risk of bacterial and viral infections. Stress the importance of always wearing a Medic Alert bracelet or carrying identification indicating name, medical problems, prescribed medications, and phone number. Stress the importance of complying with follow-up care.

References

Broyles, B.E. (2005). *Medical-Surgical Nursing Clinical Companion.* Durham, NC: Carolina Academic Press.

Corbet, J.V. (2004). *Laboratory Tests and Diagnostic Procedures with Nursing Diagnoses* (6th ed.). Upper Saddle River, NJ: Prentice Hall.

Gahart, B.L. and Nazareno, A.R. (2005). *2005 Intravenous Medications.* St. Louis: Mosby.

Heitz, U. and Horne, M.M. (2005). *Mosby's Pocket Guide Series: Fluid, Electrolyte and Acid-Base Balance* (5th ed.). St. Louis: Mosby.

Huether, S.E. and McCance, K.L. (2004). *Understanding Pathophysiology* (3rd ed.). St. Louis: Mosby.

Ignatavicius, D.D. and Workman, M.L. (2006). *Medical-Surgical Nursing across the Health Care Continuum* (5th ed.). Philadelphia: W.B. Saunders.

Spratto, G.R. and Woods, A.L. (2005). *2005 Edition: PDR Nurse's Drug Handbook.* Clifton Park, NY: Thomson Delmar Learning.

CASE STUDY 5

Pheochromocytoma

GENDER
- F

AGE
- 56

SETTING
- Health care provider's office

ETHNICITY/CULTURE
- Black American, West Indian descent

PREEXISTING CONDITIONS
- History of cigarette smoking

COEXISTING CONDITIONS
- Hypertension

LIFESTYLE
- RN

COMMUNICATION

DISABILITY

SOCIOECONOMIC STATUS
- Middle

SPIRITUAL/RELIGIOUS
- Nondenominational

PHARMACOLOGIC
- Furosemide (Lasix)
- Acetaminophen (Tylenol)
- Propranolol HcL (Inderal)
- Prazosin HcL (Minipress)

PSYCHOSOCIAL
- Anxiety

LEGAL

ETHICAL

ALTERNATIVE THERAPY

PRIORITIZATION
- Decrease release of epinephrine and norepinephrine
- Stabilize blood pressure

DELEGATION
- RN
- Client education

MODERATE

THE ENDOCRINE SYSTEM

Level of difficulty: Moderate

Overview: This case involves a thorough assessment of the client's condition, including all current medications she is taking. It involves history and physical examination to gather appropriate data to aid in confirming a diagnosis. The nurse must use critical-thinking skills to prioritize care in the event hypertensive crisis develops.

Client Profile

Ms. P is a 56-year-old female who is seen at her primary health care provider's office after experiencing severe headaches. The nurse at the health care provider's office initiates the initial interview. Ms. P's vital signs are:

- Blood pressure: 250/110
- Pulse: 114, rapid and regular
- Respirations: 20
- Temperature: 98.4° F

An electrocardiogram (EKG) is ordered and reveals sinus tachycardia. Ms. P denies other medical problems but admits to years of cigarette smoking, which she stopped 15 years ago. Ms. P reports wearing glasses for distance reading but denies blurred vision. Medication history reveals furosemide (Lasix) 50 mg PO daily, amlodipine (Norvasc) 10 mg PO daily, propranolol HcL (Inderal) 40 mg PO two times per day, and acetaminophen (Tylenol) 650 mg PO PRN headache. She reports occasional constipation and uses increased roughage in the diet, which helps ease defecation. Her parents and siblings are alive and well. Ms. P is referred to the community hospital emergency department (ED) because of the elevated blood pressure.

Case Study

On arrival at the ED, Ms. P's vital signs are:

- Blood pressure: 250/100
- Pulse: 120, rapid and regular
- Respirations: 18
- Temperature: 98.4° F

She is transferred to a telemetry unit and is seen by a physician assistant (PA), who completes a history and physical while avoiding vigorous abdominal palpation. Ms. P is transferred to a medical unit and the following order prescribed: nitroprusside sodium (Nitropress) 0.5 mg/kg per minute stat via infusion pump. Serum lab tests ordered are: sodium (Na), potassium (K+), glucose and urine glucose, 24-hour urine collections for vanillylmandelic acid (VMA), computed tomography (CT) scan of the adrenal gland, and abdominal imaging techniques. The results of the serum labs reveal:

- Sodium (Na): 145 mEq/L
- Potassium (K+): 4 mEq/L
- Glucose: 130 mg/dL
- Positive glucosuria

The 24-hour urine collections result reveal slight elevation in metanephrine and catecholamines, the CT scan identifies an adrenomedullary tumor on the left adrenal gland, measuring 0.5 cm, but abdominal imaging techniques are negative for metastasis of the tumor. An endocrinology consult is ordered for a team conference to determine surgical interventions. After the health care provider reviews the current labs and diagnostic findings, a diagnosis of pheochromocytoma is made. The health care team decides to begin treatment of the presenting symptoms while waiting for the endocrinology consult. The treatment plans are discussed with Ms. P Her blood pressure is currently 130/80, and her pulse is 102 and regular. She denies headache at this time. The registered dietitian discusses the dietary plan of care with Ms. P. The endocrinologist reviews the collected data, and determines that Ms. P can be monitored on an outpatient basis, and orders repeat CT scan and abdominal X-rays for three months from today's date. Ms. P will be discharged to home within 24 hours and will have follow-up visits with her primary health care provider.

Questions and Suggested Answers

1. **Discuss the incidence, prevalence, risk factors, and pathophysiology of pheochromocytoma.** Pheochromocytomas are rare. They may occur at any age, but peak incidence is between ages 40 and 50 years. They affect men and women equally. Because of the high incidence of pheochromocytomas in family members, the client's family members should be alerted and screened for this tumor. Fewer than 10% of the tumors are malignant. Risk factors include smoking, drugs that may increase catecholamine release, such as histamines, some anesthetics (such as halothane), atropine, and opiates of steroids. The pathophysiology of the tumor involves hypersecretion of catecholamines into the circulatory system, which trigger a paroxysm related to excesses of those hormones. There is intense a-receptor-mediated peripheral vasoconstriction, causing cool, moist hands and feet, and facial pallor. There is marked elevation of systolic and diastolic blood pressures when the catecholamines are released, and tachycardia results from epinephrine hypersecretion.

2. **Discuss clinical manifestations of pheochromocytoma.** Hypertension is a major manifestation, and headache is reported in 80–90% of the complaints. However, the typical triad of symptoms comprises headache, diaphoresis, and palpitations. The causes of hypertension experienced by the client with pheochromocytoma should be accurately determined since the treatment for pheochromocytoma-induced hypertension is managed with specific classifications of drugs. Blood pressures may be extremely elevated, such that they are life threatening and may cause severe complications, such as cardiac dysrhythmias, dissecting aneurysm, stroke, and acute renal failure. Hyperglycemia may result from conversion of liver and muscle glycogen to glucose by epinephrine secretion, requiring insulin to maintain normal blood glucose levels.

3. **Discuss assessment and diagnostic findings of pheochromocytoma.** If the "five Hs" (hypertension, headache, hyperhidrosis [excessive sweating], hypermetabolism, and hyperglycemia) occur with sympathetic nervous system overactivity, pheochromocytoma is suspected, because their presence has high specificity and sensitivity for the tumor, but absence of hypertension excludes the diagnosis. A 24-hour urine specimen is collected for determining free catecholamines such as metanephrines (MN) and VMA. The tests are combined so as to increase the accuracy of the diagnosis. If these tests are inconclusive, a clonidine suppression test is usually performed. Total plasma catecholamine (epinephrine and norepinephrine) concentration is measured with the client supine and at rest for 30 minutes. Normal plasma values of epinephrine are 100 pg/mL; normal values of norepinephrine are generally less than 100–550 pg/mL. Values of epinephrine greater than 400 pg/mL or norepinephrine values greater than 2,000 pg/mL are considered diagnostic for pheochromocytoma. If the results of the plasma and urine tests of catecholamines are inconclusive, a clonidine suppression test may be performed. If the release of catecholamines is not suppressed, the diagnosis of pheochromocytoma is indicated. Imaging studies such as CT scan, magnetic resonance imaging (MRI) and ultrasound may be done to localize the tumor and to determine whether more than one tumor is present. The neurologist may order ^{131}I-metaiodobenzylguanidine (MIBG) scintigraphy to determine the location of the tumor and to identify chromaffin tissue throughout the adrenal gland.

4. **Discuss nursing diagnoses to pheochromocytoma.**

   - High risk for injury R/T altered cardiovascular, renal, or cerebral perfusion caused by hypertension – Nursing interventions will focus on placing the client on continuous telemetry, assessing for signs and symptoms related to angina, congestive heart failure, and dysrhythmias, reporting and documenting appropriately. Administering medications as prescribed, and evaluating their effectiveness or need for modification of prescribed dosage. Evaluating the client's neurologic status and maintaining a quiet environment.
   - Pain R/T headache – Nursing interventions will focus on pain assessment and management. Administering of analgesic as prescribed, and monitoring blood pressure to determine the cause of the headache.
   - Knowledge deficit R/T condition, treatment, and health maintenance – Nursing care will include informing client of the status or progress of the problem, and prescribed care and benefits. Inform the client

about the need for periodic follow-up appointments to observe for return of normal blood pressure and plasma and urine levels of catecholamines.

The following are prescribed:

- Prazosin HcL (Minipress) 1 mg PO daily with gradual increase to 6 mg PO daily
- Propranolol HcL (Inderal) 40 mg PO two times per day
- Furosemide (Lasix) 50 mg PO daily
- Acetaminophen (Tylenol) 650 mg PO PRN headache

5. **What are the purposes for the prescribed orders?** *Prazosin HcL* is an alpha-adrenergic blocking agent that lowers blood pressure by permanently binding to alpha-1-adrenergic receptors resulting in a decreased response to stimulation of the sympathetic nervous system. Adrenergic blockade at the alpha-adrenergic receptors leads to vasodilation, reduction of peripheral vascular resistance, resulting in decreased blood pressure. *Propranolol HcL* is a beta-adrenergic blocking agent that lowers supine and standing blood pressures but is prescribed for Ms. P to reduce and stabilize her heart rate. It reduces and stabilizes heart rate by blocking cardiac effects of beta-adrenergic stimulation, which reduces the force of the heart's contraction and depresses automaticity of the sinus node. *Furosemide* is a potent loop diuretic that lowers the blood pressure by inhibiting reabsorption of sodium and chloride primarily in the loop of Henle and also in proximal and distal renal tubules, resulting in decrease in intravascular volume. The diuretic effect of furosemide results in loss of sodium and water excretion, which will help to normalize the serum sodium and maintain the blood pressure.

6. **What are the most common adverse effects, drug-to-drug, drug-to-food/herbal interactions of the prescribed medications?** The most common adverse effects of *prazosin HcL* include marked hypotension (with the first dose, which is the reason for the gradual increase in dosing), dizziness, drowsiness, headache, fatigue, paresthesias, depression, palpitations, syncope, tachycardia, nausea and vomiting, edema, and dyspnea. The most common adverse reactions of *propranolol HcL* include confusion, fatigue, drowsiness, bradycardia, paresthesia of the hands, and impotence. It must be used with caution unless combined with an alpha-adrenergic blocking agent, such as prazosin. The most common adverse reactions of *furosemide* are hypokalemia, dehydration, hypochloremia, hypomagnesium, hyponatremia, hypovolemia, and metabolic alkalosis. With prazosin HcL, drug-to-drug interactions can occur with simultaneous use of antihypertensive agents, diuretics, beta-adrenergic blocking agents, and nifedipine which will increase the antihypertensive effects of prazosin HcL. Severe postural hypotension can result with the concurrent use of propranolol and verapamil. Clonidine may decrease the antihypertensive effects of prazosin. No clinically significant drug-to-food/herbal interactions have been established. Drug-to-drug interactions may occur with the simultaneous use of propranolol HcL and phenothiazines and beta-adrenergic agents, which may cause hypotension. The concurrent use of phenobarbital or rifampin may decrease propranolol's effects due to increased liver breakdown. Use with gabapentin may result in paroxysmal dystonic movements of the hands and use with haloperidol may cause severe hypotension. Methimazole or propylthiouracil may increase propranolol effects. Simultaneous use with rizatriptan may increase peak levels of rizatriptan due to decreased rizatriptan metabolism. The concurrent use of cimetidine may decrease propranolol clearance, increasing its adverse effects. Additive bradycardia may occur with digoxin. The simultaneous use of antacids decreases propranolol absorption. Use with furosemide increases propranolol levels. Smoking may increase propranolol HcL clearance and decrease its effects. There are no clinically significant drug-to-food/herbal interactions established. With furosemide, drug-to-drug interactions may occur with the simultaneous use of antihypertensives and nitrates which may increase hypotension. Concurrent use with other diuretics, piperacillin, amphotericin B, stimulant laxatives, and corticosteroids, may increase the risk of hypokalemia. The simultaneous use with aminoglycosides increases the risk of ototoxicity, and warfarin or thrombolytic agents simultaneous use with furosemide may increase the effectiveness of anticoagulants. Charcoal will decrease absorption of furosemide from the gastrointestinal (GI) tract and hydantoins decrease its diuretic effects. Use with propranolol increases plasma propranolol levels.

7. **Discuss pre-operative preparation for surgical intervention for pheochromocytoma.** Surgical resection of the tumor usually with adrenalectomy is the treatment of choice. If tumors are present in both adrenal glands, bilateral adrenalectomy may be present. The client's preparation includes control of blood pressure and blood volumes; usually carried out over seven to ten days. The client usually undergoes volume expansion with isotonic sodium chloride solution, and phentolamine or phenoxybenzamine (Dibenzyline) may be used. The client needs to be well hydrated before, during, and after surgery to prevent hypotension. Because manipulation of the tumor during surgical excision may cause release of stored epinephrine and norepinephrine, with marked increases in blood pressure and changes in heart rate, nitroprusside sodium (Nitropress) and alpha-adrenergic blocking agents may be required during and after surgery. Intravenous administration of corticosteroids (methylprednisolone sodium succinate [Solu-Medrol]) may begin the evening before surgery and continue during the early postoperative period to prevent adrenal insufficiency.

8. **Discuss surgical management of pheochromocytoma.** Routine preparation is done and informed consent is verified before anesthesia is administered. Both an experienced anesthesiologist and an experienced surgeon are crucial for the procedure. During the surgery, intravenous phentolamine, a rapid-acting alpha-adrenergic antagonist, is used, along with intravenous beta blockers, such as esmolol, to normalize the blood pressure. Postoperative care during the first 24–48 hours requires vigilant nursing assessment. The client is closely monitored for adrenal insufficiency, hypotension, hemorrhage, and shock. Accurately monitor urine output and blood pressure to determine impending shock and consequent renal shutdown. The client's dressing is checked frequently for bloody drainage, because if the client is bleeding internally for even brief periods, an abdominal hematoma can develop resulting in paralytic ileus (indicated by abdominal pain, distention, severe nausea, vomiting, and diminished or absent bowel sounds), or nonmechanical bowel obstruction. Pain assessment and management should be appropriately implemented, although opioid analgesic can cause hypotension.

9. **Discuss client education for pheochromocytoma.** The client should comply with prescribed medications. Blood pressure monitoring should be done on a daily basis and unusual headaches and abnormal blood pressure readings reported promptly to the health care provider. Follow-up care with health care provider is important to evaluate effectiveness of prescribed medications, or the need for modification. The need to continue to have serum potassium levels monitored should be stressed, and foods high in potassium should be discussed and written out as appropriate for the individual client.

References

Broyles, B.E. (2005). *Medical-Surgical Nursing Clinical Companion*. Durham, NC: Carolina Academic Press.

Corbet, J.V. (2004). *Laboratory Tests and Diagnostic Procedures with Nursing Diagnoses* (6th ed.). Upper Saddle River, NJ: Prentice Hall.

Gahart, B.L. and Nazareno, A.R. (2005). *2005 Intravenous Medications*. St. Louis: Mosby.

Heitz, U. and Horne, M.M. (2005). *Mosby's Pocket Guide Series: Fluid, Electrolyte and Acid-Base Balance* (5th ed.). St. Louis: Mosby.

Huether, S.E. and McCance, K.L. (2004). *Understanding Pathophysiology* (3rd ed.). St. Louis: Mosby.

Ignatavicius, D.D. and Workman, M.L. (2006). *Medical-Surgical Nursing across the Health Care Continuum* (5th ed.). Philadelphia: W.B. Saunders.

Spratto, G.R. and Woods, A.L. (2005). *2005 Edition: PDR Nurse's Drug Handbook*. Clifton Park, NY: Thomson Delmar Learning.

Sweeney, A.T. (July 2005) "Pheochromocytoma." Available at www.emedicine.com/med/topic1816.htm.

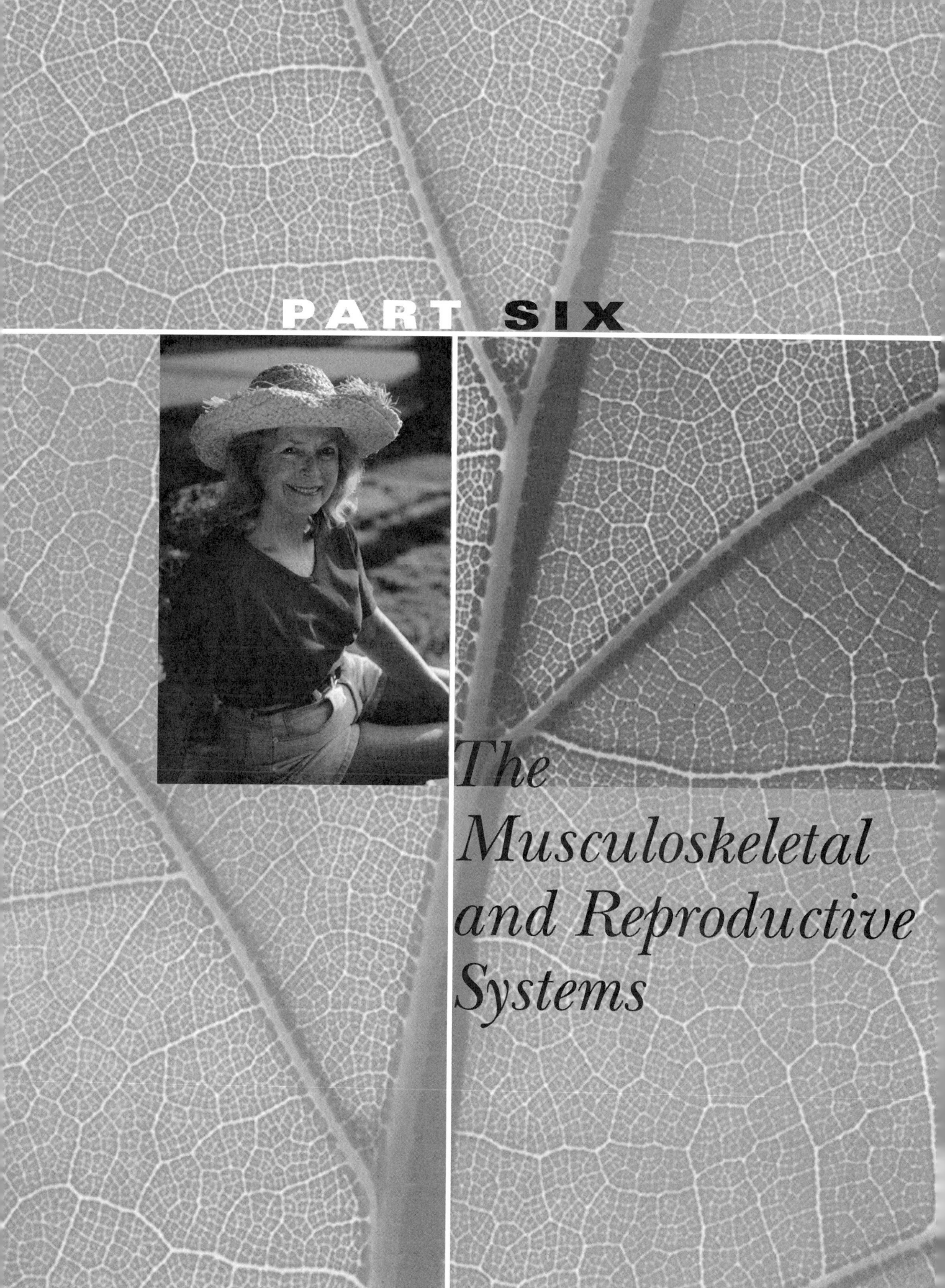

PART SIX

The Musculoskeletal and Reproductive Systems

CASE STUDY 1

Cervical Cancer Stage IA

GENDER
- F

AGE
- 25

SETTING
- Women's well clinic of a medical center

ETHNICITY/CULTURE
- Native American

PREEXISTING CONDITIONS
- HPV infection

COEXISTING CONDITIONS
- Squamous intraepithelial lesion

LIFESTYLE
- Unemployed college student
- Lives with sister

COMMUNICATION

DISABILITY

SOCIOECONOMIC STATUS
- Low

SPIRITUAL/RELIGIOUS
- Nondenominational

PHARMACOLOGIC
- Codeine sulfate

PSYCHOSOCIAL
- Anxiety
- Fear

LEGAL

ETHICAL

ALTERNATIVE THERAPY
- Meditation

PRIORITIZATION
- Encourage verbalization of feelings
- Prepare for cryosurgery

DELEGATION
- RN
- Client education

EASY

THE MUSCULOSKELETAL AND REPRODUCTIVE SYSTEMS

Level of difficulty: Easy

Overview: The case involves a thorough and sensitive assessment of the client's condition, taking into account the client's cultural views on health, wellness, and treatment. The nurse must use communication skills that will enhance trust and optimize the nurse–client relationship.

Client Profile

Ms. R is a 25-year-old female college student who is seen in the women's health clinic of a medical center due to complaints of spotting between menstruation. Ms. R is 5'5" and weighs 120 pounds.

Case Study

Ms. R reports to the nurse practitioner (NP) on initial interview that her most recent Papanicolau test (Pap) test is positive and that she had an appointment to see her family health care provider but missed the scheduled date, and the health care provider is away on personal business with an indefinite time of return. She admits to be being sexually active with the same partner for the past five years. Her reason for coming to the women's clinic is due to "spotting between menstruation" at the time of her last menstrual cycle. However, she is not "spotting" at the time of this visit. Her vital signs on admission are:

Blood pressure: 124/78
Pulse: 78 and regular
Respirations: 18
Temperature: 98.6°F

After continuing the history and physical, the NP discusses the need for further diagnostic evaluation, and when it is ascertained that Ms. R understands the need for the presented evaluation, the NP does a pelvic examination, a colposcopy, and an endocervical curettage. After the procedures, specimens are sent to the lab for analysis. Ms. R's vital signs are repeated and reveal:

Blood pressure: 128/80
Pulse: 80
Respirations: 18
Temperature: 98.6°F

The NP gives Ms. R an appointment for follow-up visit and informs her that at the time of that visit, the results of the colposcopy and endocervical curettage will be discussed with her.

Questions and Suggested Answers

1. **Discuss the etiology and pathophysiology of cervical cancer.** Carcinoma of the cervix is predominantly squamous cell cancer (10%) are adenocarcinoma. It is now less common because of early detection by Papanicolau (Pap) smear, yet it is still the third most common female reproductive cancer and affects a large percentage of women in the United States each year. Etiologies include multiple sex partners, smoking, and chronic cervical infection. The pathophysiology is seen with the progression from normal cervical cells to dysplasia and then to cervical cancer, which is related to repeat injuries to the cervix. It is an insidious disease with relationship to the human papilloma virus (HPV), and women who smoke have a 50% higher risk for developing cervical cancer than non-smokers.

2. **Discuss cultural and ethnic considerations of cervical cancer.** Cervical cancer has a higher incidence among Hispanic, black American, and Native American women than white women. Mortality rates from cervical cancer are more than twice as high among black American women as among white women.

3. **Discuss clinical manifestations of cervical cancer.** Precancerous changes are symptomatic, but leukorrhea and intermenstrual bleeding eventually occur. The discharge is usually thin and watery but becomes very dark and foul smelling as the disease advances, suggesting the presence of infection. Vaginal bleeding is initially spotting,

but as the tumor enlarges, bleeding becomes heavier and more frequent. Pain is a late symptom followed by weight loss, anemia, and cachexia.

4. **Discuss diagnostic studies use to confirm cervical cancer.** Pap smear, the Schiller iodine test, colposcopy, and cervical biopsy are used to diagnose cervical cancer. The *Pap smear* tests for malignant cells in the uterus. It is usually performed five to six days after menstruation, and the client should avoid sexual intercourse or douching before the test. A small amount of secretion is obtained from the cervix by means of swabbing the exterior of the cervix with an applicator. The smears are placed on dry slides and immediately sprayed with a fixative. It is done to examine the cells from the cervix and usually detects abnormal cells. The results of the Pap smear are reported by classification (Class I through V). The *Schiller iodine test* involves application of iodine solution to the cervix. Normal tissues stain dark brown, but abnormal tissues fail to pick up the color. A *cervical biopsy* of the uterine cervix uses a colposcopy. Multiple biopsies are usually obtained at specific sites with biopsy forceps. A *colposcopy* is the direct visualization of the vagina and cervix by means of a special binocular microscope and light system to identify the extent of cervical lesions.

The following are prescribed:

- Contact the clinic if you are experiencing excessive bleeding, discharge, or abdominal pain.
- Return to the clinic in one month for discussion on the results of the specimens sent to the lab.
- Codeine sulfate 15 mg PO q6h PRN

5. **What is the purpose for the prescribed medication?** *Codeine sulfate* relieves the discomfort that may occur after the colposcopy and endocervical curettage. Codeine sulfate works by binding to delta receptors resulting in analgesia.

6. **What are the most common adverse reactions, drug-to-drug, drug-to-food/herbal interactions of the prescribed medication?** The most common adverse reactions of *codeine sulfate* are confusion, sedation, hypotension, constipation, nausea, and vomiting. Drug-to-drug interactions may occur with the simultaneous use of monoamine oxidase (MAO) inhibitors. Additive central nervous system (CNS) depression may occur with the simultaneous use of alcohol, antidepressants, antihistamines, and sedating/hypnotics. Simultaneous use with buprenorphine, butorphanol, nalbuphine, or pentazocine may precipitate opioid withdrawal in physically dependent clients. Drug-to-herbal interactions may occur with the simultaneous use of kava, valerian, skullcap, chamomile, and hops, which can increase CNS depression. There are no clinically significant drug-to-food/herbal interactions established.

7. **Discuss surgical management for cervical cancer.** If conservative measures are not helpful, surgery may be necessary to relieve pain and enhance the possibility for pregnancy. The surgical procedure selected depends on the individual client. A *gynecologic laparoscopy* may be used to fulgurate (cut with high-frequency current) endometrial implants and to release adhesions. The procedure involves the use of general anesthesia, and the client is placed in a modified lithotomy position with the head tilted downward. The external genitalia are cleansed with an antiseptic solution and draped. A uterine manipulator is inserted through the vagina and cervix and then into the uterus to permit organs such as the ovaries, fallopian tubes, and uterus to be moved for better visualization. The abdomen is cleansed with antiseptic solution and sterile drapes positioned around the incision site. A small incision is made and a pneumoperitoneum created, and a pneumoperitoneum needle inserted to deliver carbon dioxide for insufflation. The needle is removed and a trocar and a laparoscope are inserted through the incision. The pelvic organs are visualized, examined, tissues samples collected, and therapeutic procedures performed as needed. The scope is then withdrawn, carbon dioxide evacuated via the trocar, the trocar is removed, the uterine manipulator is removed, the skin incision is closed, the perineum cleansed and a pad is applied to the perineum to prevent drainage to the skin. Nursing priorities after the procedure include placing the client in telemetry, monitoring for reaction to anesthetic agent such as tachycardia, bradycardia, hyperpnea, hypertension, allergic reaction, or hypotension. The nurse should report complaints of unusual abdominal pain or bleeding since both may be due to laceration during the procedure.

8. **Discuss the clinical stages of cervical cancer.**

    Pre-invasive: Stage 0 – The carcinoma is in situ; cancer is limited to epithelial layers, with no evidence of invasions.

    Invasive: Stage I – Carcinoma is strictly confined to the cervix. *Stage Ia* – Microinvasive identified only microscopically. *Stage Ia1* – Invasion no greater than 3 mm in depth and no greater than 5 mm and no wider than 7 mm. *Stage Ia2* – Invasion greater than 3 mm and no greater than 5 mm and no wider than 7 mm. *Stage Ib* – Clinical lesions confined to cervix or preclinical lesions greater than Stage Ia. *Stage Ib1* – Clinical lesions no greater than 4 cm in size. *Stage Ib2* – Clinical lesions greater than 4 cm in size. *Stage II* – Carcinoma extends beyond the cervix but not onto the pelvic wall. *Stage IIa* – Vaginal extension only. *Stage IIb* – Paracervical extension with or without vaginal involvement. *Stage III* – Carcinoma extends to one or both pelvic walls. Involves lower third of vagina. One or both ureters obstructed by the tumor as seen on intravenous (IV) urogram. *Stage IIIa* – No extension onto the pelvic wall. *Stage IIIb* – Extension onto the pelvic wall or hydronephrosis or non-functioning kidney, or both. *Stage IV* – Extension of carcinoma beyond the true pelvis. Clinical involvement of the mucosa of the bladder or rectum. *Stage IVa* – Spread of carcinoma to adjacent organs. *Stage IVb* – Spread to distant organs.

9. **Discuss client education for cervical cancer.** The client should comply with clinic appointment, inform her partner of her current medical condition, use condom at all times when having sexual activity, and have an annual Pap smear or as per primary health care provider's instructions. Cervical cancer stage IA is limited to the cervix. However, if it goes undiagnosed and untreated, it could lead to invasive cervical cancer, which is the third most common cause of death related to reproductive cancers. Because stage Ia cervical cancer occurs mainly in young women, with peak incidence of dysplasia occurring in their mid-twenties, nurses should be vigilant with primary prevention starting at the elementary school age with sexual activity clearly defined and explained. Primary prevention will hopefully generate more awareness of the risk factors of this type of cancer in an effort to decrease its incidence and prevalence in future years.

References

Black, J.M. and Hawks, J.H. (2005). *Medical-Surgical Nursing: Clinical Management for Positive Outcomes.* Philadelphia: W.B. Saunders.

Broyles, B.E. (2005). *Medical-Surgical Nursing Clinical Companion.* Durham, NC: Carolina Academic Press.

Corbet, J.V. (2004). *Laboratory Tests and Diagnostic Procedures with Nursing Diagnoses* (6th ed.). Upper Saddle River, NJ: Prentice Hall.

Gahart, B.L. and Nazareno, A.R. (2005). *2005 Intravenous Medications.* St. Louis: Mosby.

Huether, S.E. and McCance, K.L. (2004). *Understanding Pathophysiology* (3rd ed.). St. Louis: Mosby.

Ignatavicius, D.D. and Workman, M.L. (2006). *Medical-Surgical Nursing across the Health Care Continuum* (5th ed.). Philadelphia: W.B. Saunders.

Spratto, G.R. and Woods, A.L. (2005). *2005 Edition: PDR Nurse's Drug Handbook.* Clifton Park, NY: Thomson Delmar Learning.

CASE STUDY 2

Closed Femoral Head Fracture (Intracapsular Fracture)

GENDER
- M

AGE
- 32

SETTING
- Hospital

ETHNICITY/CULTURE
- Black American/West Indian

PREEXISTING CONDITIONS

COEXISTING CONDITIONS

LIFESTYLE
- Professional painter

COMMUNICATION

DISABILITY

SOCIOECONOMIC STATUS
- Middle

SPIRITUAL/RELIGIOUS
- Methodist

PHARMACOLOGIC
- Morphine sulfate (Duramorph)
- Enoxaparin sodium (Lovenox)
- Docusate sodium (Colace)

PSYCHOSOCIAL
- Anxiety
- Pain

LEGAL
- Worker's compensation should be available until client returns to work.

ETHICAL

ALTERNATIVE THERAPY

PRIORITIZATION
- Stabilize extremity
- Assess and manage pain
- Assess neurological status of lower extremities

DELEGATION
- RN
- CNA
- Client education

THE MUSCULOSKELETAL AND REPRODUCTIVE SYSTEMS

Level of difficulty: Easy

Overview: This case first involves assessment of all major body systems for life-threatening complications, including head, thoracic, and abdominal injuries. The case involves assessment of pain and assessment of the skin for intactness, color, temperature, movement, sensation, pulses, and capillary refill. The triage nurse uses critical thinking to appropriately prioritize care of clients with hip dislocation in a busy emergency department (ED). The certified nursing attendant (CNA) can take vital signs and monitor the client for signs of bleeding, such as restlessness, or unusual findings on the skin (e.g., bruising) and inform the nurse.

Client Profile

Mr. P is a 32-year-old painter who is brought to the ED via emergency medical services (EMS) after falling from a ladder while painting a building under contract by his employer. He is 5'9" and weighs 150 pounds.

Case Study

On arrival to the ED, Mr. P is alert, oriented to time, person, and place, but is voicing intolerable pain in the right thigh with slight movement and moderate pain over his entire back. He denies known allergies to foods or drugs or the use of herbals. Vital signs reveal:

Blood pressure: 130/80
Pulse: 90
Respirations: 20
Temperature: 98.6°F

He is medicated with morphine 10 mg IM for pain as prescribed. Serum labs done in the ED reveal:

Hematocrit (Hct): 36%
Hemoglobin (Hgb): 14%
Serum calcium: 9 mg/dL
Serum phosphorous: 4 mg/dL

Mr. P is transferred from the stretcher that he is brought in on to a ED bed. His right leg remains immobilized by a long backboard. An EMS personnel provides the triage nurse with a detailed report of physical findings and neurovascular status of the injured extremity on arrival to the injury site. The ED health care provider arrives and after gathering additional pertinent history, the health care provider examines Mr. P for other bony injuries and a careful knee examination is also done. Mr. P is transferred to the orthopedic unit, weighed on a bedscale, then placed on bed rest. A complete assessment is done, including assessment of abrasions and other injuries. An EKG shows normal sinus rhythm, and a chest X-ray is negative for rib fracture or diaphragmatic damage. A venography is negative for pulmonary embolism. A pulse oximeter is initiated with a noted oxygen saturation of 98%. At a later time during the shift, a computed tomography (CT) of the spine, pelvis, hip, and leg is done and reveals an intact spine and pelvis, dislocation of the femoral head, and soft tissue damage of the leg and thigh, but no pre-existing disorders. After the multidisciplinary team reviews the data of diagnostic studies and physical findings, a diagnosis of closed femoral head dislocation is made, and plans for surgery are discussed with Mr. P. He is informed that no food or fluids should be taken (NPO) after a scheduled time in preparation for the surgical procedure. A closed reduction/internal fixation of the femoral head is scheduled. An intravenous (IV) line is initiated with IV solution of 0.9% sodium chloride at 125 mL/hr, and a trapeze is placed over the bed with instructions given to Mr. P on its purpose and use.

Questions and Suggested Answers

1. **Discuss the different types of fractures, including the closed fracture.** A fracture is a disruption or break in the continuity of the structure of the bone. Traumatic injuries account for the majority of fractures, although some fractures are secondary to a disease process (pathologic fractures). There are various types of fractures. A closed fracture is also referred to as a simple fracture, which is an uncomplicated fracture with intact skin over the fracture site. That means the bone does not protrude through the skin. An avulsion fracture is fracture of bone resulting from strong pulling effect of tendons or ligaments at the bone attachment. A comminuted fracture is a fracture with more than two fragments, with the smaller fragments seeming to be floating when viewed on X-ray. A displaced, overriding fracture involves a displaced fracture fragment that

is overriding the other bone fragment, with the periosteum disrupted on both sides. A greenstick fracture is an incomplete fracture with one side splintered and the other side bent. Impacted fracture is a comminuted fracture in which more than two fragments are driven into each other. An intra-articular fracture is a fracture extending to the articular surface of the bone. A longitudinal fracture is an incomplete fracture in which the fracture line runs along the longitudinal axis of the bone. The periosteum is not torn away from the bone. An oblique fracture is a fracture in which the line of the fracture extends in an oblique direction. Pathologic fracture is a spontaneous fracture at the site of a bone disease. Spiral fracture is a fracture in which the line of the fracture extends in a spiral direction along the shaft of the bone. A stress fracture is a fracture that occurs in normal or abnormal bone that is subjected to repeated stress, such as from jogging or running. A transverse fracture is a fracture in which the line of the fracture extends across the bone shaft at a right angle to the longitudinal axis.

2. **Discuss clinical manifestations of clients with closed femoral head fracture.** *Acute pain* is caused by soft tissue damage and is compounded by muscle spasms, swelling, and impaired sensation (numbness). *Altered tissue* perfusion may occur due to a deep vein thrombus that has impaired circulation. *Impaired physical mobility* because of the pain and fracture of the extremity. The client will need immobilization of the fractured extremity. *Alteration in sensory perception* such as tactile sense because of the possibility of nerve injury from the initial trauma.

3. **Discuss the potential complications of a closed femoral head fracture.** Because the femoral head and neck lie within the joint capsule and are not covered in periosteum, they do not have a large blood supply. Therefore, these fractures, when they occur, are usually evidenced by fragment and may further decrease blood supply. The decrease in blood supply increases the risk of *nonunion* and *avascular necrosis*. *Nonunion* fracture is one that is never completely heals; therefore, this type of fracture is at risk for pathological fracture, and pseudoarthrosis (false joint). Nonunion fractures are commonly treated with bone grafts. In most cases of bone grafting, chips of bone are taken from the client's iliac crest or other site and are packed or wired between the bone ends to facilitate union. Allografts from cadavers, which are frozen or freeze-dried and stored under sterile conditions in a bone bank, may also be used. *Avascular necrosis (aseptic necrosis, osteonecrosis)* refers to death of bone tissue due to lack of blood supply. Surgical interventions for avascular necrosis include total hip arthroplasty or hemiarthroplasty for older persons, and osteotomy or an arthrodesis for younger adults. An osteotomy may involve either a block osteotomy in which a section of a bone is excised, cuneiform osteotomy, in which a wedge of a bone is removed, and a displacement osteotomy, in which a bone is redesigned surgically to alter alignment or weight-bearing stress areas. Osteotomy procedures require the use of a walker or crutches. If arthrodesis (ankylosis) is to be done, the procedure involves surgical induced fixation of the joint to relieve the pain and provide support to the extremity. Arthrodesis may require the use of a body cast.

4. **Discuss the use of crutches instead of a walker for this client.** Crutches are used for persons with limitations of lower extremity function, but who have full use of upper extremities. Walkers are used for persons who have weakness in both upper and lower extremities or for older persons with hip problems, arthritis, or neuromuscular disease. Mr. P is a candidate for the use of crutches.

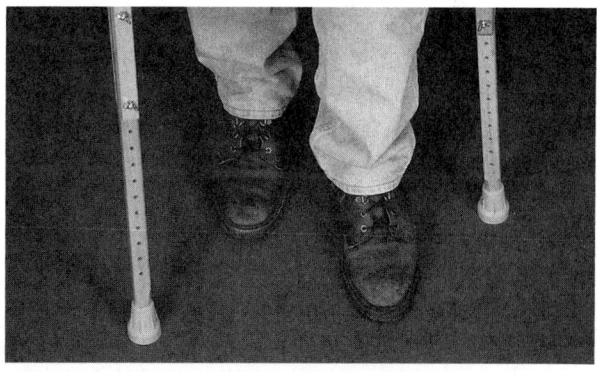

Crutch-walking, four-point gait

5. **Discuss the teaching guidelines for crutch walking.** The client should be instructed to wear shoes that will not slip, such as rubber-soled shoes. The physical environment should be free of hazards such as throw rugs and wet floors. The client should never walk with the crutches if he feels dizzy or light-headed. The client should not exceed the weight-bearing limitations given by the health care provider, and should not attempt stairs unless instructions have been given, and demonstration of the use of crutches on stairs. The client should use crutches that have been properly sized with axillary and handgrip pads in place and rubber caps covering the tips of both crutches. The client should use both armrests of a chair when rising from a sitting position, so that the chair does not tip over.

6. **What are common nursing diagnoses for clients with closed femoral head fracture?**

    - Acute pain R/T soft tissue damage, muscle spasm, and mobility of extremity
    - Risk for peripheral neurovascular dysfunction
    - Impaired physical mobility R/T disruption in bone structure and pain
    - Deficient knowledge R/T condition, treatment, rehabilitation, and health maintenance

7. **What are expected outcomes for clients with closed femoral head fracture?**

    Problem: Acute pain
    Expected outcome: Denies experiencing pain greater than 5 on a 0-to-10 pain scale. Requests pain medication every six hours instead of every four hours as prescribed.

    Problem: Paresthesias and numbness in lower extremity
    Expected outcome: Denies paresthesias or numbness. Pulses remain strong and equal at all pulse points.

    Problem: Immobility of lower extremity
    Expected outcome: Has full or improved range of motion in the extremity. Able to turn without assistance. Has smooth, coordinated movements.

The following are prescribed:

- Complete bed rest
- Morphine sulfate (Duramorph) 1–2 mg IV PRN for pain
- Enoxaparin sodium (Lovenox) 100 mg/1 mL SC daily
- Docusate sodium (Colace) 100 mg PO three times per day

8. **What are the purposes for the prescribed orders?** *Complete bed rest* prevents further injury to the broken bone, and soft tissue. *Morphine sulfate* is a schedule II opioid analgesic that relieves pain and promotes comfort by binding with delta receptors and decreasing the perception of pain in the central nervous system (CNS), thus, promoting analgesia. *Enoxaparin sodium* prevents clot formation, which decreases the risk for deep vein thrombosis, which is a critical occurrence with hip dislocation. Enoxaparin sodium is a low-molecular-weight heparin effective in preventing clot formation because it binds to antithrombin IIa in the coagulation activities, causing blood-clotting time to increase so as to prevent or slow further development of thrombolic condition. *Docusate sodium* is a stool softener that prevents constipation related to decreased immobility, and the high risk for constipation related to opioid medications such as morphine. It prevents constipation due to its detergent action that has emulsifying and wetting properties that permits water and fats to penetrate and soften stools for easier passage.

9. **What are the most common adverse reactions, drug-to-drug, drug-to-food/herbal interactions for the prescribed medications?** The most common adverse reactions of intravenous *morphine sulfate* are pruritus, confusion, sedation, and constipation. Drug-to-drug interactions may occur with the simultaneous use of CNS depressant drugs, which will increase sedation. The concurrent use of clomipramine, barbiturates, tricyclic antidepressants, and antihistamines will increase CNS depression. Simultaneous use with buprenorphine, nalbuphine, butorphanol, or pentazocine may decrease analgesia. The concurrent use with cimetidine will decrease the metabolism and may increase the effects. The simultaneous use of MAO inhibitors may

precipitate hypertensive crisis. Drug-to-herbal interactions may occur with simultaneous use of kava-kava, valerian, and St. John's Wort. The most common adverse reaction of **enoxaparin sodium** is bruising at the site of injection, especially if the agent is not administered at a 90-degree angle. This also decreases enoxaparin's action. Drug-to-drug interactions may occur with the simultaneous use of aspirin or warfarin, which can increase risk of hemorrhage. Drug-to-herbal interactions may occur with the simultaneous use of garlic, ginger, gingko, feverfew, and horse chestnut, which may increase risk of bleeding. The most common adverse reaction of **docusate sodium** is diarrhea. Drug-to-drug interactions are seen with the simultaneous use of mineral oil, which may increase systemic absorption. There are no clinically significant drug-to-food/herbal interactions established.

10. **Discuss the discharge plans for the client following mobilization of the closed femoral head fracture.** The primary nurse and the social worker ascertain that the client can move independently and safely before discharge. The social worker will determine the need for home health aide (HHA) for an appropriate period of time. Educate the client about safety and fall prevention. Provide health care resource information for literature on safety in the workplace. The primary nurse will teach the client the importance of taking prescribed pain medications before pain becomes severe, and about common adverse effects to look for and what actions to take if they occur. The importance of follow-up care is emphasized during discharge planning.

References

Beebe, R. and Funk, D. (2005). *Fundamentals of Basic Emergency Care* (2nd ed.). Clifton Park, NY: Thomson Delmar Learning.
Black, J.M. and Hawks, J.H. (2005). *Medical-Surgical Nursing: Clinical Management for Positive Outcomes*. Philadelphia: W.B. Saunders.
Broyles, B.E. (2005). *Medical-Surgical Nursing Clinical Companion*. Durham, NC: Carolina Academic Press.
Deglin, J.H. and Vallerand, A.H. (2005). *Davis's Drug Guide for Nurses* (9th ed.). Philadelphia: F.A. Davis.
Gahart, B.L. and Nazareno, A.R. (2005). *2005 Intravenous Medications*. St. Louis: Mosby.
Huether, S.E. and McCance, K.L. (2004). *Understanding Pathophysiology* (3rd ed.). St. Louis: Mosby.
Ignatavicius, D.D. and Workman, M.L. (2006). *Medical-Surgical Nursing across the Health Care Continuum* (5th ed.) Philadelphia: W.B. Saunders.
Lilley, L.L., Harrington, S., and Synder, J.S. (2005). *Pharmacology and the Nursing Process* (4th ed.). St. Louis: Mosby.
Smeltzer, C.S. and Bare, B.G. (2004). *Textbook of Medical-Surgical Nursing* (10th ed.). Philadelphia: Lippincott Williams & Wilkins.
Spratto, G.R. and Woods, A.L. (2005). *2005 Edition: PDR Nurse's Drug Handbook*. Clifton Park, NY: Thomson Delmar Learning.

CASE STUDY 3

Osteomyelitis of Left Foot

GENDER
- M

AGE
- 64

SETTING
- Hospital

ETHNICITY/CULTURE
- White American

PREEXISTING CONDITIONS
- Status-post femoral-popliteal bypass

COEXISTING CONDITIONS
- Peripheral vascular disease

LIFESTYLE
- CPA

COMMUNICATION
- English

DISABILITY
- Decreased mobility

SOCIOECONOMIC STATUS
- Middle

SPIRITUAL/RELIGIOUS
- Lutheran

PHARMACOLOGIC
- Ticarcillin disodium/clavulanate potassium (Timentin)

PSYCHOSOCIAL
- Anxiety
- Depression

LEGAL

ETHICAL

ALTERNATIVE THERAPY

PRIORITIZATION
- Antibiotic therapy
- Promote wound healing

DELEGATION
- RN
- Client education

THE MUSCULOSKELETAL AND REPRODUCTIVE SYSTEMS

Level of difficulty: Easy

Overview: This case involves assessment of the client's present problems. The nurse must be knowledgeable about osteomyelitis and the need for immediate medical and nursing interventions to prevent systemic complications and chronic osteomyelitis. The case involves pain management and antibiotic administration with knowledge of unintended effects of analgesic and antibiotic medications, and interventions for these effects.

Client Profile

Mr. Y is a 64-year-old certified public accountant who was discharged from the hospital three weeks ago after amputation of the left great toe related to complete loss of circulation in his extremity. Mr. Y is married and has a 28-year-old daughter in college. His wife is an elementary school teacher. He and his family own a three-bedroom co-op in a newly developed neighborhood.

Case Study

Mr. Y's past medical history includes hypertension and arterial insufficiency. He is status-post (S/P) femoral-popliteal bypass three weeks ago. His family history includes diabetes mellitus (mother) and hypertension and peripheral vascular disease (father). Mr. Y reports that both he and his wife have good health insurance and that he receives a salary while recuperating from surgery. However, he says he is concerned about the continuation of his salary, which is dependent on the length of time the infection will take to heal. Vital signs are:

Blood pressure: 140/94
Pulse: 94
Respirations: 20
Temperature: 101.4°F

The entire foot is tender and warm to touch. There is a moderate amount of mildly odorous drainage coming from the wound. The nursing history and physical examination is completed by the nurse, after which the health care provider reviews the data, asks the client about history of allergies, which the client denies. The health care provider continues the history and physical examination, and a specimen from the infected site is sent to the lab for analysis. The following diagnostic studies are ordered: radionuclide bone scan of the left foot, and a magnetic resonance imaging (MRI), blood culture and gram stain, culture and sensitivity of the wound, white blood cell (WBC) count with differential, and erythrocyte sedimentation rate (ESR). The bone scan reveals infection of the bone marrow, and the MRI identifies calcification of the bones of the foot and provides definitive diagnosis for osteomyelitis. The blood culture and gram stain are positive for P. aeruginosa and Staphylococcus aeruginosa. WBC with differential reveals:

White blood cell (WBC) count: 13,000/mm^3
Neutrophils: 82%
Eosinophils: 4%
Basophils: 2%
Lymphocytes: 43%
Monocytes: 8%
Erythrocyte sedimentation rate (ESR): elevated, 90%

After the multidisciplinary team reviews the diagnostic studies, a diagnosis of osteomyelitis of the left foot is confirmed; the findings are discussed with the client; and plans for surgical debridement are decided upon by the team and Mr. Y. The debridement is done and the surgical plan is to implement high doses of parenteral antibiotics initially followed by oral antibiotics and serial bone scans. Specific orders are written for the surgical team to change the wound dressing during daily rounds.

Questions and Suggested Answers

1. **Discuss the pathophysiology of osteomyelitis.** Osteomyelitis is a pyrogenic infection of the bone, bone marrow, and surrounding tissue. Aerobic gram-negative bacteria alone or mixed with gram-positive organisms are often found. The infecting organisms can invade by indirect or direct entry. After gaining entrance to the bone by way of the blood, the microorganisms then lodge in an area of bone in which circulation is slow.

Chronic osteomyelitis is either a continuous, persistent problem (a result of inadequate acute treatment) or a process of exacerbations and remission.

2. **Discuss groups of persons in whom osteomyelitis is most difficult to manage.** Obesity is a serious health risk and has been associated with increased risk of mortality and morbidity. The mechanisms behind the obesity co-morbidities are not completely understood, but it is clear that the insulin resistance that is typical of truncal obesity is also associated with hypertriglyceridemia. Both the obesity and the hypertriglyceridemia interfere with tissue perfusion. If bone injury occurs and blood supply is impaired, over a period of time, infection of the bone will develop. Persons who are malnourished, or have a history of alcoholism or liver failure are the most difficult because of their immunocompromised status.

3. **Discuss indirect and direct osteomyelitis.** The *indirect entry* (hematogenous) of microorganisms in osteomyelitis most frequently affects growing bone in boys less than 12 years old, and is associated with their higher incidence of blunt trauma. Adults with vascular insufficiency disorders (e.g., diabetes mellitus) and genitourinary and respiratory infections are at higher risk for a primary infection to spread via the blood to the bone. The pelvis and vertebrae, which are vascular-rich sites of bone, are the most common sites of infection. *Direct entry* osteomyelitis can occur at any age when there is an open wound (e.g., penetrating wounds, fractures) and microorganisms gain entry to the body.

4. **Discuss the organism that is the most common cause of osteomyelitis.** The organism that is the most common cause of osteomyelitis is Staphylococcus aureus. It is a nonmotile gram-positive bacterium that is normally found on the skin and in the throat. However, life-threatening staphylococcal infections may arise within hospitals, and are frequently responsible for osteomyelitis and other infectious diseases. Staphylococcus aureus infections have become increasingly more difficult to treat due to the development of resistance to penicillin-related antibiotics. These bacteria are called *methicillin-resistant Staphylococcus aureus* (MRSA).

5. **Discuss the clinical manifestations of acute and chronic osteomyelitis.** *Acute osteomyelitis* refers to the initial infection or an infection of less than one month in duration. The systemic clinical manifestations include fever, night sweats, chills, restlessness, nausea, and malaise. Local manifestations include constant bone pain that is unrelieved by rest and worsens with activity. The clinical manifestations of chronic osteomyelitis include constant bone pain and swelling, tenderness, and warmth at the infection site.

6. **Discuss common nursing diagnoses for clients with osteomyelitis.**

   - Acute pain R/T inflammatory process secondary to infection – The nurse should prioritize care by focusing on the client's complaint of pain, assessing location, and intensity of the pain with the use of a pain scale. Analgesics should be implemented on time as scheduled, and the client should be instructed to request pain medication before the pain becomes too severe. Elevation of the extremity will reduce swelling, if present, and promote comfort.
   - Impaired physical mobility R/T pain – The nurse should assist the client as needed to reduce the client's frustration with impaired mobility, and to prevent injury. Assistive devices (e.g., long-handed shoehorn, socks helpers, pick-up stick) should be used to increase independence in activities of daily living.
   - Ineffective therapeutic regimen management R/T lack of knowledge regarding long-term management of osteomyelitis – The nurse must provide information and instruction regarding wound care, aseptic technique, and dressing disposal to reduce the risk of cross-contamination and encourage wound healing. The nurse should also review drug regimen including schedule, name, dosage, purpose, and side effects, because long-term antibiotic therapy is required.

The following are prescribed:

- Ticarcillin disodium/clavulanate potassium (Timentin) 3.1 g IV q4h
- 0.9% NaCL at 100 mL per hour
- Vitamin A (Aquasol A) 15,000 IU daily
- Vitamin C (ascorbic acid) 500 mg PO two times per day
- ESR, hemoglobin, WBC, albumin levels

7. **What are the purposes for the prescribed orders?** *Ticarcillin disodium/clavulanate potassium* is an extended-spectrum penicillin and beta-lactamase inhibitor used to treat bone infections. It destroys the organisms, halting the infectious process by interfering with synthesis of mucopeptides essential to formation and integrity of bacterial cell wall, resulting in the death of organisms. Intravenous therapy is to aid with hydration status and as an adjunct to antibiotic therapy. *Vitamin A* is a fat-soluble vitamin supplement that enhances wound healing by providing collagen synthesis, and improving immune response. *Vitamin C* is a water-soluble vitamin supplement that enhances wound healing and capillary wall integrity by increasing collagen formation and protecting mechanisms of the immune system, which supports wound healing. The *ESR* helps to assess the client's inflammatory status, and the infectious and necrotic process in relationship to antibiotic management. This is seen with elevation of the levels if the infectious process continues in the presence of the antibiotic therapy, or it decreases and returns to normal when the infectious process responds effectively to the antibiotic regimen. The *hemoglobin* reveals the blood's oxygen-carrying capacity and helps determine the significance of oxygen to the involved tissues. An *elevated WBC count* indicates infection and helps with the management of wound care. The *albumin levels* indicate the nutritional status of the client and the need for modification of treatment.

8. **What are the most common adverse reactions, drug-to-drug, drug-to-food/herbal interactions for the prescribed medications?** The most common adverse reactions of *ticarcillin disodium/clavulanate potassium* are diarrhea, risk of anaphylaxis, epigastric distress, nausea, vomiting, hypernatremia, hypokalemia, headache, rashes, and phlebitis at the infusion site, especially if infused too rapidly through a peripheral site. Drug-to-drug interactions may occur with the simultaneous use of oral contraceptives and ticarcillin disodium/clavulanate potassium and oral contraceptives, decreasing the effectiveness of the contraceptive agents. The concurrent use with probenecid decreases renal excretion and increases serum levels, and there is a synergistic effect when used with amikacin or gentamycin. As with other bacteriocidal antibiotics, its actions may be antagonized by bacteriostatic agents such as erythromycin, tetracyclines, and chloramphenicol. If used with beta-adrenergic blocking agents, the risk of allergic reactions increases. The risk of bleeding is increased if used concurrently with heparin, alteplase, anistreplase, nonsteroidal anti-inflammatory agents (NSAIDs), aspirin, dextran, dipyridamole, and plicamycin. The concurrent use with methotrexate decreases methotrexate elimination and increases the risk of serious toxicity. There are no clinically significant common adverse reactions of *vitamin A* established. There are no clinically significant drug-to-drug, drug-to-food/herbal interactions established. There are no clinically significant adverse reactions of *vitamin C* established. Drug-to-drug interactions may occur with the simultaneous use of oral anticoagulant, which may inhibit *ascorbic acid* uptake by leukocytes and tissues, and ascorbic acid may diminish the effects of disulfiram.

9. **Discuss discharge instructions for the client with osteomyelitis.** If the client is discharged to home with an unhealed wound that has approximated at the edges without odor or drainage, the client may be instructed in the use of a transparent film dressing, which provides a moist environment that promotes granulation tissue. The client should monitor the wound site for swelling or pain and report these findings to the primary health care provider. The client should complete antibiotics as prescribed, and keep scheduled appointments. The client should maintain weight, decrease the amount of salt used in the diet, exercise, and monitor blood pressure.

References

Black, J.M. and Hawks, J.H. (2005). *Medical-Surgical Nursing: Clinical Management for Positive Outcomes*. Philadelphia: W.B. Saunders.

Broyles, B.E. (2005). *Medical-Surgical Nursing Clinical Companion*. Durham, NC: Carolina Academic Press.

Gahart, B.L. and Nazareno, A.R. (2005). *2005 Intravenous Medications*. St. Louis: Mosby.

Huether, S.E. and McCance, K.L. (2004). *Understanding Pathophysiology* (3rd ed.). St. Louis: Mosby.

Ignatavicius, D.D. and Workman, M.L. (2006). *Medical-Surgical Nursing across the Health Care Continuum* (5th ed.). Philadelphia: W.B. Saunders.

Spratto, G.R. and Woods, A.L. (2005). *2005 Edition: PDR Nurse's Drug Handbook*. Clifton Park, NY: Thomson Delmar Learning.

CASE STUDY 4

Osteoarthritis

GENDER
- F

AGE
- 58

SETTING
- Community health clinic

ETHNICITY/CULTURE
- Black American

PREEXISTING CONDITIONS
- Post menopause

COEXISTING CONDITIONS
- Father has severe OA of the hands

LIFESTYLE
- Laundromat manager

COMMUNICATION

DISABILITY

SOCIOECONOMIC STATUS
- Low

SPIRITUAL/RELIGIOUS
- Baptist

PHARMACOLOGIC
- Aspirin (acetylsalicylic acid)
- Antacid (TUMS)
- Celecoxib (Celebrex)
- Calcium carbonate (Os-Cal)
- Capsaicin (Zostrix)

PSYCHOSOCIAL
- Mood changes
- Difficulty adjusting to limitation of use of hands

LEGAL

ETHICAL
- Client should have the right to use alterntive therapy with prescribed medications.

ALTERNATIVE THERAPY
- Vegan diet
- Ginseng
- Cayenne pepper

PRIORITIZATION
- Pain management

DELEGATION
- RN
- LPN
- Client education

MODERATE

THE MUSCULOSKELETAL AND REPRODUCTIVE SYSTEMS

Level of difficulty: Moderate

Overview: This case involves a thorough assessment of the client's condition and current over-the-counter and herbal medications. It involves careful inspection and palpation of joints for symmetry, size, shape, color, appearance, and pain, and the use of arthritis disability and discomfort scales to assess the client's functional level for the past week to help determine assistance needed for activities of daily living (ADL). The licensed practical nurse (LPN) can reinforce teaching, after the registered nurse (RN) has initiated it, and continue with assessment procedures.

Client Profile

Ms. C is a 58-year-old female who is seen at the community health clinic for routine annual evaluation. Ms. C is 5'5" and weighs 150 pounds. The LPN is assigned to take her vital signs, which are:

Blood pressure: 140/84
Pulse: 84
Respirations: 18
Temperature: 98.6°F

Case Study

On initial interview by an RN, Ms. C reports increase in dull, aching pain around the joints of the digits of both hands. Observation of the hands finds evidence of early manifestations of Heberden's and Bouchard's nodes. On further assessment, she reports the use of aspirin to help relieve pain, and antacids (TUMS), to decrease the discomfort in her stomach, which she believes is due to the constant use of aspirin. Continued gathering of data reveals lack of exercise and years of "vegan" diet, but the use of herbs and nuts as supplements. After the RN completes the history and physical, Ms. C is seen by a nurse practitioner (NP) who corroborates data gathered by the nurse, discusses the findings with Ms. C, then orders serum labs to help confirm the presenting symptoms and subjective data. Serum labs are ordered and reveal:

White blood cell (WBC) count: 10,0000 mm^3
Red blood cell (RBC) count: 4.5 million/mm^3
Hemoglobin (Hgb): 13 g/dL
Hematocrit (Hct): 38%
Platelet count (PLT): 250,000 cells/mm^3
Calcium: 8.4 mg/dL
Sodium (Na): 135 mEq/L
Potassium (K+): 4.4 mEq/L

Rheumatoid factor, antinuclear antibody, and erythrocyte sedimentation rate (ESR) are elevated. The labs are reviewed and the client is referred to the community hospital for a magnetic resonance imaging (MRI) of the hands and spine. Ms. C is to return home and have the diagnostic test completed as scheduled, and to continue with follow-up care at the clinic. Ms. C undergoes MRI of the hands and spine, which reveals degenerative changes, especially in the spine. The health care provider discusses the laboratory findings and the result of the MRI with Ms. C, and a diagnosis of osteoarthritis (OA) is confirmed. The health care provider discusses the plan of care for OA, and the following medications are prescribed for her: aspirin (acetylsalicylic acid), topical capsaicin (Zostrix), celecoxib (Celebrex), and calcium (Os-Cal). Ms. C is seen by an RN in the clinic who reviews the prescribed medications with her and allows her to ask questions pertaining to the plan of care as discussed by the health care provider. After dialogue between the client and nurse, Ms. C informs the nurse that she will fill the prescriptions at a pharmacy in her community. A follow-up clinic appointment is scheduled for her, and she leaves the clinic.

Questions and Suggested Answers

1. **What is your understanding of the above situation?** Although the causative mechanism for OA at the cellular level has not been well identified, it is believed that the disease may be genetic or familial. Clients with OA report a family history of the disease, which supports a possible genetic cause, especially for women who have the nodal type of arthritis. Ms. C's history of OA may be directly related to genetic origin.

2. **What are some women's health considerations for OA?** Before 50 years of age, more men than women suffer from OA. The disease is much more common in women, especially black women, after 50 years of age; the reason for this difference is not known. Women are more prone to hand involvement, especially in the distal and proximal interphalangeal joints of the fingers, which often produces painful, bone nodes. Women also have a greater number of affected joints compared with men, but men have more hip involvement.

3. **What is the significance of Heberden's and Bouchard's nodes and their relationship with OA?** Herberden's and Bouchard's nodes are deformities of the joints of the hands seen in clients with OA. Heberden's and Bouchard's nodes are abnormal cartilaginous or bony enlargement of a distal interphalangeal joint of a finger, which usually occurs in degenerative disease of the joint such as seen in OA. Heberden's nodes are located on the distal interphangeal joints as an indication of osteophyte formation and loss of joint space. Bouchard's nodes are located on the proximal interphangeal joints, indicating similar disease as Heberden's nodes. Both types of nodes are often red, swollen, and tender, with visible disfigurement. These deformities will affect the client's ADLs, therefore, the use of assessment tools and discomfort scale can be useful in determining the client's functional level and indicate what assistance the client needs to complete the listed activities.

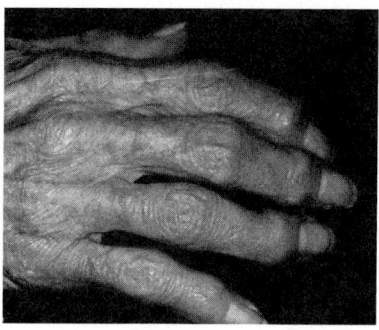

Osteoarthritis

4. **What are common nursing diagnoses for the client with OA?**

   - Chronic pain R/T muscle spasm, cartilage deterioration, or joint inflammation
   - Self-care deficit (partial) R/T pain, fatigue, and immobility
   - Impaired physical mobility R/T pain and muscle atrophy
   - Deficient knowledge R/T condition, treatment, and home care

5. **Discuss nonpharmacologic measures that can be used for clients with OA.** Some nonpharmacologic measures that can be used for OA are rest, positioning, weight control, transcutaneous electric nerve stimulation (TENS), and complementary and alternative therapies. *Weight control* is one of the measures the client may use to alleviate pain or discomfort. However, according to the National Arthritis Foundation, there is no "arthritic diet," but a well-balanced diet is recommended, and gradual weight loss for obese clients may lessen the stress on weight-bearing joints, decrease pain, and slow joint degeneration. *TENS* is particularly helpful for vertebral involvement. It involves the delivery of an electric current through electrodes applied to the skin surface over the painful region, at trigger points, or over a peripheral nerve. However, successful self-management of this modality requires that the client is able to hold the TENS unit to achieve pain relief. ***Complementary and alternative therapy*** includes acupuncture, tai chi, therapeutic touch, music therapy, and imagery. Acupuncture is the insertion of very fine needles into the skin at specific locations to restore energy balance, but it is most widely used for pain and is proven effective in treating chronic or degenerative pain such as with arthritis. The purpose is to influence physiological, emotional, and psychological functions in the mind and body. Tai chi is a holistic movement therapy that is a traditional Chinese martial art that is a mind-body exercise. The goal of this therapy is to integrate body movements, mind concentration, muscle relaxation, and breathing to achieve the desired outcome. Therapeutic touch is the use of hands on or near the body with the intention to heal. It consists of five steps: centering, assessing the energy field, clearing and

mobilizing the client's energy field, directing energy for healing, and balancing the energy field. In centering, the practitioner quiets oneself and focuses attention on the client with the intention to heal. In clearing and mobilizing, the practitioner holds his or her hands two to four inches from the client's body and moves the hands with the palms facing the client, from head to foot in a sweeping motion. The practitioner then places his or hands on the client and energy is directed toward the client. Finally, the practitioner seeks to balance the energy in the client by using head-to-toe clearing motions with the intention of smoothing the energy of the client. Therapeutic touch has been used to reduce anxiety, reduce pain, improve the immune system, and improve functional ability. Music therapy is a multisensorial technique that involves the hands, voice, emotions, mind, and spirit. Music therapy has two branches: active and passive. In the active therapy, instruments are used to correspond to all sensory organs so as to obtain suitable motor and emotional responses. In passive music therapy, listening to specific music and or sounds may be done in order to relax, stimulate, motivate, or soothe the body and mind. Imagery is the formation of a mental representation of an object, place, event, or situation that is perceived through the senses. The scientific base for using imagery relates to the reduction of stress, which is mediated through psychoneuroimmune interactions. Imagery can be used to reduce pain, reduce nausea and vomiting, decrease anxiety, and promote comfort during various types of treatments. Cayenne pepper, which is the source of capsaicin products, and omega-6 fatty acid, one of the body's essential fatty acids, are used to relief the discomfort found with OA. Glucosamine sulfate is a natural product found in bone cartilage has been used to relieve pain and possibly slow the progression of OA.

6. **What is the role of the physical therapist for clients with OA?** The role of the physical therapist includes provision of special heat treatments, such as paraffin dips, diathermy (electrical current) and application of sound waves with the use of ultrasonography.

The following are prescribed:

- Aspirin (acetylsalicylic acid) 1 g PO three times per day
- Capsaicin (Zostrix) apply to affected areas three to four times per day only
- Celecoxib (Celebrex) 200 mg PO two times per day
- Calcium (Os-Cal) 1 g PO in the morning and at bedtime

7. **What are the purposes for the prescribed medications?** *Capsaicin* is a topical analgesic that relieves arthritic pain by blocking substance P, a slow-chronic neurotransmitter of Type C nerve endings. The spinal cord secretes substance P transmitter, which is released slowly, building up in concentration over a period of seconds or even minutes, therefore, there is a "lag" in pain sensation, resulting in decrease in pain for the client. *Celecoxib* is a non-steroidal anti-inflammatory COX-2 inhibitor that relieves pain by blocking the COX-2 enzymes that occur at sites of inflammation. It spares the COX-1 that produces prostaglandins that help regulate normal cell activity, including protecting the lining of the gastrointestinal (GI) tract. The drug therefore relieves pain by decreasing the inflammatory response at the joints, but also prevents adverse effects of the GI system from developing. *Os-Cal* is a calcium supplement that helps to improve mild calcium deficiency. It is prescribed for morning and at bedtime because the body most readily utilizes it when the client is in a fasting state and immobile.

8. **What are the most common adverse reactions of the prescribed medications?** The most common adverse reactions of *capsaicin* are burning, stinging, and redness at the site of application. Although there are no common adverse reactions of *celecoxib* established, some of the following occur at a frequency of 0.1% or greater: dyspepsia, diarrhea, abdominal pain, constipation, and GI bleeding. The most common adverse reactions of *calcium replacement (Os-Cal)* are constipation and flatulence. Intravenous use may manifest arrhythmias and phlebitis.

9. **Discuss the drug-to-drug and drug-to-food/herbal interactions of the prescribed medications.** There are no clinically significant drug-to-drug, drug-to-food/herbal interactions established for *capsaicin*. Drug-to-drug interactions may occur with the simultaneous use of *celecoxib* and aspirin, increasing the risk of GI ulceration

and bleeding. Antacids decrease the absorption of celecoxib, thus decreasing its effects. The simultaneous use with lithium and warfarin may increase drug levels, especially in the elderly. The simultaneous use with fluconazole and ketoconazole may increase celecoxib levels. If used concurrently with ACE inhibitors, there may be a decreased antihypertensive effect. There are no clinically significant drug-to-food/herbal interactions established. With *calcium supplements (Os-Cal)* drug-to-drug interactions may occur with the simultaneous use of digoxin, which may increase digoxin toxicity. Chronic use with antacids in clients with renal insufficiency may lead to milk-alkali syndrome or metabolic alkalosis. Oral Os-Cal, when used simultaneously with tetracyclines, fluoroquinolones, phenytoin, and iron salts, may increase their absorption. Concurrent use with diuretics (thiazide) may result in hypercalcemia, and if used simultaneously with sodium polystyrene sulfonate, may decrease serum potassium. Drug-to-food interaction may occur with the simultaneous use of cereals, spinach, or rhubarb to decrease the absorption of calcium supplements.

10. **Design a specific pain management for the client with OA.**

    - Consider cultural influences on pain response.
    - Evaluate with the client and the health care team the effectiveness of past pain control measures.
    - Teach the use of nonpharmacologic techniques before and after painful activities.
    - Promote adequate rest and sleep to facilitate pain relief.
    - Utilize a multidisciplinary approach to pain management, when appropriate.
    - Monitor client's satisfaction with pain management at specified intervals.
    - Compliant use of prescribed medications, heat, and cold.

11. **What specific information should a nurse provide for the client who is discharged to home about topical capsaicin?** After application of the topical medication, the client may experience a burning sensation for a short period of time. The client should use plastic gloves for application, and to prevent burning of the eyes or other areas of the body, the client should wash her hands immediately after the application. Remind the client that the drug is for external use only and not to apply tight bandages to the site. Regular use of three to four times daily is necessary for desired effects. If the pain worsens, the client should inform her health care provider.

References

Broyles, B.E. (2005). *Medical-Surgical Nursing Clinical Companion.* Durham, NC: Carolina Academic Press.

Corbet, J.V. (2004). *Laboratory Tests and Diagnostic Procedures with Nursing Diagnoses* (6th ed.). Upper Saddle River, NJ: Prentice Hall.

Deglin, J.H. and Vallerand, A.H. (2005). *Davis's Drug Guide for Nurses* (9th ed.). Philadelphia: F.A. Davis.

Gahart, B.L. and Nazareno, A.R. (2005). *2005 Intravenous Medications.* St. Louis: Mosby.

Huether, S.E. and McCance, K.L. (2004). *Understanding Pathophysiology* (3rd ed.). St. Louis: Mosby.

Ignatavicius, D.D. and Workman, M.L. (2006). *Medical-Surgical Nursing across the Health Care Continuum* (5th ed.). Philadelphia: W.B. Saunders.

Kuhn, M.A. (April 2002). "Herbal Remedies: Drug-Herb Interactions." *Critical Care Nurse* 22(2): 22–30.

Lewis, S.M., Heitkemper, M.M., and Dirksen, S.R. (2004). *Medical-Surgical Nursing: Assessment and Management of Clinical Problems* (6th ed.). St. Louis: Mosby.

Munzo, C. and Luckman, J. (2005). *Transcultural Communication in Nursing* (2nd ed.). Cliftion Park, NY: Thomson: Delmar Learning.

Spratto, G.R. and Woods, A.L. (2005). *2005 Edition: PDR Nurse's Drug Handbook.* Clifton Park, NY: Thomson Delmar Learning.

CASE STUDY 5

Breast Cancer

GENDER
- F

AGE
- 40

SETTING
- Hospital

ETHNICITY/CULTURE
- Black American

PREEXISTING CONDITIONS

COEXISTING CONDITIONS
- Abscess of the left breast at age 16
- Mother and brother died of breast cancer

LIFESTYLE
- Elementary school teacher
- Uses oral contraceptives

COMMUNICATION

SOCIOECONOMIC STATUS
- Middle income, but may need supplemental financial support

SPIRITUAL/RELIGIOUS
- Baptist

PHARMACOLOGIC
- Doxorubicin HcL (Adriamycin)
- Cyclophosphamide (Cytoxan)
- Docetaxel (Taxotere)
- Tamoxifen citrate (Nolvadex)
- Ondansetron HcL (Zofran)

PSYCHOLOGICAL
- Anxiety
- Denial
- Fear

LEGAL

ETHICAL
- The client has the right to choose treatment.
- Is the family able to cope with the present stressors?

ALTERNATIVE THERAPY
- Prayer
- Herbal medications

PRIORITIZATION
- Careful and accurate breast history interview
- Active listening

DELEGATION
- Advanced practice nurse for clinical breast examination
- Client education

THE MUSCULOSKELETAL AND REPRODUCTIVE SYSTEMS

Level of difficulty: Difficult

Overview: This case involves a thorough assessment of the client's condition, including past medical history, family history of cancer including breast cancer, past surgical history, prescribed medications, and herbal supplements the client is currently taking. It requires empathy and the ability to identify with the client's feelings.

Client Profile

Mrs. W is a 40-year-old married client who is seen in the doctor's office for routine examination because she felt a lump in the upper outer quadrant of her left breast during breast self-examination (BSE). Mrs. W is 5'9" and weighs 194 pounds. During a thorough breast examination, a painless mass that is hard, irregular in shape, and nonmobile in the upper outer quadrant is detected by the health care provider. Her reproductive history reveals one child, age seven years. She reports that her menstrual cycle began at the age of 12. She had used oral contraceptives for several years before her child was conceived. Mrs. W also reports a breast biopsy at the age of 16 for an abscess of the left breast. Her family history includes her mother and a brother who died of breast cancer. Her father, who is 90 years old, and her older sister, who is 42 years old, are both well.

Case Study

Mrs. W is referred for mammography at the community hospital. The mammography is done and reviewed by a radiologist. Mrs. W is later seen by her primary health care provider at his office. The results are discussed, and she is scheduled for diagnostic studies (ultrasound of the left breast and Tru-Cut Core breast biopsy) at a hospital that specializes in oncology. Mrs. W leaves the health care provider's office concerned because of her family history of breast cancer. The diagnostic studies are done and confirm the diagnosis of early stage II cancer of the left breast. Mrs. W is seen by her primary health care provider and an oncologist who discuss her plan of treatment, which will include administration of medication at the hospital and also at home. Mrs. W is admitted to the hospital for treatment for breast cancer and is informed that she will be discharged to home on Tamoxifen citrate (Nolvadex). Her vitals are:

Blood pressure: 134/84

Pulse: 86

Respirations: 18

Temperature: 98.4° F

Questions and Suggested Answers

1. **Discuss the various histopathologic types of cancers.** Breast cancer is the most common malignancy in women in the United States and is second only to lung cancer as a cause of death. Various histopathologic types of breast cancer exist, with various prognoses. These include infiltrating ductal carcinomas (colloid, inflammatory, Paget's disease, medullary, papillary, and tubular) with frequency of occurrence 70–80%, infiltrating lobular carcinoma 10–15%, and noninvasive carcinoma, such as ductal carcinoma in situ with 4–6% frequency of occurrence. Paget's disease is a breast malignancy characterized by a persistent lesion of the nipple and areola with or without a palpable mass. Itching, burning, bloody nipple discharge with superficial erosion, and ulceration may be present. Nipple changes are often diagnosed as an infection or dermatitis, which can lead to treatment delays. Diagnosis is good when the cancer remains in the nipple only. Inflammatory breast cancer is the most malignant form of all breast cancers, yet is rare. It is an aggressive and fast-growing cancer. The skin of the breast looks red, feels warm, and has a thickened appearance that is often described as resembling an orange peel (peau d'orange). Sometimes the breast develops ridges and small bumps that look like hives. The inflammatory changes, often mistaken for an infection, are caused by cancer cells blocking lymph channels. Metastases occur early and widely, with radiation, chemotherapy, and hormone therapy more likely used than surgery.

2. **Discuss etiologies for breast cancer.** A number of factors are thought to relate to the cause of breast cancer. Hereditary or genetically-related susceptibility, hormonal regulation, environmental factors, such as chemical

pesticide and radiation exposure, are believed to play a role in the development of breast cancer. Some risk factors place women at higher risk than men, such as gender, with women having 99% of breast cancer cases. Major breast cancers are found in postmenopausal women. Family history with breast cancer in a first-degree relative, particularly when premenopausal or bilateral, increases the risk. Gene mutations (BRCA-1 or BRCA-2) play a role in 5–10% of breast cancer cases. Personal history of colon cancer, endometrial cancer, and ovarian cancer are also risk factors.

3. **Discuss cultural and ethnic considerations for breast cancer.** Black American women have lower survival rates from breast cancer than white women, even when diagnosed at an early stage. Black women are diagnosed at a later stage of breast cancer than white women, but this fact alone does not account for the higher mortality rate. White women have a higher incidence of breast cancer than non-whites, and breast cancer is the most commonly diagnosed cancer among Hispanic women. Hispanic women, especially Mexican Americans, have the lowest rate of cancer screening of any ethnic group, and tend to have larger, more advanced tumors, which may relate to their higher mortality rate compared with white women. Hispanic women are also more likely to be diagnosed at a later stage of breast cancer than white women. Although the incidence of breast cancer among Navajo women is no greater than their non-native peers (Hispanic white, non-Hispanic white, black American, and Asian Pacific Islander women), their five-year survival rate is among the poorest of all ethnic groups in New Mexico.

4. **Discuss clinical manifestations for breast cancer.** Clinical manifestation of breast cancer is usually evidenced as a single lump often in the upper, outer quadrant of the breast because it is the location of most of the glandular tissue. There may be nipple discharge that is usually unilateral and may be clear or bloody. Nipple retraction may occur and peau d'orange may occur due to the plugging of dermal lymphatics.

5. **Discuss diagnostic studies used to confirm breast cancer.** *Mammography* with the primary purpose being to detect breast tumors that are not palpable by physical examination. However, some actual cancers may not appear on mammography or may appear as benign. *Ultrasonography* (ultrasound) of the breast is done in conjunction with mammography since some actual cancers may not appear on mammography or may appear as benign. It is also able to distinguish fluid-filled cysts from tumors of the breast. *Axillary lymph node palpation* includes examination of five sets of lymph nodes (pectoral [anterior] nodes, midaxillary [central] nodes, subscapular [posterior] nodes, brachial [lateral] nodes, and infraclavicular [subclavicular] nodes). On palpation, breasts should be firm without masses, lumps, tenderness, nipples without discharge, axillae smooth, and nodes non-palpable. *Tru-Cut Core breast biopsy* removes the core tissue of the breast that is strongly suggestive for malignancy. It is a procedure that is documented as 95% accurate in diagnosing breast tumors.

6. **Discuss common nursing diagnoses for breast cancer.** *Anxiety* related to the diagnosis of cancer. The nurse should encourage the woman to talk about feelings and diagnosis of cancer to promote successful resolution of fear and establish effective coping mechanisms. The nurse should provide opportunity for significant others to discuss situation and learn about support groups to help decrease concern and anxiety. The nurse should provide information about signs and symptoms to report to health care provider (i.e., new persistent problems such as changes of the breast). *Risk for disturbed body image disturbance* related to disease process. The nurse should assess degree of self-esteem disturbance so appropriate interventions can be initiated. Assist the client to verbalize feelings and encourage open communication with significant others to improve self-image.

The following are prescribed:

- Doxorubicin HcL (Adriamycin) 30 mg/m² IV for four cycles
- After the four cycles of doxorubicin, start cyclophosphamide (Cytoxan) 4 mg/kg IV over seven days
- Ondansetron HcL (Zofran) 24 mg PO 30 minutes before cyclophosphamide therapy
- Premedicate client with dexamethasone (Decadron) 8 mg two times per day × five days, starting one day prior to docetaxel (Taxotere)

7. **What are the purposes for the prescribed medications?** ***Doxorubicin HcL*** destroys rapidly proliferating cells and slowly developing carcinomas. The intravenous method provides system benefits and four cycles of the drug will appropriately destroy the cancerous cells. Doxorubicin HcL destroys rapidly proliferating cells and slowly developing ones by blocking effective DNA and RNA transcription. ***Cyclophosphamide*** destroys rapid proliferating cells and slowly developing carcinomas. It works by blocking the synthesis of DNA, RNA, and protein of the cells, resulting in development of proliferating and slowly developing cells. ***Cyclophosphamide*** is administered after doxorubicin HcL, because doxorubicin HcL causes severe bone marrow suppression and cytoxan is an alkylating agent with reactions that take place at any time during the cell cycle and has potent adverse effects such as blood dyscrasias. Administering both drugs simultaneously could cause severe adverse reactions. ***Docetaxel*** binds to the microtubule network of the cells that is essential for interphase and mitosis of the cell cycle, preventing the normal functioning of the cells, thereby inhibiting mitosis in the cells. ***Ondansetron HcL*** prevents nausea and vomiting associated with cancer chemotherapy. When zofran is administered before chemotherapeutic agents, it causes the release of serotonin from the receptors located in the vagus nerve in the gastrointestinal (GI) tract. When they are released, the nerve terminals send signals to serotonin receptors in the chemoreceptor trigger zone (CTZ) to block the sensation of nausea and vomiting.

8. **What are the most common adverse reactions, drug-to-drug, drug-to-food/herbal interactions of the prescribed medications?** The most common adverse reactions of ***doxorubicin*** are stomatitis, severe myelosuppression, complete alopecia, cardiotoxicity, and skin reaction due to prior radiation. Drug-to-drug interaction is seen with simultaneous use of barbiturates, which may decrease the effects of doxorubicin, warranting an increase of the dose. Drug-to-drug interaction may also occur with other drugs that suppress bone marrow. There are no clinically significant drug-to-food/herbal interactions established. The most common adverse reactions of ***cyclophosphamide*** are nausea, vomiting, neutropenia, and reversible alopecia. Drug-to-drug interaction is seen when used simultaneously with doxorubicin HcL with a noted increase in cardiac toxicity. There are no clinically significant drug-to-food/herbal interaction established. The most common adverse reactions of ***methotrexate*** are headache, ulcerative stomatitis, glossitis, gingivitis, leukopenia, and thrombocytopenia. Drug-to-drug interaction may occur with the simultaneous use of chloramphenicol, probenecid, folic acid, and cholestyramine. Drug-to-food/herbal interaction may occur with the simultaneous use of echinacea, which may increase the risk of hepatotoxicity. The most common adverse reactions of ***ondansetron HcL*** are headache, sedation, and diarrhea. Drug-to-drug interactions may occur with the simultaneous use of rifampin, which may decrease the serum level of ondansetron HcL. There are no clinically significant drug-to-food/herbal interactions established.

9. **Discuss common sites of breast cancer recurrence and metastasis.** ***Local recurrence*** is identified on the skin, and is usually firm, with discrete nodules, occasionally pruritic, usually painless. ***Regional recurrence*** is in the lymph nodes with enlarged nodes in axilla or supraclavicular area, usually non-tender, superior vena caval obstruction from enlarged supraclavicular nodes, and pain in the shoulder and arm of the affected side.

10. **Discuss client education for breast cancer.** The client should continue with monthly BSE and have clinical breast examination and screening mammography annually. Encourage the client to make lifestyle changes to help lower the risk for metastasis. Exercise is one example of lifestyle changes that will reduce the progression, because exercise decreases body fat, thereby reducing the amount of free estrogen stored in body fat which is one of the risk factors of breast cancer.

References

Black, J.M. and Hawks, J.H. (2005). *Medical-Surgical Nursing: Clinical Management for Positive Outcomes*. Philadelphia: W.B. Saunders.

Broyles, B.E. (2005). *Medical-Surgical Nursing Clinical Companion*. Durham, NC: Carolina Academic Press.

Corbet, J.V. (2004). *Laboratory Tests and Diagnostic Procedures with Nursing Diagnoses* (6th ed.). Upper Saddle River, NJ: Prentice Hall.

"Core Biopsy as Alternative to Fine Needle Aspiration Biopsy in Diagnosis of Breast Tumors." Available at http://theoncologist.alphamedpress.org.

Gahart, B.L. and Nazareno, A.R. (2005). *2005 Intravenous Medications.* St. Louis: Mosby.

Huether, S.E. and McCance, K.L. (2004). *Understanding Pathophysiology* (3rd ed.). St. Louis: Mosby.

Ignatavicius, D.D. and Workman, M.L. (2006). *Medical-Surgical Nursing across the Health Care Continuum* (5th ed.). Philadelphia: W.B. Saunders.

Johansen, A.M. (2005). "Breast Cancer Chemoprevention: A Review of Selective Estrogen Receptor Modulators." *Clinical Journal of Oncology Nursing* 9(3): 317–320.

Robinson, F., Sandoval, N., Baldwin, J., and Sanderson, P.R. (2005). "Breast Cancer Education for Native American Women: Creating Culturally Relevant Communications." *Clinical Journal of Oncology Nursing* 9(6): 689–692.

Simpson, C., Herr, H., and Courville, K.A. (October 2004). "Concurrent Therapies That Protect Against Doxorubicin-Induced Cardiomyopathy." *Clinical Journal of Oncology Nursing* 8(5): 497–501.

Spratto, G.R. and Woods, A.L. (2005). *2005 Edition: PDR Nurse's Drug Handbook.* Clifton Park, NY: Thomson Delmar Learning.

CASE STUDY 6

Myasthenia Gravis

GENDER
- M

AGE
- 30

SETTING
- Hospital

ETHNICITY/CULTURE
- Black American

PREEXISTING CONDITIONS

COEXISTING CONDITIONS
- Respiratory tract infection
- Emotional stress

LIFESTYLE
- Law school student
- Lives with parents

COMMUNICATION

DISABILITY
- Activity intolerance related to muscle weakness and fatigue

SOCIOECONOMIC STATUS
- Low

SPIRITUAL/RELIGIOUS
- Baptist

PHARMACOLOGIC
- Pyridostigmine (Mestinon)
- Prednisone (Deltasone)
- Azathioprine (Imuran)

PSYCHOSOCIAL
- Anxiety
- Depression

LEGAL
- Financial support, depending on extent of medical interventions

ETHICAL

ALTERNATIVE THERAPY

PRIORITIZATION
- Airway patency
- Aspiration precaution

DELEGATION
- RN
- Client education

THE MUSCULOSKELETAL AND REPRODUCTIVE SYSTEMS

Level of difficulty: Difficult

Overview: This case involves a thorough assessment of the client's condition with specific focus on complaints of fatigability. It involves current exposure to infectious agents or current infectious problems. The nurse must use critical-thinking skills to prioritize care for the client in a busy emergency department (ED). Questions pertaining to medications and herbal supplements should be a significant part of the history that is taken.

Client Profile

Mr. T is a 30-year-old law student living at home with his parents. He is expected to graduate at the end of the current semester. Prior to entry into the ED, Mr. T reports having been on amoxicillin as prescribed by his primary health care provider for respiratory infections three weeks ago. Mr. T returned to college after completing the course of amoxicillin but reports feeling unusually tired and was easily fatigued after a two-hour lecture class.

Case Study

In the ED, Mr. T complains of muscle weakness of the eyes and eyelids, has difficulty speaking, and reports noticing that chewing and swallowing were difficult but nonspecific during break period at 10:00 AM. The ED health care provider is notified and immediately responds to the triage nurse's report. Vital signs are:

- Blood pressure: 120/80
- Pulse: 78
- Respirations: 16
- Temperature 98.4°F

History and physical are done and find ptosis (drooping of the eyelids) and weakness of facial muscles. Normal pupillary responses to light and accommodation are present. The following diagnostic tests are ordered: serum T_3, T_4, serum protein electrophoresis, and acetylcholine receptor antibodies (AChR) level. The results of the tests reveal: T_3: 205 ng/dL, T_4: 15 ug/dL, serum protein electrophoresis is negative for rheumatoid arthritis, systemic lupus erythematosus and polymyositis, and the AChR level is elevated (1.2 mmol/L). The findings are discussed with Mr. T and his parents as per his approval, and myasthenia gravis (MG) is diagnosed. Mr. T will be discharged to home in 48 hours. He and his parents are involved in an interdisciplinary team discussion before discharge: speech-language pathologist in collaboration with the primary RN, a registered dietitian, and an occupational therapist. The client will return to the clinic in two weeks for reevaluation of medication regimen.

Questions and Suggested Answers

1. **Discuss the incidence and pathophysiology of MG.** The incidence of MG in the United States is estimated to be 14 per 100,000 people, resulting in 40,000 cases in the United States population annually. It is the most common disorder of the neuromuscular junctions and, although it is a rare disease, it may begin at any age, from before 10 years of age to after 60 years of age. The peak of onset is between 20 and 30 years of age. Women are affected three times more often than are men and symptoms in men usually appear after the age of 50. MG is a chronic autoimmune motor disorder with no effect on sensation or coordination. it is a disease of the neuromuscular junction of the voluntary and striated muscles. Normally, a chemical impulse precipitates the release of acetylcholine from vesicles on the nerve terminal at the myoneural junction. Continuous binding of acetylcholine to the receptor site is required for muscular contraction to be sustained. In MG, autoantibodies directed at the acetylcholine receptor sites impair transmission of impulses across the myoneural junction, which causes fewer receptors to be available for stimulation. As a result, nerve impulses are not transmitted to the skeletal muscles and the antibodies accelerate the degeneration of the acetylcholine (ACh) receptors. The result is weakness of voluntary muscles that escalates with continued activity. These antibodies are found in 80–90% of the people with MG. The blood cells and thymus gland produce the antibodies that cause the acetylcholine to be ineffective in producing action potential in the muscle groups (Broyles, 509) resulting in fatigue and weakness primarily in muscles innervated by the cranial nerves, as well as in skeletal and respiratory muscles. The disease process can progress from mild to generalized weakness that may lead to death related to respiratory failure because of the inability of the neuromuscular junctions to transmit enough signals from the

nerve fibers to the muscle fibers. The overall cause of MG is the development of immunity by the client against his or her own acetylcholine-activated receptors (AChR) in the muscle end plate membranes. Therefore, they are too weak to stimulate the muscle fibers.

2. **Discuss clinical manifestations of MG.** The initial manifestation of MG usually involves the ocular muscles. Diplopia (double vision) and ptosis (drooping of the eyelids) are common. However, the majority of the clients also experience weakness of the muscles of the face and throat (bulbar symptoms) and generalized weakness. The weakness of the facial muscles will result in a bland facial expression. Laryngeal involvement produces dysphonia (voice impairment) and increases the client's risk for choking and aspiration. Generalized weakness affects all the extremities and the intercostal muscles, resulting in decreasing vital capacity and respiratory failure.

3. **Discuss assessment and diagnostic findings of MG.** An anticholinesterase test is used to diagnose MG. Anticholinesterase agents stop the breakdown of acetylcholine, and in doing so, increase acetylcholine availability. Edrophonium chloride (Tensilon) is injected intravenously, 2 mg at a time to a total of 10 mg. Thirty seconds after injection, facial muscle weakness and ptosis should resolve for about five minutes. This immediate improvement in muscle strength after the administration of Tensilon represents a positive test and usually confirms the diagnosis. Atropine 0.4 mg should be available to control the side effects of edrophonium, which include bradycardia, sweating, and cramping.

4. **Discuss complications of MG.** *Myasthenic crisis (MC)* is a complication of MG. It is an exacerbation of the disease process characterized by severe generalized muscle weakness and respiratory and bulbar weakness that may result in respiratory failure. The most common precipitator of MC is infection, but undermedication is a major cause. If MC is diagnosed, neostigmine methylsulfate (Prostigmin) is administered intramuscularly or intravenously until the client is able to swallow oral anticholinerase medications. Neuromuscular respiratory failure is the critical complication of the crisis, and because the weak respiratory muscles cannot support inhalation, respiratory support and airway protection are key interventions when caring for the client in crisis. Therefore, endotracheal intubation and mechanical ventilation should be anticipated and be readily available. *Cholinergic crisis* results from overmedication, which causes depolarization block of acetylcholine. It does not improve or deteriorate with the administration of edrophonium. The overmedication causes acute exacerbation of muscle weakness.

5. **Discuss differences and care of the client with myasthenic crisis and cholinergic crisis.** The *priority care* for myasthenic crisis is implementing medication as prescribed promptly, maintaining adequate respiratory function, and holding of cholinesterase inhibiting drugs. The *priority care* for cholinergic crisis is holding of cholinergic drugs until cholinergic effects decrease, providing optimum ventilatory support, and administering IV atropine as prescribed. Respiratory distress and varying degrees of dysphagia (difficulty swallowing), dysarthria (difficulty speaking), eyelid ptosis, diplopia, and prominent muscle weakness are symptoms of myasthenic and cholinergic crisis. Providing ventilatory assistance takes precedence in the immediate management of the client with myasthenic crisis, with ongoing assessment for respiratory failure, monitoring pulmonary function parameters (e.g., vital capacity, inspiratory volume) to track the progression of impaired respiratory function. Arterial blood gas (ABG) is done to determine the need for oxygen therapy or airway clearance (suctioning), nasogastric tube (NGT) for tube feedings, and for implementing the use of a mechanical ventilator appropriately.

6. **Discuss plasmapheresis and its relationship to MG.** Plasmapheresis is an adjunctive therapy for clients with refractory MG. It is the process by which plasma is separated from formed elements of blood. The plasma is discarded and the packed red cells are joined with albumin, normal saline, and electrolytes and returned to the client. The purpose is to remove plasma proteins containing antibodies that are believed to cause MG. Although plasmapheresis improves the symptoms in 75% of clients, its potential complications include myasthenic or cholinergic crisis, and at times hypovolemia. Therefore, muscle strength should be assessed before and after the procedure, with particular attention paid to vital capacity, swallowing ability, diplopia, and ptosis

to evaluate the effectiveness of the treatment. Intravenous immune globulin (IVIG) has recently been shown to be nearly as effective as plasmapheresis in controlling symptom exacerbation.

7. **Discuss surgical management of MG.** *Thymectomy* (surgical removal of the thymus gland) produces antigen-specific immunosuppression and results in clinical improvement. It can decrease or eliminate the need for medication. The entire gland must be removed for optimal clinical outcomes, and the transsternal thoracic surgical approach is used. After the surgery, the client is transferred to an intensive care unit, and special focus is given to respiratory function. If the entire gland is removed, it may take a year for the client to benefit from the procedure, due to the long life of circulating T cells.

The following are prescribed:

- Pyridostigmine (Mestinon) 60 mg PO daily
- Prednisone (Deltasone) 2 mg/kg/day × one week
- Azathioprine (Imuran) 1 mg/kg/day as maintenance dose

8. **What are the purposes for the prescribed medications?** *Pyridostigmine bromide* is a cholinergic anticholinesterase that improves muscle tone by enhancing neuromuscular impulse transmission by preventing degradation of ACh by the enzyme acetylcholinerase (AChE). When degradation is prevented, increase in the response of the muscles to nerve impulses and improvement in muscle strength occurs. NOTE: Pyridostigmine bromide must be administered exactly on time! *Prednisone* is a glucocorticoid and is used to reduce remission, control and improve symptoms, and in doing so suppress the inflammatory process which is a precipitating factor for the development of MG. *Azathioprine* slows the rate of occurring symptoms by inhibiting DNA, RNA, and normal protein synthesis of the abnormal cells involved in MG. Because there is a delay in response to azathioprine, both prednisone and azathioprine are usually administered simultaneously, with the intent of tapering prednisone when the effects of azathioprine are evident.

9. **What are the most common adverse reactions, drug-to-drug, drug-to-food/herbal interactions of the prescribed medications?** The most common adverse reactions of *pyridostigmine bromide* are dizziness, headache, abdominal cramps, nausea, vomiting, diarrhea, miosis, excessive salivation, and sweating. The most serious adverse effect is an anticholinergic crisis. Drug-to-drug interactions may occur with the simultaneous use of pyridostigmine and muscle relaxants, aminoglycosides, anesthetics, procainamide quinidine, mecamylamine, polymyxin, magnesium, corticosteroids, and antidysrrythmics, which may antagonize the effects of pyridostigmine. Pyridostigmine will decrease the action of gallamine, metocurine, pancuronium, tubocurarine, and atropine. Decamethonium and succinylcholine will increase the action of pyridostigmine. There are no clinically significant drug-to-food/herbal interactions established. The most common adverse reactions of *prednisone* are depression, euphoria, hypertension, nausea, decreased wound healing, ecchymoses, fragility, hirsutism, petechiae, adrenal suppression, muscle wasting, osteoporosis, and cushingoid appearance. With prednisone, drug-to-drug interactions may occur with the simultaneous use of barbiturates, cholestyramine, colestipol, theophylline, phenytoin, and rifampin, which increase prednisone's metabolism, requiring an increased dose of prednisone. Alcohol, salicylates, indomethacin, amphotericin B, digoxin, cyclosporine, and diuretics increase the action of prednisone. Decreased effects of anticoagulants, anticonvulsants, antidiabetic agents, ambenonium, neostigmine, isoniazid, toxoids, vaccines, anticholinesterases, salicylates, and somatrem are seen with concurrent use of prednisone with these agents. The simultaneous use of amphotericin B and diuretics increases potassium loss. Neostigmine and pyridostigmine simultaneous use with **prednisone** may cause severe muscle weakness in clients with MG. The simultaneous use of grapefruit juice may increase the serum levels. Prednisone-related potassium loss will increase if used with aloe, buckthorn, rhubarb, and senna. The most common adverse reactions of *azathioprine* are immunosuppression (leukopenia, thrombocyctopenia, and macrocytic anemia), nausea, vomiting, diarrhea, fever, and malaise. With ACE inhibitors, blasalazid, mesalamine, and sulfasalazine, they may cause increased risk of leukopenia. The use of azathioprine with prolonged corticosteroids therapy may cause muscle wasting. Azathioprine may increase the serum levels of cyclosporine and methotrexate and it decreases the effects of anticoagulants and

tubocurarine and other nondepolarizing neuromuscular blocking agents. There are no clinically significant drug-to-food interactions established, but azathioprine should not be used with echinacea.

10. **Discuss client education for MG.** The client and significant other(s) (S/O) should be provided with information about MG, both written and verbal. They should be aware of adverse reactions of both anticholinerase drugs and steroids, and emphasis should be placed on the importance of taking anticholinerase medications on time. The client and S/O should be made knowledgeable that if the medication is not taken on time, difficulty in swallowing due to weakness will develop. Written instructions on how to distinguish myasthenic crisis from cholinergic crisis should be given, and the importance of seeking medical attention promptly should be stressed. The client should be taught strategies to conserve energy, such as determining the best times for rest periods throughout the day. Frequently used items should be readily available and in easy reach. If the client drives a motor vehicle, encourage him to apply for a handicapped license plate to minimize walking from parking spaces. The client should sit upright when eating, with the neck slightly flexed to facilitate swallowing. Soft foods in gravy or sauces can be swallowed more easily, and may be prepared this way. If choking occurs frequently, the client should inform the health care provider, who may suggest pureeing foods to a pudding consistency. Suctioning equipment should be available at home, and client and S/O should be instructed how to use it. If ptosis of the eyelids occur, instruct the client to tape the lids closed for short intervals, and regularly instill artificial tears. Patching one eye may help with double vision. The client should always wear a medical alert bracelet and carry identification at all times. Follow-up care is mandatory to monitor progress of the disease.

References

Broyles, B.E. (2005). *Medical-Surgical Nursing Clinical Companion.* Durham, NC: Carolina Academic Press.
Corbet, J.V. (2004). *Laboratory Tests and Diagnostic Procedures with Nursing Diagnoses* (6th ed.). Upper Saddle River, NJ: Prentice Hall.
Deglin, J.H. and Vallerand, A.H. (2005). *Davis's Drug Guide for Nurses* (9th ed.). Philadelphia: F.A. Davis.
"FDA Approves Stavelo™ for treatment of Parkinson's Disease." (December 2005). From http://www.pharma.us.novartis.com.
Gahart, B.L. and Nazareno, A.R. (2005). *2005 Intravenous Medications.* St. Louis: Mosby.
Guyton, A.C. and Hall, J.E. (2006). *Textbook of Medical Physiology* (11th ed.). Philadelphia: W.B. Saunders.
Howard, J.F. (January 2005). "Myasthenia Gravis – A Summary." Available at www.myasthenia.org/information/summary.htm.
Huether, S.E. and McCance, K.L. (2004). *Understanding Pathophysiology* (3rd ed.). St. Louis: Mosby.
Ignatavicius, D.D. and Workman, M.L. (2006). *Medical-Surgical Nursing across the Health Care Continuum* (5th ed.). Philadelphia: W.B. Saunders.
"Parkinson's Disease: Challenges, Progress, and Promise." (July 2005). Available at ww.ninds.nih.gov/disorders/parkinsons_disease/parkinsons_research.htm.
Spratto, G.R. and Woods, A.L. (2005). *2005 Edition: PDR Nurse's Drug Handbook.* Clifton Park, NY: Thomson Delmar Learning.